the Better sex™

GUIDE TO

EXTRAORDINARY LOVEMAKING

QUIVER

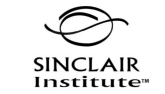

SINCLAIR
Institute™

BY THE CREATORS OF
BETTER SEX VIDEOS®

www.bettersex.com®

the Better

sex™

GUIDE TO

EXTRAORDINARY LOVEMAKING

Text © 2009 Sinclair Institute and Yvonne K. Fulbright, Ph.D.
Photography © 2009 Quiver

First published in the USA in 2009 by
Quiver, a member of
Quayside Publishing Group
100 Cummings Center
Suite 406-L
Beverly, MA 01915-6101
www.quiverbooks.com

13 12 11 10 09   1 2 3 4 5

ISBN-13: 978-1-59233-352-3
ISBN-10: 1-59233-352-4

Library of Congress Cataloging-in-Publication Data
Fulbright, Yvonne K.
  The better sex guide to extraordinary lovemaking / Sinclair Institute and Yvonne K.
Fulbright.
     p. cm.
  ISBN-13: 978-1-59233-352-3
  ISBN-10: 1-59233-352-4
  1. Sex instruction--Popular works. 2. Sex--Popular works. I. Sinclair Intimacy Institute.
II. Title.
  HQ31.F847 2009
  613.9'6--dc22
                                                    2009021134

All photography by Richard Avery with the exception of pages 210, 211, 252, 255, 257,
    259, 263, and 265 by Lucia Scarlatta.
Illustrations by Robert Brandt
Sinclair Institute review by Susan Yeager Montani

Visit www.bettersex.com

Printed and bound in Singapore

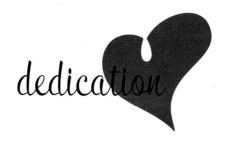

dedication

Dedicated to those who support our efforts and continued journey
to educate and empower millions of people with our sexual
health message through Sinclair's films and books.

"Sexual health is a state of physical, emotional, mental, and social wellbeing
related to sexuality: it is not merely the absence of disease, dysfunction,
or infirmity. Sexual health requires a positive and respectful approach to
sexuality and sexual relationships, as well as the possibility of having
pleasurable and safe sexual experiences, free of coercion, discrimination,
and violence. For sexual health to be attained and maintained, the sexual
rights of all persons must be respected, protected, and fulfilled."

—World Association for Sexual Health

contents

step one: DESIRE

step two: AROUSAL

step three: ORGASM

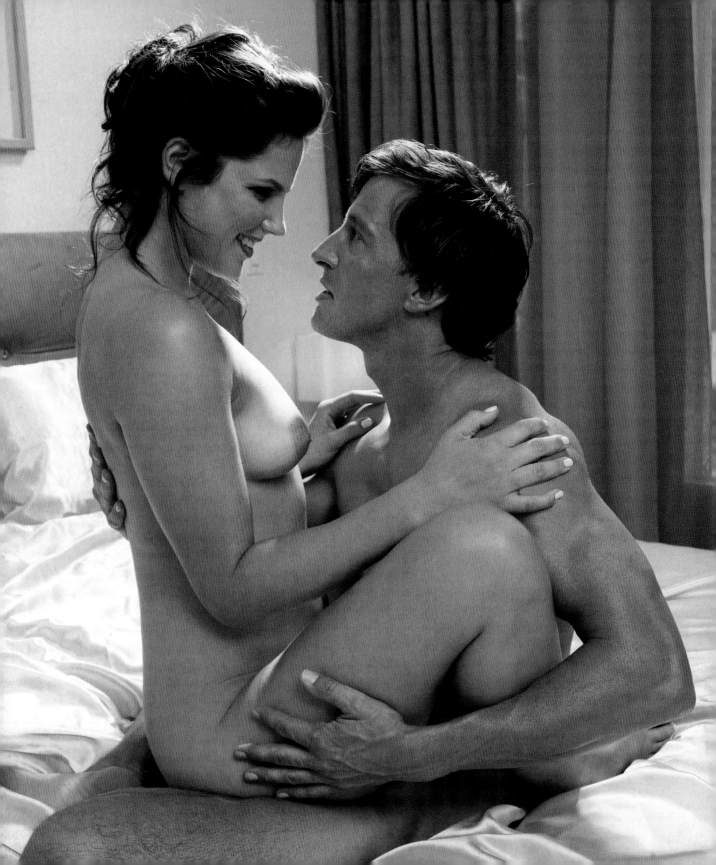

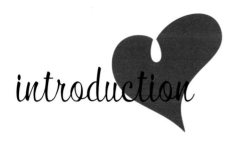

introduction

A Better Sex Life, Now!

SEXUAL ECSTASY IS AS EASY AS ONE, TWO, THREE, WITH
THE SINCLAIR INSTITUTE'S SIMPLE THREE-STEP PROGRAM:

DESIRE, AROUSAL, ORGASM.

OF ALL THE JOURNEYS we embark upon as human beings, the quest for more satisfying
sex is by far the most thrilling, heart-pounding, and intriguing exploration. Such an
erotic expedition is, after all, the most personal, provocative, and passion-inducing
pursuit you can undertake in your lifetime. Whether we make the journey with a lover
or solo, it is a path like no other, helping us to understand our psyche and soul, our
urges, our need to connect with others, and our selves.

Amazing sex is no small undertaking. That's not to say, however, that the Sinclair
program presented in this work cannot be mastered by the erotically inclined. Jam-
packed with research-backed information, this sex primer was written by a qualified
sex expert, who is thrilled to guide you through your process of sexual education and
exploration. So whether your intimacy inquest involves ideas for seduction and sex
play, advice on intensifying arousal, instruction on how to best make love, exposure
to some non-vanilla forms of sex, or the secrets to renewing wilting ardor, know that
this sex manual was penned with all of your needs and desires in mind.

"*Love is the ultimate state, where compassion prevails
and kindness rules. Your work is to discover your
world and then with all your heart give yourself to it.*"

—BUDDHA

This quintessential hotter-sex guide covers every aspect of sexual activity needed to become sex savvy, from the basics, such as anatomy, mutual masturbation, and positions, to more advanced or envelope-pushing forms of sexual expression, such as role-playing, anal sex, Internet sex, and fetishes. It is for anyone—whether novice or master, timid or adventuresome—longing to:

- Have more sex
- Revamp and improve your sex life
- Feel more connected to your partner
- Truly understand sexual response and how the physiological, psychological, and spiritual all interact
- Avoid or overcome sexual disorders that can trump your game
- Up your sexual repertoire safely and responsibly
- Comprehend human sexual nature
- Explore your sexual potential with adventure after adventure
- Realize your utmost propensity for pleasure

The last point bears repeating: This is for anyone longing to realize his or her utmost propensity for pleasure. This promising classic seeks to provide you frankly with the information, tools, and skills you need to fuel desire, ravish your own and each other's bodies, have red-hot sex, and communicate effectively for mutual sexual fulfillment and ecstasy. It also examines both the causes and solutions to common sexual issues that can plague lovers, offering preventative measures to avoid these plagues at any point in your life cycle or relationship.

Powered by major scientific research findings, the significance of which are highlighted throughout, this work helps you and your lover understand one another, giving great attention to gender differences when appropriate. The better-sex program herein is intended for those both in need of crucial, basic information and those desiring a deeper understanding of more complex concepts. There are a number of features designed to help you master the basics—and go beyond them to refine your sensual skills and titillation talents, including:

- "SEXercises" to explore your sexual nature
- "The Science of Sex" fact sections
- "Sexpertise" tips for better lovemaking
- "Sexual Q&A" sidebars answering frequently asked questions
- "In the Bedroom" activities that will help you better connect with your partner
- "Sexual Homework" to practice what you learn in each chapter

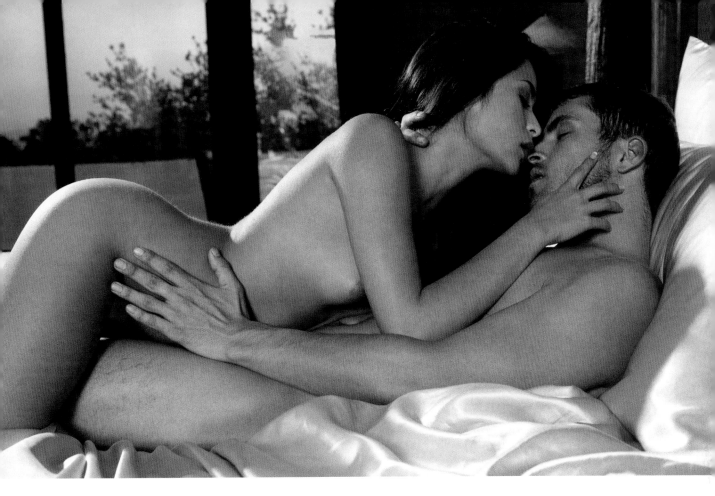

You'll find questions for you and your lover, questions meant to be not only thought-provoking but also meant to cultivate reflection and a greater awareness of your capacity for sexual desire and response. Explicit photos and illustrations throughout will further inspire your erotic activities, realistically equipping you with the artistry, maneuvers, and key elements needed for stimulating pleasure zones and realizing your maximum arousal ability, most notably released in the form of orgasm.

YOUR BETTER-SEX GUIDE

The Sinclair Institute is recognized as a leading source of sex-education videos and sexual health products for individuals and couples who want to improve the quality of intimacy and sex in their relationships. Since 1991, Sinclair has been helping millions of viewers maintain long-lasting, intimate relationships with the ingredients for a lifetime of great sex. More than five million videos alone have been sold in more than twenty-four countries. Guided by the Sinclair advisory board, a diverse team of well-known professional sex educators, researchers, and therapists, these instructional films provide the most accurate, up-to-date sexual-health information available today. They help facilitate a sometimes difficult conversation with your partner about sexual needs and desires. Institute programs have won numerous awards and have received international recognition from organizations that promote sexual health. But the real reward is hearing over and over again from our viewers about increased intimacy and joy in their relationships, as is our hope for this book.

As a member of the Sinclair team, I feel it is an honor to write this much-needed and important sex-education manual. As an AASECT-certified (American Association of Sexuality Educators, Counselors, and Therapists) and academically trained sex educator and sexologist, I have been helping individuals and couples for well over a decade—in the classroom, via the Internet, on the radio, on TV, and through my sex columns, articles and books—to understand and improve their sex lives. In answering people's questions and concerns, I know well the highs and lows of seeking sexual enlightenment, of wanting sexual intimacy that's more fulfilling, exhilarating, fusing, and problem-free. As we hear daily, many are hungering for incredible sex. This work holds the keys to that very longing.

All of us at the Sinclair Institute hope that this work book will become a significant resource for you, and your lover, as your strive for maximum sexual satisfaction. It is our hope that this book will be ranked as your ultimate sex guide, acting as both a catalyst to unlocking your unrealized sexual potential and as a stepping stone to discovering increased pleasure and intimacy in your relationship.

HOW THIS BOOK IS ORGANIZED

The Sinclair Institute's three-step program is actually modeled after the major components of the human sexual-response cycle. The "sexual response cycle" is a term that encompasses a pattern of events that a person typically goes through when physically and/or mentally stimulated. First named and researched by sexologists William Masters and Virginia Johnson in the 1960s, this cycle originally consisted of four phases that are progressive and, at times, overlapping.

According to this cycle, when your body responds to sexual stimulation, it feels arousal before experiencing a stage known as the plateau phase—or a heightened stage of arousal—before culminating with orgasm, and finally concluding in resolution. In the 1970s, Dr. Helen Singer Kaplan added the desire component to the cycle, at the very beginning, for a five-phase model. It is the five-phase model that has been largely used by sexologists, sex therapists, and other professionals ever since.

Rooted in the sexual-response cycle, this work explores the physiological, psychological, and spiritual functions that take place primarily at the desire, arousal, and orgasm stages, enabling you to capitalize on everything sex researchers currently know about human sexual response and how it impacts your relationship and degree of intimacy. In offering a three-step program, this Sinclair Institute book is divided into three major parts: Desire, Arousal, and Orgasm.

Step One: Desire

In Step One—Desire—you will learn about the nature of sexual desire, namely lust and libido, and how sexual cravings, or a lack thereof, impact your and your partner's ability to bask in sex play. The sexual psychology of each gender is explored to help you amplify your amorous efforts and to please your partner even more. Sexual knowledge makes for sexual prowess and power. So in this section, you'll get a complete review of the essential basics, from sexual anatomy, to understanding desire, to fantasy to tricks for turning on your partner.

Step Two: Arousal

In Step Two—Arousal—I'll address the nature of sexual excitement and add fuel to your sexual fire. In amping up your arousal quotient and sexual creativity, we'll cover various forms of sex play, including kissing, foreplay, sexual intercourse, oral sex, and erotic power-play, as well as oft-undiscovered, sensitive sweet spots for building sexual tension. Step-by-step techniques and tips for these different forms of sexual intimacy will be delivered to further enhance your lovemaking skills and ability to excite any part of the body, especially the ones most critical for climax.

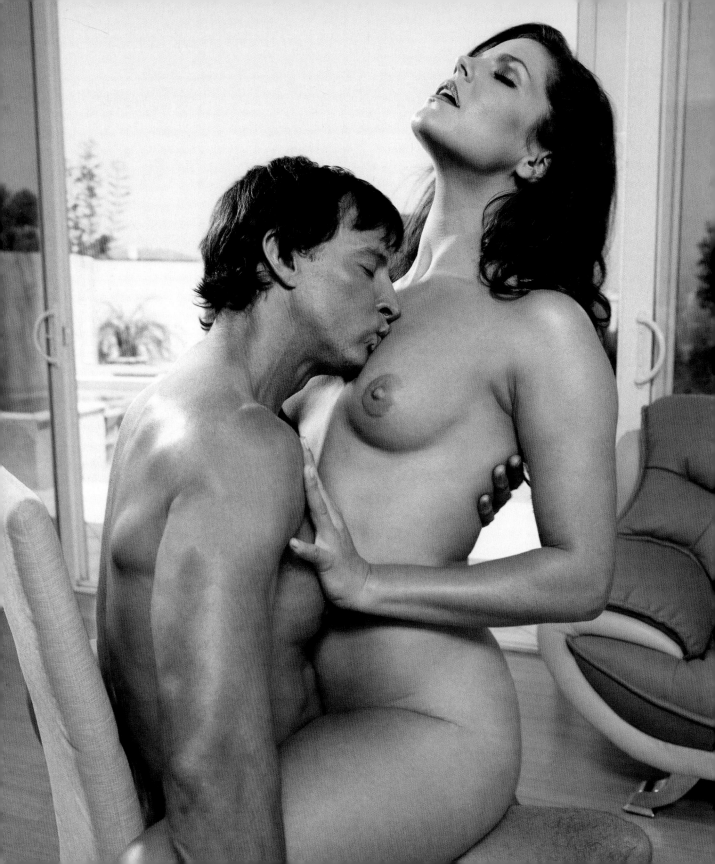

Whether licking, love-biting, massaging, fingering, stroking, sucking, or loving, this section is packed with tantalizing tips galore to help you disarm your lover and maximize your sexual gratification. Stressing sexual creativity, trust, communication, and the importance of intimacy for a happier sex life, Part Two dishes out ideas for variety, fun, and investigation, helping you dodge issues that can afflict romantic relationships. Crucial hot spots and the top ten sexual positions for orgasmic lovemaking are given special attention as are "forbidden" pleasures that can make for even greater sexual bliss.

Step Three: Orgasm

Part Three—Orgasm—delivers all of the critical information you need to know about climax. Here you'll learn the nature of orgasms, how to overcome orgasmic difficulties, and how to have the sweetest, and more frequent, orgasms. In seeking peak sexual response, we will also delve into Eastern approaches to sexual enlightenment. Sensual, sexy, mind-body-soul teachings from traditions such as Tantra will all be explored for further discovering what is most sexually satisfying for you and your lover.

While working your way through this book, it is important to realize that every person's sexual response is unique, with different stimuli eliciting different responses. Your reactions may not be as neatly compartmentalized as the sexual-response cycle model nor necessarily flow in one direction. The exercises, methods, and means to discovery all have, however, the ability to bring you to a euphoric state at any point in your sexual response.

Enjoyable sex for a lifetime is one of the greatest gifts you can give yourself, your lover, and your relationship. Realizing that such "sexploration" will require, at times, patience, understanding, compassion, commitment, and heart, *The Better Sex Guide to Extraordinary Lovemaking* seeks to equip you with the knowledge necessary in overcoming any challenges and the confidence to explore with expertise.

The ability to have thrilling sex doesn't boil down to how to touch someone "here" in "this" way. It is far more complex—and fun—than that. This book seeks to be the alchemy of sex for you, equipping you with the knowledge you need to take your sex life from mediocre to magnificent. The passion pilgrimage you're about to embark upon promises to reap substantial rewards if you let it, having the potential to send you—and your lover—to the depths of your sexual souls.

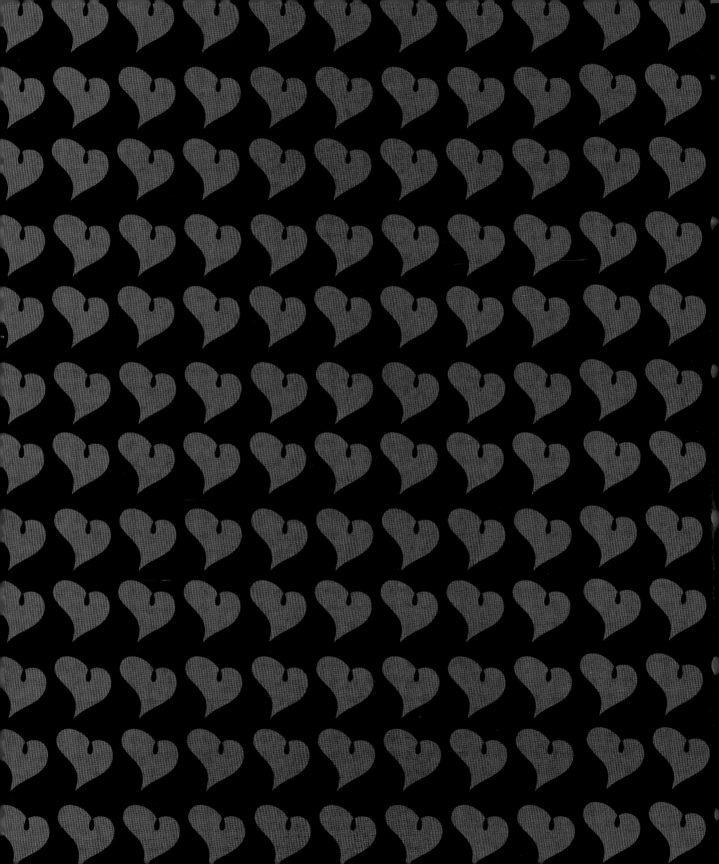

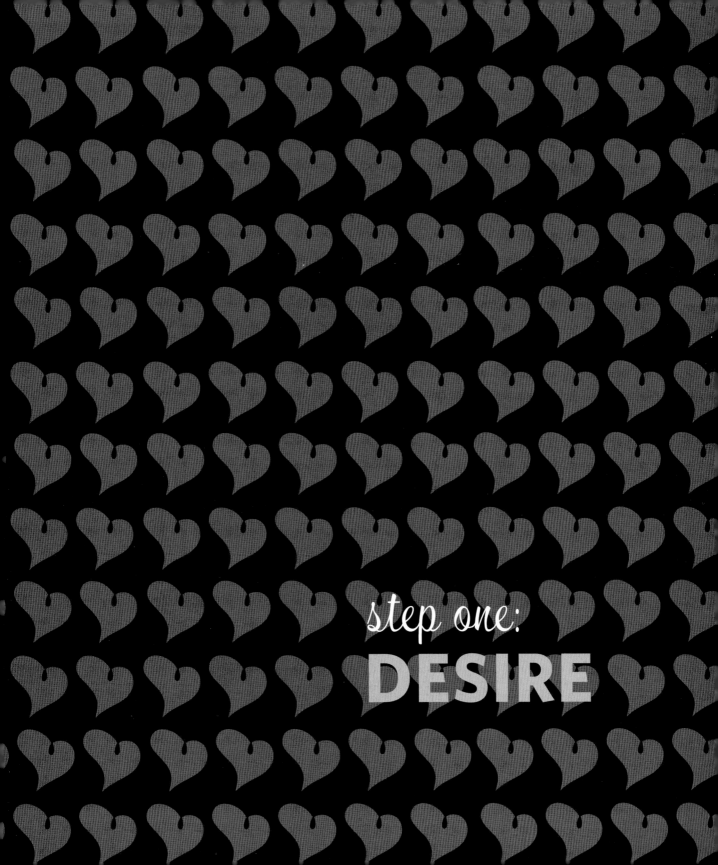

step one:
DESIRE

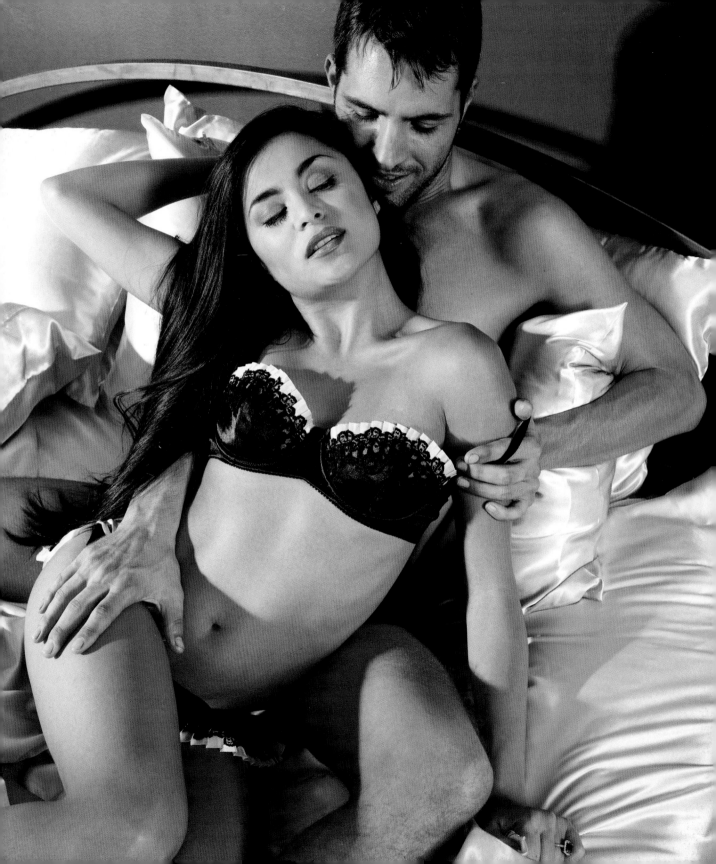

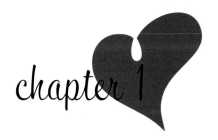

Learn the Nature of Desire to Understand How to Please Yourself and Your Partner

SEXUAL DESIRE. Simply hearing the term is foreplay in and of itself. The phrase captures all the imagination can dish out for sexual allure, from the obscene and dirty, to the piquant and energizing, to the engrossing and exciting. The term is loaded, and the sexual urge such desire envelopes has a hold on all of us, fostering fantasy, fear, or a famishing fervor for more.

Often captured as Eros, the Greek god of lust and love, our drive for sexual intimacy is our creative urge to live and love passionately. This sexual love has historically been regarded as a life-preserving instinct of sorts, an impulse that gratifies some of our most basic human needs, ultimately protecting and preserving the body and mind. When energized by sexual desire, we feel motivated to pursue that which we long for. When submerged in the insistent sexual impulse of eroticism, our intimate relationships thrive as we feel alive and sexually connected with our partner and ourselves. Sexual desire is among the strongest of the forces that motivate human behaviors. The sexual gratification it can lead to is one of the greatest pleasures we humans know.

"A sexual journey that begins in physical desire and delight can end in wisdom."

Being sexual is a core part of being human. As human beings, we are sexual beings, with sexuality, sexual response, and sexual desire central components to our existence. While humans have long struggled to fully embrace and celebrate these sensual elements of the self, there is no denying that one of our fundamental creative impulses involves experiencing desire—and a longing to tune in to our sexual desires.

As we begin our journey toward more satisfying sex, understanding desire as its own entity, separate from arousal, is necessary in grasping our sexual nature. Sexual desire can be induced by intentional or unintentional physical excitation, sexual objects, experiences, fantasies, dreams, wishes, interest, or spontaneous excitement. Whether due to an image, thoughts, memory, scent, sound, or sensory source, sexual desire fuels lust, that intense, unbridled craving for sexual gratification. This primitive, unpredictable human feeling can take us by surprise, or we can actively seek to kindle it. That kindling is made easier or more complicated by your attitudes, mood, and health, and those of your partner, as well as the opportunities available. It is a very subjective experience.

This basic biological longing for sexual release is also closely linked to our innate psychic energy known as the libido. Derived from primordial biological urges, our libido, or sex drive, propels us to express our yen for sexual pleasure. Our sexual desire is the conscious impulse of our libido, our recognition of a longing or hope for something that promises sexual, sensual enjoyment or satisfaction.

On a biological level, such desire serves the important purpose of prompting humans to seek out and engage in sexual activity, having implications for reproduction and survival of our species. Thus, many men and women believe that biological and hormonal processes influence and cause sexual desire. And indeed, research is continually affirming that hormones do play some part in the timing and magnitude of desire.

Exercise 1.1: Sexual Pondering

In your own private space, ponder the following questions. Feel free to jot down your thoughts in a notebook. Really take your time doing this exercise, letting your mind go anywhere about anything.

1. What kinds of objects, physical sensations, foods, memories, and/or interests stimulate your sexual desire?
2. When was the last time you felt pure, sweet lust, to the point you could barely control yourself? Who or what hurled you into this untamable state?

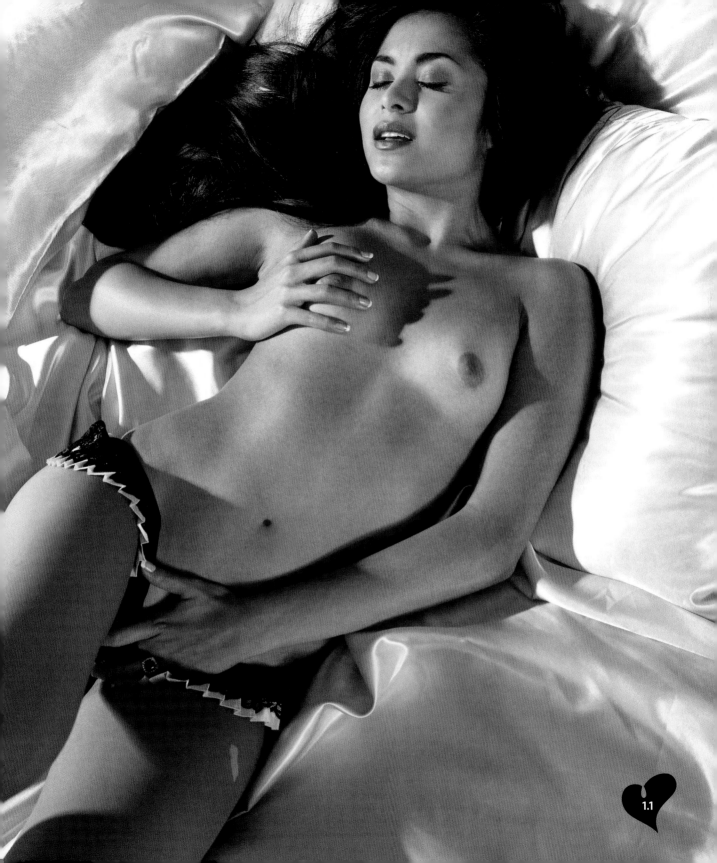

3. Has your sexual desire ever felt more driven by instinct than anything? What was it like to finally revel in your pleasure? What needs did this pleasure-seeking fulfill for you?
4. How can you re-create any of the memories you just gave to the above?

Now get together with your partner, and take turns completing the following sentences.

- For me, the optimal environment for sex would be . . .
- My optimal physical and emotional state for sex involves being or feeling . . .
- Best sex, for me, is dependent upon my relationship being . . .

THE DESIRE FOR SEXUAL VARIETY

For years, evolutionary psychologists have been researching our desire for sexual variety when it comes to both long-term and short-term mating strategies. A 2003 international study involving more than sixteen thousand people across ten major world regions confirmed that sex differences in the desire for sexual variety are culturally universal. The investigation, led by David Schmitt, Ph.D., of Bradley University, revealed that, married or single, heterosexual or gay, men have a significantly greater desire for a larger number of sexual partners than do women. Furthermore, of the men and women who were actively pursuing short-term mates, more than 50 percent of men, but less than 20 percent of women, desired more than one sexual partner in the next month. Previous research conducted by Schmitt and David Buss, Ph.D., at the University of Michigan, also found that men tend to more actively seek short-term relationships than women and require less time than women in getting to know their partners before sleeping with them.

THE
SCIENCE OF *Sex*

According to sex researcher Rosemary Basson, M.D., a woman's motivation to be sexual often stems from her intimacy needs. In an effort to increase emotional intimacy with her lover, a woman will deliberately find or be receptive to sexual stimuli that have the potential to be sexually arousing.

The Role of Testosterone in Sexual Desire and Response

Lust is primarily associated with the hormone testosterone in both men and women. Levels fluctuate with every day, week, and year, and throughout the lifecycle. Testosterone levels are further influenced by one's sex and a number of other biological, psychological, and social factors, as well as the quality and dynamics of the person's sexual relationship. While men have five times more testosterone than women, a female's testosterone receptors are more sensitive than a male's. While often regarded as the male hormone, it is important to realize that testosterone impacts both sexes during sexual activity.

The Rise and Fall of Testosterone

Some researchers hold that male sexual desire is, on average, stronger and more constant from hour to hour and day to day than a female's since men's testosterone levels are steadier. For females, testosterone increases around ovulation, with many women experiencing increased sexual desire and libido around the time an egg is released from the ovary. Studies cited in sources such as the Personality and Social Psychology Bulletin have indicated that women are likelier to masturbate, initiate sex, fantasize about sex, wear provocative clothing, and frequent singles bars around the time of ovulation more than any other time of the month. Research in selected papers of the Fifth World Congress of Sexology has further reported that women with high versus lower levels of circulating testosterone, in general, have higher levels of vaginal blood flow response to erotic stimuli thanks to this hormone.

Overall, men and women with higher circulating levels of testosterone tend to engage in more sexual activity, including masturbation. Male athletes who inject testosterone, too, experience increased sexual thoughts, morning erections, sexual encounters, and orgasms. On the flip side, low levels of testosterone dampen one's sex drive, resulting in fewer fantasies, masturbatory activities, and sex. While often chalked up as problematic, low testosterone may serve a purpose at times. According to a 2001 study out of the Mayo Clinic, as a man becomes increasingly attached to his family, his testosterone level goes down. With the birth of his child, in particular, fathers experience a significant decline in levels of testosterone, including when he holds the baby.

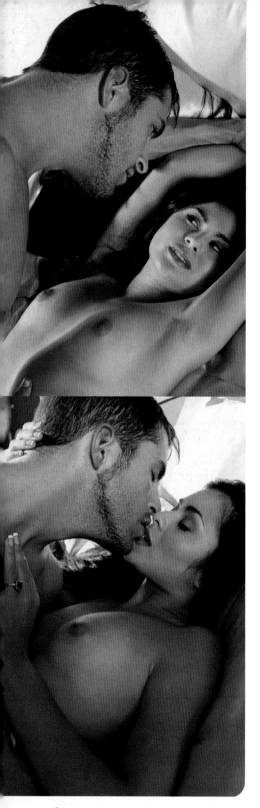

$\mathscr{S}\mathscr{e}$Xercise 1.2: Testosterone Analysis

Contemplate the following, and then share your response with your lover:

1. How would you rate your testosterone level . . .
   a. Strong—I desire lots of sex and enjoy my fair share of masturbating.
   b. Average—My libido gets my attention regularly, and I become easily aroused when I tune into my sexual desire.
   c. Low—My sex drive doesn't feel powerful in that I seldom experience sexual thoughts or the desire to be sexually intimate, including with myself.

2. Are there times of the day, week, or month that your testosterone levels seem heightened, such as . . .
   a. In the morning, when you first get up?
   b. When you're ovulating?
   c. Other?

3. How can you and your lover take advantage of these higher testosterone moments?

TUNE INTO THE SEX CYCLE

As summarized in Personality and Social Psychology Bulletin, research is continually confirming that a woman's fertility cycle influences her motives for sexual behavior. To date, we know that women prefer different characteristics in a potential male sex partner when she's at midcycle (meaning peak fertility) than when she's at low fertility. It is also at this time that she, in general, shows a greater preference for men who are more attractive, symmetrical, and masculine. At midcycle, women also tend to experience:

- An increase in frequency of sexual intercourse and self-stimulation
- More interest in erotic materials, from which she can become more easily aroused at this time
- More sexual desire, arousal, and fantasy
- Orgasm more readily
- Sexual jealousy

Research out of the University of Texas, Austin, has further found that postmenopausal women are likelier than premenopausal women to report love/emotional bonding cues as desire motivators.

Women who cheat are also likely to do so during the fertile phase of their cycle. In capitalizing on a woman's cyclic variations in sexual desire, couples should work to take advantage of these times when she's likelier to be in the mood! Women can lead this effort in keeping a fertility-cycle journal for three months or so, noting her degree of sexual desire on a daily basis and charting the times of the month she feels the most aroused. Couples can then aim to plan romantic rendezvous around these times, blissfully basking in her heightened sexual feelings and orgasmic response.

YOUR BRAIN ON SEX

Now, testosterone is not a solo player in one's zeal for sexual intimacy. The brain itself hosts a smorgasbord of neurotransmitters that impact a human's sexual thirst. These chemical messengers are involved in all aspects of our being: the physical, psychological, and emotional. You know them well. Neurotransmitters bring on the experiences of pain or pleasure, rage or contentment, depression or euphoria, and aggression or intimacy and bonding. Hence, you can see how they ultimately stimulate or inhibit sexual desire, arousal, and performance in influencing moods, emotions, and even personality traits that can affect our sex lives. When it comes to sex and love, dopamine, norepinephrine, and serotonin have proven themselves to be the major players.

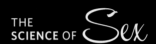

THE SCIENCE OF *Sex*

Research, such as that published in the journal *Social Forces*, continually finds, too, that males with higher testosterone levels marry less often, are more abusive in their marriages, and divorce more regularly.

SEXUAL Q&A: MALE SEXUAL PEAK

Is there any truth to the notion that males reach their sexual peak in their late teens/early twenties?

A male's libido peaks in his late teens/early twenties, when testosterone levels are highest. His hormone levels are high since he is growing and becoming more sexually mature, with testosterone having a major influence on his sexual cognitions and responses. Levels of free testosterone have been shown, for example, to predict the frequency of sexual thoughts in adolescent boys.

While a male reaches a hormonal "peak" at this time, his body does continue to produce testosterone for the rest of his life. And some men maintain quite an active libido well into their senior years, having some of the best sex of their lives at older ages. This is because, despite the fact that maintaining erection and reaching orgasm may come more readily in their younger years, many men come to know more rewarding sex with age. They know that such sex is about having better relationships, a greater familiarity with the body, better ejaculatory control, and the understanding that the enjoyment of sex goes far beyond its physical pleasures.

Dopamine: Brain researchers believe that sexual desires may be indirectly related to elevated levels of dopamine, which inspires and motivates pleasure pursuits, particularly in individuals who are madly in love. This chemical cousin of amphetamines helps us to enjoy sex and look forward to sexual activity, influencing our pleasure by:

- Helping us to perceive and respond to our senses
- Impacting our emotions and primitive drives
- Partially enabling muscle movement and regulating functions such as breathing
- Firing up our neurons
- Reinforcing sexual desire
- Impacting the rush of pleasure we feel with orgasm
- Increasing a sexual experience's intensity and a person's sexual energy

If you're looking to up your dopamine drive, this neurotransmitter can be elevated via a high-protein, low-carbohydrate diet, nutritional supplements, acupuncture, exercise, touch, fantasy, and sex itself. Prescription drugs such as Wellbutrin raise dopamine levels in the brains of people who are depressed, and these drugs can stimulate lust and improve one's sex drive. Wellbutrin is thought to work by boosting the activity of dopamine receptors in the brain.

Norepinephrine: A chemical derived from dopamine, norepinephrine is also thought to stimulate testosterone production, in turn stimulating one's sex drive and contributing to a "lover's high." It is further thought to indirectly boost sex by enhancing mood and promoting emotional states conducive to lovemaking. Norepinephrine is a neurotransmitter used by the nervous system to increase sexual activity and interest.

Serotonin: This neurotransmitter appears to promote sexual responsiveness in controlling negative emotions and removing tension and anxiety that can inhibit sexual arousal. Serotonin fights depression and helps to prevent premature ejaculation by delaying orgasm. It facilitates warmth, intimacy, and optimism.

Yet while seemingly a positive contributor for sex, when it comes to serotonin, there is such a thing as too much of a good thing. Increased levels of serotonin have been found to impact sexual desire through decreased libido and impaired ejaculation in those using antidepressants. While it is thought that such sexual problems are due to Selective Serotonin Reuptake Inhibitors (SSRI) drugs, a.k.a. antidepressants, acting specifically to increase serotonin activity, what exactly happens to cause sexual side effects is unknown. For some individuals, such dilemmas can be resolved by lowering the SSRI dosage or by changing antidepressant brands, under a physician's guidance.

Know His Body

A male's seminal fluid may contribute to romantic passion thanks to neurotransmitters. It has been reported that semen contains dopamine and norepinephrine as well as tyrosine, an amino acid needed to manufacture dopamine. Ejaculate also contains testosterone, which elevates sex drive. Researchers are currently investigating how a woman is affected by the seminal fluid deposited in her vaginal canal during sexual intercourse. In 2002, investigators at State University of New York at Buffalo found that females whose lovers used condoms scored higher on tests for depression than those who did not use protection. Researchers believe that hormones from a male's semen may be absorbed into the body through the vagina, boosting a woman's mood.

Know Her Body

Female sexual desire is also stimulated by her ovaries and adrenal cortex (the outer portion of the adrenal gland, which is located on top of each kidney), both of which secrete androgens. The release of this hormone may result in increased genital skin sensitivity and direct action on her spinal cord, brain, and neurotransmitters, all of which coordinate in getting her turned on. Overall, a female's sexual response is regarded as more complex than that of the male.

PRIMED FOR SEX? YOU BE THE JUDGE . . .

Pioneering sex researchers have held that sexual experiences begin with desire. It is this appetite for sex that manifests and coaxes an individual to seek out a partner, pursue an encounter, and engage in sex acts. According to the sexual-response cycle presented by sex researchers William Masters and Virginia Johnson in the 1960s, and later by Helen Singer Kaplan in the 1970s, desire leads to sexual arousal. Yet new findings are suggesting that the experience of desire may not be such a precursor to sexual arousal but rather an afterthought of sorts. Arousal may just precede desire, since desire may be the brain's reaction to a sensation that triggers arousal by a subliminal or physical stimulus such as a touch on the hand.

Researchers at the University of Amsterdam have concluded that the body appears to be primed for sex before the mind even has time to react. Sexual desire isn't always a conscious process. It appears, rather, to emerge from sexual stimulation or the activation of one's sexual system. In investigating sexual responsiveness, Dutch researchers found that the body is practically instantly activated when exposed to sexual imagery. The more intense the sexual images, the stronger the electric signals emitted by the participants' involuntary responses. Investigators concluded that sexual responsiveness can be launched or intensified by stimuli we're not even aware of.

So, in understanding the nature of your desire, sexual desire may be best placed after arousal. Interestingly enough, this would be more in accordance with other recent research neurobiologists have conducted, which indicates that there is a pattern in human awareness in other areas of life. Before we are conscious that we want to do something—opening a book, for instance—the brain regions needed to perform the activity are already fired up. This challenges the idea that we humans are proactive deciders in our desires. Regardless of which comes first, our main concern in this section is how to power up your sex drive to its fullest for better sex.

Love vs. Sex

Humans can easily distinguish feelings of desire from romance, as these experiences are associated with different constellations of brain regions. This was demonstrated by Helen Fisher, Ph.D., and her colleagues at Rutgers University when comparing brain patterns of those in love versus those not in love. In a study in 2002, men were asked to watch three types of videos: one erotic, one relaxing, and one on sports. In analyzing the findings of their brain scans, Fisher found that the brain patterns produced by watching each of these visuals were different from those found in brain scans of her subjects who were not in love.

Lust at First Sniff: Pheromones

A hotter sex life could be right under your nose. Actually, it may be in your nose. While there has been no convincing evidence to date, some neuroscientists believe that an olfactory nerve, coined "Nerve O," is involved in processing human pheromones, which are odorless, invisible chemical substances that may trigger sexual response. "Nerve O," the endings of which are in the nasal cavity, has fibers that go from the human vomeronasal organ (VNO) directly to sex and emotion regions of the brain, bypassing the brain's olfactory cortex. According to neurologist Dr. Alan Hirsch, there is a direct connection between the olfactory bulb at the top of your nose and the septal nucleus of the brain (erection center).

While research is still trying to sort through how pheromones work exactly, researchers believe that these highly individualized scented hormones, detected subconsciously by our olfactory systems, help humans to identify a potential partner's sexual cues, influencing mating, bonding, and caring for offspring. Incredibly, this unsuspecting "aphrodisiac" of sorts is the product of armpit sweat that has been broken down by bacteria. These hormones are related to the apocrine glands of the skin and glandular secretion and flora present in moist areas of the body, such as the feet, mouth, and genitals.

With smell being our most powerful sense in many regards, a person's odor can affect whom he or she has sex with and how often. As reported in the Archives of Sexual Behavior, males exposed to a synthesized human male pheromone have reported higher levels of sexual intercourse, petting, affection, and kissing. They're also likelier to be sleeping with a romantic partner.

Thus, all indicators show that humans are actually biologically programmed to prefer the scent of some possible lovers over others, especially when it comes to reproduction. With just one whiff, basic drives, feelings, and thoughts can be triggered, with your nose delivering instant indicators if you're aroused. The ultimate goal in one's subconscious ability to detect odors is to learn more about a potential mating partner's major histocompatibility complex (MHC), a set of genes that—if dissimilar to yours—boost your offspring's immune system, ultimately helping the infant to better resist disease.

"He Just Smells So Good . . ."

The desire for opposite immune systems was confirmed in the "sweaty t-shirt study," conducted by Swiss researcher Claus Wedekind and colleagues in 1995. Female participants were asked to smell plain cotton tees that were worn by male participants who had not used scented soaps or deodorant for two nights. Results revealed that opposites attract, with women preferring men whose immune systems were different from their own. Those men whose immune systems were too similar to that of a female participant were regarded as unpleasant. Such is important when considering the consequences.

Research by geneticist Carol Ober and colleagues at the University of Chicago has found that couples with high levels of chemicals in common are likely to have fertility problems such as miscarriage. Research at the University of New Mexico has further found that the women who have similar chemical makeups as their lovers are also likely to encounter infidelity, or to at least strongly consider such. Couples who are more dissimilar, on the other hand, have a better chance of successfully procreating and remaining monogamous. The 2006 article in Psychological Science reported that women were happiest with their sex lives when their immune systems were not similar to their male partners; women whose immune system genes are more similar to their partner's report greater dissatisfaction with their sex lives. Pheromones may also enhance a female's mood and have an alleviating effect on any depression and stress she's experiencing.

THE
SCIENCE OF *Sex*

The word "pheromone" comes from the Greek words pherein, meaning "to carry," and hormone, meaning "to excite." They are also known as "ectohormones," meaning they are chemical messengers transported outside of the body that have the potential to evoke particular responses or behaviors.

"She Just Smells So Good . . . "

While women are often credited for sniffing their way to a better mate for reproduction, 2001 research out of the University of Texas, Austin, has found that men are quite capable of using a female's body odor to detect ovulation. Male study participants were asked to rate t-shirts worn by female participants during three consecutive nights of their late follicular (ovulatory) phase of the menstrual cycle. Researchers then compared reactions to these shirts with ratings these same men gave t-shirts worn by the women during the luteal (nonovulatory phase). They found that the men rated the scent of t-shirts from the follicular phase as sexier and more pleasant. Researchers concluded that women look and smell more attractive to men at certain times of the month.

WHAT'S LOVE GOT TO DO WITH IT?

Up to this point, we have focused namely on the biologically driven aspect of sexual desire. Yet Mother Nature is only one piece of the puzzle when it comes to human sex drive and sexual response. While biological mechanisms play a huge role in active or nonexistent sexual desire, emotional, psychological, and spiritual factors come heavily into play, as well.

Sexual desire involves your entire being. It is inseparable from your mental and spiritual energies, which are, in many cases, what ultimately turn you on. Even when physically aroused, you can still "check out" of a lust-filled moment if you are unable to become mentally and emotionally stimulated. These additional components, which go into making up your sexual energy, must be romanced, too.

Most books on sexuality—aside from those focusing on Tantric sex, sacred sex, or the Kama Sutra—largely ignore sexual energy. Yet this aspect of sexual intimacy is what makes for fantastic sex. This powerful force of nature goes far beyond sex drive, revealing itself in much of who we are, how we behave, and what we stand for. Sexual energy is what fuels sexual desire and response, making sex acts not just things we "do," but enthralling expressions—and exchanges—of ourselves. All of us house sexual energy. In satisfying sex, we harness it.

Anybody can have sex. Plenty of people want no more than raw physical sex resulting in climax. Yet even the idea of casual sex resounds more with people when it is cast as a "meaningful fling." Most women and men want, or come to eventually want, something more than the physical in getting into bed with someone. Most people know that the best of sex involves much more than the libido. It's about connection, love, passion, care, sincerity, empathy, and compassion, among a host of other feel-good characteristics. Sexual

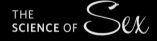

THE
SCIENCE OF *Sex*

Our sense of smell is so powerful that neurologist Alan Hirsch found that one-quarter of patients who had lost their sense of smell developed a sexual dysfunction. In being the strongest of our five senses, smell is highly involved in sexual attraction, function, and pleasure.

desire and intimacy need to involve those and so much more, or else it's hard for many individuals to feel desire, arousal, and satisfaction. For many lovers, sexual intimacy is mostly about:

Emotional safety

Emotional security entails being in a healthy, committed relationship, one where you feel confident and good about your union and your partner. Such a relationship is often defined as having honest, sound communication; feeling heard and understood; being able to disclose your innermost thoughts; feeling supported and supportive; keeping promises and being reliable; and being able to depend on one another. Lovers are able to reveal their complex selves—the good and the bad—histories included, and truly be there for each other.

Being present

Being present means discovering meaning in your relationship, in each other, and in your intimacy. You focus on the "now" and don't live in the past or be too focused on what will happen in the future. You enjoy the moment and are attentive to one another. When you have sex, it isn't about rushing toward a goal like orgasm; instead, it's about enjoying the entire ride.

Having a loving space in which to explore
your dreams and sexual imagination

Even the most familiar of lovers can feel vulnerable to the power and safety dynamics involved in sharing private fantasies, wishes, and dreams. When you take such a risk, you want to feel affirmed and liberated. You want to be able to appreciate a balance of safety and excitement as you explore expanding desire in all of its realms. You feel that you are able to reveal yourselves without fear of judgment or criticism. You feel respected and accepted unconditionally as you expose some of your most private thoughts and desires, sexual or otherwise.

Finding love, connection, and healing with
one another, with nature, or with a higher power

Humans desire love, affection, and sensual fusion. In desiring sex, we long to make love. We yearn to hear sweet nothings. We want to fuse heart, body, and soul. We value touch, talk, togetherness, thought, realism, idealism, passion, devotion, and feeling known through and through. Lovemaking is a gift to be shared with each other and a way to become one with the universe.

Feeling like an equal

Healthy relationships are built on equality, harmony, and reciprocity. So if you sabotage your relationship by expecting sex, being controlling, or by getting jealous or possessive, you, in effect, kill desire. You can't strive for superb sex unless you feel valued and nurtured. As friends and lovers, you must take turns giving, receiving, and being selfless, when sexually intimate and not. Neither of you can be dominated or made to feel less than worthy. Good lovers are a team who love and respect one another, in bed and out.

Being stimulated beyond the physical

Beyond initial physical, sexual attraction, you eventually want more out of your sexual liaisons. You find yourself stimulated by your lover's intellect, sense of humor, communication style, creativity, spirituality, values, optimism, thoughtfulness and consideration, interests, and so on. Sex becomes more about your relationship than about simply eye candy or even decent sex.

Keeping a relationship healthy and vital

Nurture your relationship and each other, and you'll nurture your lovemaking experience as well. You do this by complimenting each other, making time for one another, showing appreciation, giving each other attention on a regular basis, and making an effort to make your lover feel special.

Exercise 1.3: Sex Brainstorming

On a piece of paper, brainstorm all of the traits you would like to see present in your romantic relationship. You don't need to write out whole sentences. Just find a quiet moment when you can relax, undisturbed, and let the thoughts just come to you as you jot down key words. Now, look over your list. Which characteristics are present in your relationship? Which ones are lacking? How can the presence or absence of the most important factors be enhancing or hurting your sex life and sexual desire?

   If both partners are comfortable, share your lists. See where you see eye to eye on relationship characteristics and where you differ. With traits that are absent, consider ways they can be fostered in your union. What can each of you do to make sure your relationship supports those traits? With characteristics that are undesirable, how can both of you work to reduce or eliminate their impact on your union?

THE SCIENCE OF *Sex*

Research at the University of Newcastle in England has found that women using birth control pills are likelier to attract men whose chemical makeup is similar to their own. In going off of the pill, there is a chance that a woman will experience diminished attraction to her mate.

WHEN SEXUAL DESIRE WANES

Sexual desire is one of the most personal aspects of our sense of self, not only as a sexual being, but as a human being. Sexual desire is intricately linked not only to the quality of our relationships but also to our quality of life. The French have acknowledged this well, having connected sexual desire with the term élan vital, meaning "life force" or "joy in living."

Given that diminished sexual desire can impact anybody at any point in life, it is best to examine issues and circumstances that can cause it to wane before exploring the many ways you can "turn on" your sex life. Having a firm understanding of the causes of decreased sex drive and desire can help you choose and pursue your own personal better-sex plan, customizing strategies to reverse and prevent sexual-desire disorders.

Sexual desire does fluctuate throughout a person's lifetime—and that can prove painful and problematic for you and/or your relationship. When our sexual needs, wants, and wishes languish, we take it very personally. Our partners take it very personally. Yet nearly everyone will experience diminished desire at some point in life. Numerous studies have reported anywhere from 25 percent to 63 percent of women and 10 percent to 52 percent of men as experiencing diminished sexual desire. Symptoms of diminished or inhibited sexual desire include:

- Rejecting sexual advances on a regular basis
- Rarely thinking about sex
- Not getting aroused by erotic people, situations, or things
- Having sex as more of an obligation than anything
- Rarely/never initiating sex
- Adverse feelings about sex

Sexual-desire problems are quite common. Such issues are of major concern to many since relationships where one or both partners experience low libido are often characterized as dissatisfying and having poor overall adjustment. Couples in relationships grappling with this issue can be left feeling unhappy, distressed, or "abnormal."

Libido can decrease for a number of reasons, as seen in the following table, "Reasons for Low or No Sex Drive." Some are within an individual's control, whereas others require professional help.

$\mathcal{S}\mathit{ex}$PERTISE

All of these components together make for much more of a lovemaking experience with one's partner, one's self, and the universe at large, as demonstrated by Dr. Gina Ogden's ISIS Wheel of Sexual Experience. In integrating sexuality, spirituality, and more, Ogden stresses the human need to go beyond a physical connection during sex. In a U.S.-based study involving almost four thousand participants, mostly females ages eighteen to eighty-six, Ogden learned that sex is a body-mind-heart-soul experience for many. Almost half of participants needed to connect with their spiritual energy at the moment of sexual ecstasy. Of the 684 male survey respondents, 80 percent said that satisfying sex is due to feeling loved and accepted. In short, to have the best sex, you need to celebrate one another.

THE
SCIENCE OF *Sex*

Sex is a powerful motivator for and source of pleasure and joy. Research in the *Journal of Social and Personal Relationships* has found that sex is strongly correlated with extraversion, openness, and self-esteem (mainly among women). Good sex can also decrease sexual anxiety.

When it comes to women in particular, academics have identified four specific motives for why women of reproductive age have sex:

1. **Sex for intimacy.** Women long to feel close or connected to their partners, using sex as a way to express love or to strengthen the union's emotional bond. This desire tends to increase the frequency of intercourse, which is in part due to the relationship's exclusivity and the ease of partner availability. Women who have sex for this reason are more committed to their partners and are less likely to have sex outside of the relationship.

2. **Sex to intensify physical pleasure.** Women pursue sex because it feels good physically or emotionally. They also like that it's exciting and fulfills their need for adventure. These women tend to be high in sensation-seeking and having positive feelings about sex. They also report a greater need for sex and sexual desire, more frequent intercourse, more partners (particularly casual sex partners), and more risk-taking.

3. **Sex to pacify or please a partner.** Women use sex as a way to avoid negative relationship consequences. These women tend to have more negative emotional responses to sex, indicating that they are having sex to please or appease their lovers.

4. **Sex as a way of dealing with negative emotions, or as a way to affirm self-worth.**

For some women, sex is a way to cope with feelings like sadness, loneliness, and stress. It may also be a way of dealing with feelings of personal inadequacy in feeling loveable and sexually desirable. Sex is used as a way to escape, avoid, or minimize negative emotional states. These women tend to be more tolerant of casual sex and are more ambivalent about sex in general.

Interestingly enough, 2008 research out of the University of Missouri indicates that women, overall, appear to endorse intimacy motives less strongly around the time they are more fertile.

What to Do When You're Not in the Mood

Getting to the heart of chronic low or no sexual desire involves untangling myriad issues and often requires professional help. First you should seek out a physician in order to rule out any physical causes. A certified sex therapist or counselor can also help you to navigate any psychological or relational issues that affect your sex life.

Before seeking out assistance, however, take a moment to listen to your body: What's out of balance? What needs attention? What health problems are ailing you? What do you want to have happen? What is going on in the "now" that can be impacting what goes on in the bedroom?

Too Stressed Out and/or Tired for Sex

Stress and fatigue are two of the most common reasons for low or no sexual desire. The good news is that these are two of the easiest issues to resolve in many respects and are often only temporary situations. Often, your sex drive rebounds when the difficult time is over. For example, you may have the energy for sex after hiring a babysitter on a regular basis or after taking a nice long vacation, either of which can bring down your stress level and boost energy.

It is important to realize, too, that even the best of life transitions such as a new job or even the birth of a child can negatively impact sexual desire. So consider if the possible reason(s) for your diminished libido are perhaps more short-term than chronic. Can these reasons be easily remedied with simple lifestyle changes that are meant to benefit your sex life, things such as going for a twenty-minute walk instead of watching TV when exhausted? What steps can you and your partner take immediately to boost your desire and response? Recognizing and repairing the physical, psychological, and relational factors that are negatively affecting your relationship is the only way to improve a lagging libido, unless you're in a predicament that you need to tough out; needing time to mourn the loss of your cherished family pet is one such example.

SeXPERTISE

According to research in the *Journal of Personality* and *Social Psychology*, having sex for procreation purposes is true only for a small percentage of women who report this as the only reason they are having sex. In most cases of vaginal-penile intercourse, women are not trying to conceive.

 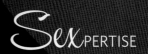

Reasons for Low or No Sex Drive

PHYSICAL

- Poor health or physical problems, including convalescence—sluggish after sickness
- Genetics
- Hormone deficiencies (e.g., low range of total testosterone)
- Medications such as antidepressants
- Overwork/exhaustion, including parenthood and nursing a newborn
- Age
- Nutritional deficits, such as low zinc, and poor diet including high-fat or too few calories consumed
- Alcohol/drug/nicotine use
- Infertility as an intimacy stressor
- Pregnancy or childbirth
- Menopause
- Contraceptives

PSYCHOLOGICAL

- Laziness, including lovers taking sex for granted
- Depression or emotional distress—feeling emotionally shut down
- Unhappiness with either self, partner, or relationship
- Feeling undesirable/body image issues
- History of sexual trauma/abuse
- Effect of having a sexual disorder
- Stress & anxiety
- Low self-esteem or poor sexual self-esteem
- Feelings of not being adequate for self or as lover
- Misconceptions of what is "normal" sexual desire
- History of poor sexual performance (e.g., poor ejaculatory control, inability to please partner, or history of erectile failure, that leads to performance anxiety)

RELATIONAL

- Reality settling in, ending unrealistic fantasies about partner/relationship
- Boredom in bedroom or sexual apathy
- Lack of or poor communication
- Fear of revealing vulnerabilities
- Chronic desire differences
- Persistent hassles and conflicts with partner—related to sex or not, or physically/emotionally abusive relationship with partner, including a history of such
- Feeling anger or resentment toward partner
- Partner desires or lack thereof
- Unskilled lover
- No longer sexually attracted to partner

SOCIAL or GENERAL

- Lack of opportunity due to other life demands
- Negative messaging that being sexually expressive is unhealthy
- Sexual ignorance
- Poor intimacy management
- Death of a loved one, including pets

Sexercise 1.4: What Does Sex Mean to You?

On your own, each partner is to answer the following questions:

1. What does sex mean to you?
2. What does it mean to have a healthy sex life?
3. What frustrates you, if anything, about societal expectations regarding your sexual desire, sexual response, and sex life?
4. Ideally, how often would you like to have sex?
5. How long would you like lovemaking sessions to last? (Note: Think beyond the actual act of sexual intercourse.)
6. Are you being realistic in the responses you have given so far?
7. How would you assess your joie de vivre (joy of living) as well as that of your partner. Why do you regard it as so?

Now, share your answers with your partner, reviewing each question one at a time and discussing your answers. Where are you on the same page? Which answers are influenced more by societal expectations than on your expectations? What excites you about what your partner has shared?

SEXUAL Q&A: HOW MUCH IS ENOUGH?

When it comes to the amount of sex I should be having, how often is normal?

Sexual desire may be a near "universal" experience, but that said, the frequency of sex is different for everyone. Sex drives vary according to the individual; what's "often" for you may be not nearly often enough for your partner. While the media may try to give us data on the "average" amount of sex people are having, this number is quite arbitrary and meaningless. Why? Because it often comes down to who was surveyed. Population samples from various studies often range in age, occupation, sexual orientation, relationship status, education, and geography, all of which can greatly impact results. Furthermore, such research often focuses on the frequency of sexual intercourse, often disregarding other forms of sexual intimacy and the matter of whether lovers are actually all that dissatisfied with the amount and type of sex they're having.

So you may have already drawn conclusions about the quality of your own sex life, based on these studies and headliners—false conclusions that can make you feel angry at yourself and/or your lover without cause. There's a lot of pressure to have sex a certain way: magically becoming aroused, lasting a long time, having an orgasm with ease, and always feeling sexually ready for a roll in the hay or for more. When you don't live up to these unrealistic expectations, you can feel dysfunctional, inadequate, abnormal, or inhibited, even if you don't have an actual problem. In avoiding the hurt, tension, relationship doubts, and confusion that can crop up, you need to navigate what's right for your sex life. You need to have heart-to-hearts on what sex, sexual desire, and a healthy sex life mean to you and your partner. In some cases, this may require working with a certified sex therapist or counselor on compatibility issues.

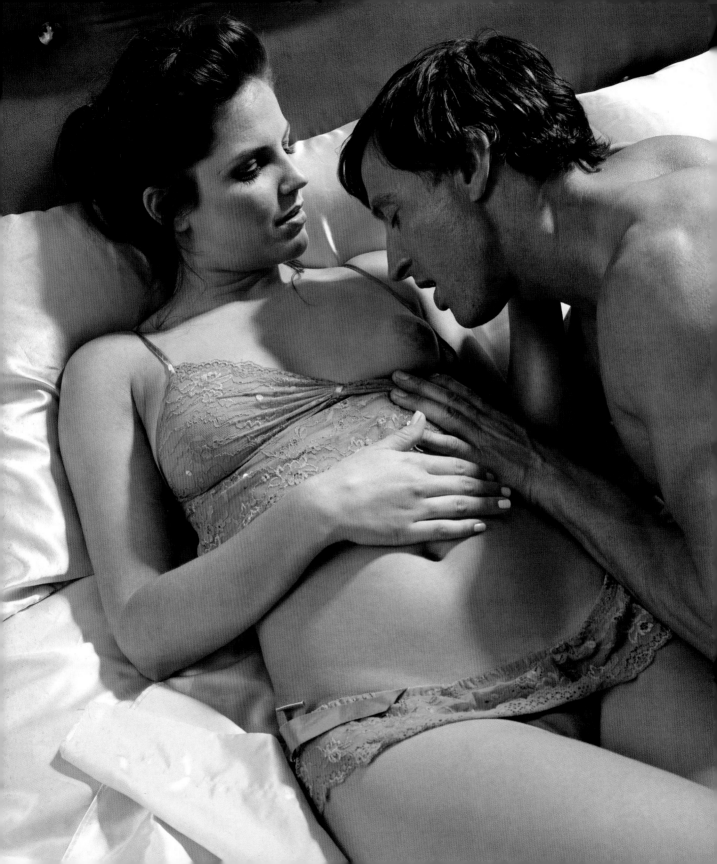

HOW SEXUALLY COMPATIBLE ARE YOU?

When it comes to sexual compatibility, the first and most important thing to realize is that it takes two to tango. You cannot simply point the finger at your partner as being the problem: He's too sexually demanding; she's too sexually inhibited, etc. In resolving incompatibility issues, whether temporary or long-term, you both need to take responsibility for finding solutions. First you'll need to examine points of possible contention, such as:

A. How sex is initiated? Is one partner always initiating? What kind of burden does that put on the initiator? What issues need to be worked through, such as the belief that the woman should always be the passive recipient of sexual advances?

B. How are you reacting to one another's desires? Are you being supportive and understanding? Are you being critical and judgmental? How is your reaction making for a hostile or positive sex environment? What can be changed about your dynamic and relationship so that both of you feel that you can share sexy thoughts or wants without fear. For example, responding to a sexual fantasy with an open mind by saying, "Thank you for sharing. I'll need to think on that since I've never truly considered how that could be a turn-on."

C. How do you deal with disappointment? Do you sulk, criticize, withdraw, or become agitated, hostile, angered, thoughtless, or even cruel when you're turned down after requesting sex or a certain type of act? Do you have any of those reactions when you give in to a request? Consider ways that you can remain positive and offer suggestions for alternative ways of being sexually intimate so that some needs are gratified.

THE SCIENCE OF *Sex*

In light of recent research on arousal preceding sexual desire, researchers at the University of Amsterdam are proposing that the answer to those suffering from low libido may be to emphasize sexy feelings or physical cues that arouse one's sexual circuitry instead of thinking sexy thoughts.

Every person's sex style is unique. In dealing with mismatched libidos, which can happen at any point in your lives together, you need to work on positive, effective communication, staying calm and confident, and not apologizing for the response and desires. Evaluate how you're listening and reacting to one another. Talk about what sex means to you, your hopes in the sexual relationship (e.g., who should take the lead, variety, the amount of foreplay, time, etc.). Finally, you need to brainstorm resolutions:

1. Figure out a compromised time frame for sexual intimacy, and conserve your energy for such, since, for many couples, the mismatch issue comes down to being sexually piqued at different times of the day. He may be more up for sex in the morning, while she is more of a night person when it comes to making love.

2. Do a "strengths analysis" of your relationship, highlighting where you are compatible and what is working. Count your sexual blessings where you can.

3. Introduce more variation in sex play. For some couples, the mismatch issue boils down to one lover being more bored than the other. So spice things up (e.g., change the location, or go sex-toy shopping).

4. Compromise. Take turns accommodating one another's desires. This is in no way encouraging you to do something that you do not want to do. More sex acts doesn't necessarily equal a greater, richer sex life. If you're uncomfortable engaging in an activity, then sex becomes problematic. Lovers should never be coerced. You can, however, engage in sex acts that may not necessarily turn you on, such as oral sex, if only in an effort to pleasure your lover. And your lover can return the favor.

BOOSTING SEXUAL DESIRE

In dealing with low or no sexual desire, professionals are quick to prescribe a drug for male clients. They've been praying for a "magic" pill to prescribe female clients for years. And while there is some value in taking medication, individuals and couples need to realize that emotional and relationship dynamics, either due to or existing prior to the dilemma, may still be at play—and that can continue to impact desire. Health behaviors, primarily diet, alcohol/drug, and exercise routine, need to be evaluated and improved. A holistic approach is in order and may involve any of the following strategies:

THE
SCIENCE OF *Sex*

According to researchers at The Kinsey Institute, evidence suggests that sexual arousal, desire, and excitement are governed by two basic, distinct operating brain channels: one that encourages sexual eagerness and another that hampers it. This may help to explain why some people become more easily turned on than others, showing that there is nothing "wrong" with you. Your level of sexual desire may just be what's right for you.

Physical Remedies for His Libido

When a male has low or no desire, prescription drugs or natural herbs may help to stimulate his libido. A number of factors play into resolving the issue, with the plan of action often based on a health practitioner's medical training (an allopathic doctor will likely choose treatment plans that differ from that of a naturopathic doctor). A physician may map out a testosterone supplementation plan, which could include pills, topical creams, lozenges, and/or injections in high or low doses. Natural male sexual enhancement products are also available, with certain ones consisting of homeopathic compounds or natural herbs. (Note: Herbal supplements are often unregulated by the U.S. Food and Drug Administration (FDA), so be sure to use such only under the guidance of a trained health professional, especially if you're using prescription drugs.)

SEXUAL Q&A: ASEXUALITY

I can't recall having ever felt sexual desire or attraction in my life. I do like to have the occasional special companion, however. It just never gets very sexual because I'm not feeling it for them in that way. Am I asexual, or do I have some kind of disorder?

Hypoactive sexual desire disorder (HSDD) is a lifelong absence and deficiency of sexual desire and sexual fantasies for sexual activity. In its primary condition, this disorder is caused by hormone imbalances or deficiency, psychological conflicts about sex, or a physical condition that disrupts the transmission of sexual messages to and from the brain. In its secondary condition, where an individual has lost interest in sex and is no longer aroused, causes include anger, stress, performance failure, anxiety, depression, and emotional difficulties. If your condition is causing you distress or interpersonal difficulties, and is not due to a psychological issue such as depression, a medical condition, or legal or illegal drug use, you should consider seeking professional help. On the other hand, you may be part of the 1 percent of the population that appears to be asexual—and that's just the way you are.

While scientific research on asexuality is limited, people who label themselves as asexual have no desire for sexual intimacy and do not experience sexual attraction, whether this was true for them at some point in their lives or not. While not desiring sex, many asexuals do, however, want relationships where their emotional and even romantic needs are met and where they are giving such in return. As with any relationship, compromise and communication are critical in the success of their relationships.

Physical Remedies for Her Libido

For women with low or no desire due to hormonal issues, hormonal balancing, which is based on feedback from a diagnostic utility test, can help put her body back on track. Some sex therapists and physicians may recommend supplements such as ArginMax, which contains ginkgo, L-arginine, ginseng, and vitamins, depending on the therapist's belief system in how to best treat the body. Studies by the manufacturer suggest that ArginMax has a positive effect on women's libido and sexual satisfaction, though this statement has not been evaluated by the FDA (the FDA does not regulate natural supplements). For ladies based in Europe, a testosterone patch is available. One thing to realize, however, is that low libido for women is rarely due to physiological causes, especially in premenopausal women.

Relational Libido Remedies

Despite any wishful thinking, you can't simply leave your other life issues at the bedroom door and expect to have a good sex life. Everything that goes on outside of your sex life works its way between the sheets, disrupting the entire relationship. And everything going on in the bedroom (or rather what's not) ripples out, affecting other parts of your life, as well. Whether low desire is due to life issues or your relationship itself, you need to examine the relationship and remove the blocks to your sexual desire. After all, it's hard to be intimate with someone whom you don't think favorably of or whom you cannot communicate with, especially if you are emotionally shut down yourself. To get back into sync with one another, practice sensual touch, role-play, and communication skills, as suggested throughout this book. Heal whatever damage has been caused by the low libido, which can include guilt, insecurity, inadequacy, and feeling unattractive, unlovable, worthless, helpless, and rejected.

Psychological Libido Remedies

You both may need to rebuild your sexual self-confidence. This involves learning how to be a more skilled lover, with a heavy focus on erotic technique. The afflicted lover also needs to counter thoughts involving "I can't," practicing self-affirming statements that will boost self-assurance and self-esteem.

$S\mathscr{ex}$PERTISE

In sorting through reasons for low or no sexual desire, consider your solo sexual practices. If you have trouble experiencing desire with a current partner but can still masturbate, have sexual fantasies, or desire sex with another individual, then your condition is more situational and relational than anything. In such cases, it is a good idea to evaluate just how content you are with your partner, your sex life, and the relationship—as well as your pain, fears, anger, doubts, resentment . . . . You then have three options: Do nothing and resign yourself to the situation; commit to letting go of negative feelings and working on relationship issues with your partner; or get out of the relationship.

Other Libido Remedies

As we delve into the next section, Arousal, you'll learn how to have more satisfying sex and how to make sure that you don't get stuck in a rut. You'll plan sensual dates, explore your wilder side, and experiment with arousers, from the "tame" to the "unconventional."

EROTOPHILIC VS. EROTOPHOBIC: WHICH ARE YOU?

"Erotophilic" means having positive attitudes toward sex. "Erotophobic" means having negative attitudes toward sex. Which describes you? Which describes your lover? Much of our ability to feel and embrace sexual desire and to react to our body's sexual responses is based on how we feel about sex and lust. People can fall anywhere in between these two extremes, especially when it comes to reacting positively or negatively to specific sexual behaviors. Being aware of this continuum is important in understanding your beliefs about the rewards of sex and relationship satisfaction. That is, if you think that sex helps maintain a good relationship, you're more apt be more satisfied with the relationship following sexual activity than someone who feels sex does not contribute to the relationship. Furthermore, you're likelier to get turned on by your desire and to embrace opportunities that allow for sexual expression.

So how do you know if you're an erotophile or erotophobe? See if you answer "yes" to one of the following quizzes more than the other.

THE EROTOPHILIC QUIZ

Do you:

- See sex as something normal and natural?
- Think that people have the right to seek out consensual sexual interactions involving mutual pleasuring?
- Have positive attitudes toward sexually explicit materials?
- Believe that sex issues need to be discussed?
- Regard sex as an act that is expressive, supportive, and bonding?
- Hold sex as something to celebrate?

If you are sex positive and feel good about your sexual self-image, you may use sexual intimacy as a way to express or achieve affection, emotional intimacy, and love—all of which, in turn, promote emotional bonding with your partner. Erotophilics' positive sexual outlook can stem from a number of things, including positive messages about sex while growing up, a partner's contagiously healthy outlook about sex, enriching sexual experiences, and sex education.

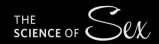

THE SCIENCE OF *Sex*

Research published in *Psychosomatic Medicine* and in *Personality and Social Psychology Bulletin* has found that middle-aged men and women who were injected with testosterone or who applied testosterone cream to parts of the body did experience increased sexual thoughts and fantasies.

THE EROTOPHOBIC QUIZ

Do you:

- Feel consumed by vulnerability, fear, and shame when thinking about sex, due to guilt, anger, disgust, blame, or self-blame?
- Avoid or deny sex?
- Have negative reactions to sexually explicit materials?
- Regard sexual intimacy, sexual discourse, and sex education as taboo?
- Feel that your views on sex can be described as repressive, restrictive, and condemning?
- Have trouble being vulnerable with another during lovemaking or are unable to express yourself?

Having an erotophobic reaction to sex may be due to any number of reasons, primarily negative sexual experience or messaging while growing up. Religious and cultural norms, mores, restrictions, and taboos around sexuality are meant to regulate our sex lives and can restrict one's sexual expression when met unchallenged. For an erotophobe who is the survivor of sexual abuse or trauma, sex has also come to represent that which is hurtful, hateful, and painful, making it extremely challenging to sexually connect with a partner.

Exercise 1.5: Define Your Sexual Past & Present

Few individuals, let alone couples, have the forum in which to process influences upon their sexual being. Plan quiet time with your lover where you can have a heart-to-heart, learning more about each other as you answer the following:

1. What feelings consume you when you think about sex?
2. Who or what taught you about sex? (You can discuss more than one resource and more than just sexual intercourse.)
3. What types of messages did you get about sex growing up? How have these messages impacted your sex life for better or for worse?
4. What sex topics or sexual behaviors evoke a negative reaction from you and why? What topics elicit a positive one and why?
5. Would you describe yourself as an erotophile or an erotophobe?
6. Would you describe your partner as an erotophile or an erotophobe?

Having a better understanding of where we come from, sexually-speaking, helps us gain a better sense of the sexual people we are today. Recognizing that we're more of an erotophobe versus an erotophile can also help us to assess any barriers that may pose a challenge to embracing more gratifying sex.

THE
SCIENCE OF *Sex*

Research by Gurit Birnbaum, Ph.D., and Omri Gillath, Ph.D., has found that those who have positive sexual self-views and who lack behavioral inhibitions about their sexuality tend to have more sexual and romantic partners and broader sexual experience when compared to people who have negative sexual self-views.

I recently became seriously involved with a young woman, and when we talked about making love for the first time, she "confessed" that she's sexually inhibited and inexperienced. She says that she needs time to tell me why and that she's working hard to embrace the desire she feels for me so that we can be intimate . . . . I don't want to push her, but in being able to better support her, I would love to know what's possibly at the heart of this. Thoughts?

Even when a person feels sexual desire and yearning, sexual inhibitions can still impact his or her ability to tune into this desire and to allow the self to let go when it comes to sexual response. While there is no way of knowing what exactly is at the root of your partner's sexual inhibition, causes for such a state include negative sex messages (e.g., from her church or family), insecurities regarding long-term virginity and sexual inexperience, shame, guilt, body loathing, the inability to reach climax, a fear of sex, a sexually repressive childhood, incidences—sexual or not— of shame or ridicule, and negative sexual experiences, including sexual abuse, sexual assault, or rape.

As you learn more from your partner, you'll get a better sense of how to be supportive to her in your sexual intimacy. Right now, being patient, understanding, and a good listener are key. Other remedies for sexual inhibitions include giving her permission to be sexual and sexually intimate, learning erotic skills for greater confidence, redirecting your lover's thinking to sexually empowering statements, and exposing yourself or your love to new forms of sexual expression and resources.

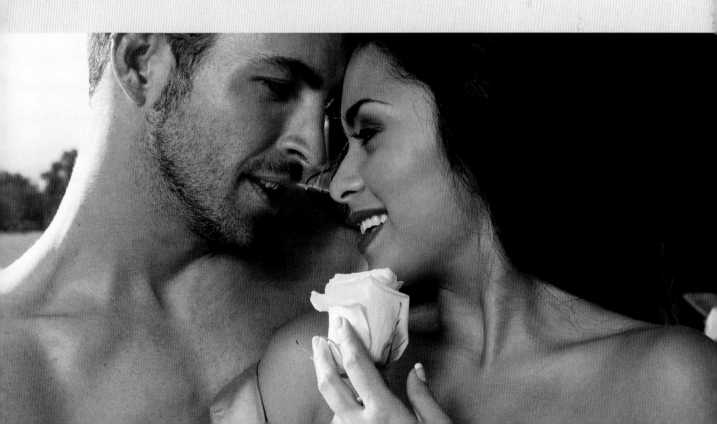

> "Love is an irresistible desire to be irresistibly desired."
>
> —ROBERT FROST

Sexual Homework

In this chapter, we looked at all of the factors that can act as facilitators or barriers to your sexual desire and ways to boost your sexual cravings. The nature of sexual desire is not only a total-body experience, but also an holistic experience—one influenced by your mental/emotional state, relationship dynamics, and society at large. In helping you to take charge of your sexual desire, in enabling you to realize the wonders of sex to the best of your abilities, the following are sexual homework assignments for your pleasuring, to be completed before you begin Chapter 2.

Private T-Shirt "Study." Explore the power of smell in your attraction for one another. Sleep one night in a t-shirt. The next night, drape the tee over your lover's face before playing with your partner's body for fifteen to forty-five minutes (or longer if you'd like!). Toy with any

your lover does the same to you. Have fun licking your partner's body, sensually rubbing yourself over different parts, or masturbating your lover. As your partner's "play thing," you are to do no more than just lie there, breathing in the t-shirt's aroma and enjoying the anticipation of what is to come next.

Meaningful Erotic Talk. We evolve as sexual beings throughout our lifetime, and with that, the meaning of sex, our wants, our needs, and our desires change. In making sure that you have the type of sex that's best for you, make sure that you're communicating about sexual intimacy. A great place to start is with Sinclair's *Lifelong Pleasures Vol. 1: Sexual Communication and Desire*. This DVD will help you and your lover understand sexual communication, the way we are all different in how we express ourselves, and how the two of you can under-

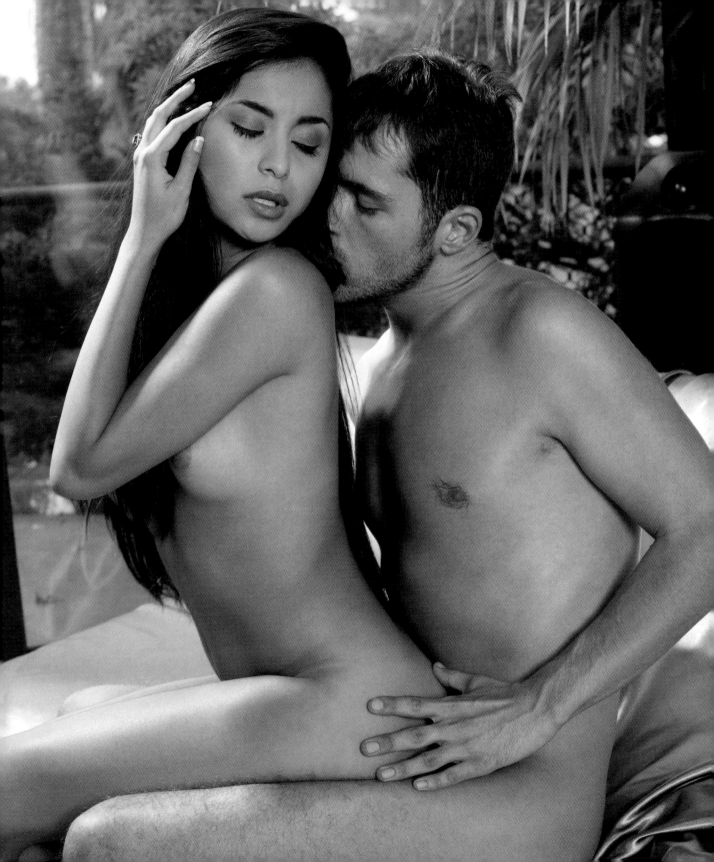

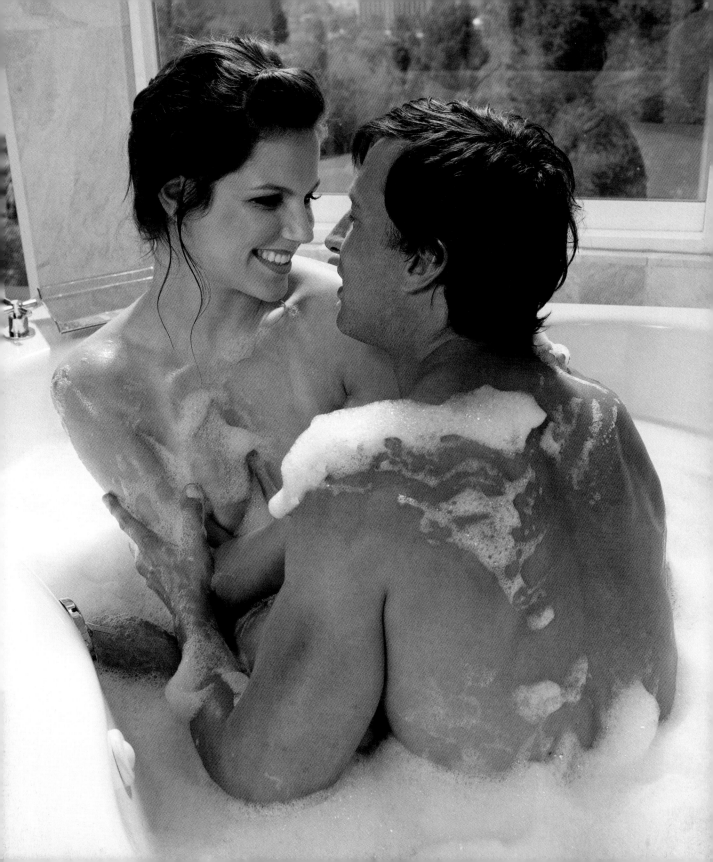

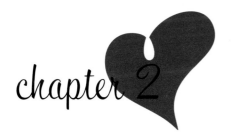

chapter 2

Turn on Your Desire to Turn on Your Sex Life

WE'RE ABOUT TO DELVE into a score of ways to amplify your sexual desire. Realize, however, that the most important component to greater sexual voracity is, by far, brainpower. It can't be said enough. Your mind is your biggest sex organ. What's between your ears is far more potent than what's between your legs.

A perfect illustration of your mind's significance is aphrodisiacs. While a handful of these agents for excitement have been proven truly effective by research, the vast majority hold their sway in no more than the power of suggestion. The tomato, for example, was considered a "love apple" by Europeans when it was first brought over from the Americas; it was thought that this, at the time exotic, fruit would spark one's libido. The Elizabethans thought the same about prunes, serving them for free in brothels to spur lust. Both scenarios show how simply thinking that something will enhance your sexual response may do just that. Your brain has that incredible of an impact on your sex life.

"The desire of the man is for the woman, but the desire of the woman is for the desire of the man."

DESIRE BEGETS DESIRE

Another very important thing to keep in mind when magnifying your sexual rapacity is that desire breeds more desire. This is both on a physiological and an emotional level. When you have sex, especially good sex, your body boosts your libido, which boosts your desire for even more sex—all of which is fueled by testosterone, the production of which is increased even more with sex. This cycle of desire makes you feel healthier and more energetic, boosting your mood and immunity and further upping your desire for more sex!

WAYS TO ENHANCE DESIRE

The first step toward enhancing your sex life and experiencing better sex is to cultivate sexual desire. This goes for both you and your lover, recognizing that the amorous efforts you make in seducing your partner are going to make you feel sexier as well.

There are a number of ways to increase your passion potential. In practicing the following exercises, you should work at your own pace. You may do each task on a daily or weekly basis or whenever the mood strikes you. Instead of making your sex sessions goal-oriented, allow yourself to get lost in the moment. Try to truly satiate how you and your partner are feeling, what the experience is like for you as a lover and as a couple. Remember, as with many travel experiences, getting there is half the fun. Making an effort to enhance your desire is going to be well worth it.

SeXercise 2.1: Strive for a Healthful Lifestyle

Being sexual with someone else means starting with the self. The healthier you are, the healthier you will be for sex. This entails exercising on a regular basis, getting an adequate amount of sleep, eating a well-balanced diet, and staying drug-free.

SEX TASK 1: Evaluate how you're taking care of your physical health. In assessing and revamping your lifestyle for a healthier you, seek to make sure that you're abiding by all of the following in taking care of your physical health:

- Aim to be smoke-free.
- Avoid excess salt, sugar, alcohol, and caffeine consumption.
- Eat a balanced diet, including whole grains, leafy vegetables, and fruits.
- Avoid foods high in saturated fat and cholesterol.
- Exercise daily for at least thirty minutes.

THE
SCIENCE OF *Sex*

Emotional arousal can make for greater sexual desire. One study in the *Journal of Sex Research* involving a movie theater found that couples who watched an emotionally arousing action movie expressed more affection than those who watched one that was less emotionally arousing. They also expressed more affection after watching the movie than they did before seeing it. For those who watched the nonaction, non-emotionally-arousing movie, there was no effect on the amount of affection expressed.

SEX TASK 2: Take care of your mental health. Be good to yourself and work on your issues, especially ones that are affecting your sex life. You can do this by seeking professional help and/or by exploring holistic forms of healing, such as energy healing, Reiki, and mantra practices. Whether you are the victim of sexual trauma or negative messaging about sexuality and your body, your history can impact what goes on in the bedroom as well as your well-being. Working with a therapist, counselor, or healer will enable you to tackle any negative thoughts, fears, stressors, guilt, anxiety, shame, or depression . . . . Freeing yourself of the shackles of hurt and negativity will help to invite a taste for sex-positive experiences.

SEXUAL Q&A: WOMEN'S SEXUAL PEAK

I'm turning 40 next month. I've heard that women reach their sexual peak in their mid- to late-thirties, so am I past my peak?

The idea that a woman reaches her sex peak—as in highest sexual desire and ability—in her thirties is based on decades-old research that showed many women in that age group were the most satisfied with their sex lives. It was immediately suspected that such results were due to biological reasons, namely reproductive ones: With their biological clocks ticking, women were being urged, undoubtedly, by Mother Nature to reproduce while they still have a chance. Researchers are still trying to confirm this hypothesis. In the meantime, many couples who buy into what may very well be a myth are not realizing their full sexual potential at other points of their lives.

Consider that social scientists have proposed that a woman's sexual peak during this time period in her life can be better attributed to social reasons than biological ones. Up until recently, most women in their thirties have been married and quite comfortable in their long-term monoga-mous unions. Being married is the factor helping those women to embrace better sex; they can do this because, as wives, they have societal permission to let go in the bedroom as never before. And there may be some truth to that. However, research does indicate that a woman can reach a sexual peak at any point in her life. For example, women report having some of the best sex of their lives after going through menopause. In having more body knowledge, in feeling sexually mature, in no longer having to worry about birth control and pregnancy, and with grown children out of their homes, these women can enjoy sex as never before.

So don't worry about whether you've reached a sexual peak. A person's sexual peak is highly individual and can happen at any point in his or her life—especially with the right mindset and a little bit of effort.

SEX TASK 3: Evaluate your medications. If you're taking prescription drugs for physical or psychological conditions such as high blood pressure, depression, high or cholesterol, evaluate your dosage. A number of medications, especially those for high blood pressure or cholesterol, can have negative side effects when it comes to your sex life. SSRIs, such as Zoloft and Prozac, as well as the birth control pills can negatively impact your level of sexual desire or ability to have an orgasm. So be sure to talk to your doctor about any medications you're on, deciding together if you should change or discontinue the prescription.

Overall, in evaluating your lifestyle and in determining where you can be taking better care of yourself holistically, you're striving for heart health and a fitter, happier you. In feeling sexier, more energetic, and desirable yourself, you'll desire sex more often when you're taking care of yourself.

$\mathcal{S}$*exercise* 2.2: Learn How to Relax

Sometimes you can't get out of your head or can't loosen up enough for loving. That's one of the many reasons why relaxation is so important. You can jump-start those all-important neurotransmitters with meditation and acupuncture, thereby reducing stress and ultimately making for wonderful sex. So make time to unwind.

SEX TASK 1: Address whatever issues are preventing you from having an opportunity to relax, and take action. For instance, you can change your commute schedule if you're typically stuck in traffic to free up "me" time; or allow yourself to be flexible as to where you can practice certain relaxation techniques, such as in your office during your lunch hour.

SEX TASK 2: Brainstorm different activities that relax you, and every now and then do them one at a time. Favorite relaxation strategies may include taking a warm bath, going for a good swim, taking a yoga class, going golfing with close friends, losing yourself in garden work, or practicing deep breathing with the sunrise.

SEX TASK 3: Be proactive in unwinding before you get to bed. Sleep is the foundation of good health—and of a good sex life. You need to make sure that you're well rested, and part of this is making sure that you're not bringing food or meals to bed (unless they're a part of sex play!), that you're not watching rousing TV shows or movies before falling asleep, and that you're taking the time to ease your body into a relaxed state for a good rest.

THE
SCIENCE OF $\mathcal{S}$*ex*

Women who exercise regularly have more active sex lives, are more easily aroused, and reach orgasm faster. A University of British Columbia study found that women who exercised for twenty minutes had greater sexual response than those who didn't exercise at all. Another study in the Electronic Journal of Human Sexuality found that, overall, men and women who exercise feel more sexually desirable, better about themselves, and more satisfied with their sex lives.

Remember, a relaxed body is more receptive to sexual touch. A relaxed mind can allow you to slip into an orgasmic state more easily. All of these can work wonders for your mind, body, and soul, including creating the "right" conditions you need for sex and seduction.

$\mathcal{S}$exercise 2.3: Seduce Your Lover

Seduction is so obvious that it's often overlooked. And that's tragic given that seducing for a lifetime is critical to bettering your sexual intimacy. Showing enthusiasm for your lover and his or her desire has a major impact on both of you. Don't take each other for granted.

SEX TASK 1: Spend quality time together. This does not mean running errands together or going on a family picnic or attending parties together. Take the time for only each other, especially leisure time that frees you of adult responsibilities.

SEX TASK 2: Regularly entice each other with romantic gestures. While lust doesn't always trigger romantic ardor, attempts at romance can invite delectable delights. Even oldies but goodies such as chocolates, flowers, or a book of love poems are sure to evoke desire.

SEX TASK 3: Immortalize your loving moments. Go through old photos, sharing your own pasts before you met as well as the memories you've created together. Record your history, highlighting how you fell in love. Start a journal, using that as motivation for good times to be had—and noted!

$\mathcal{S}$exercise 2.4: Maintain Touch

Humans thrive on touch. If we're deprived of it, we wilt much like flowers. Touch is essential for a good relationship, with sexual and affectionate touch important for both sexes. Couples who do not stay physically connected often develop an aversion to touch, which can lead to a sexless relationship. One partner may also fear the intention behind the touch if they have issues with sexual intimacy, whether currently or historically.

SEX TASK 1: Kiss, hug, and hold hands on a regular basis. You can also practice an occasional hand caress. Done in silence, this exercise involves each partner taking a turn to explore the other lover's hands. In a relaxed, candlelit space, for ten to twenty minutes, feel the texture of your partner's hands. Observe the lines, fingernails, length, shapes . . . . Close your eyes to see if this changes the way you're processing the energy coming off of the hands. Gently massage the tendons. Absorb the energy and warmth. Think about how those hands have made you happy.

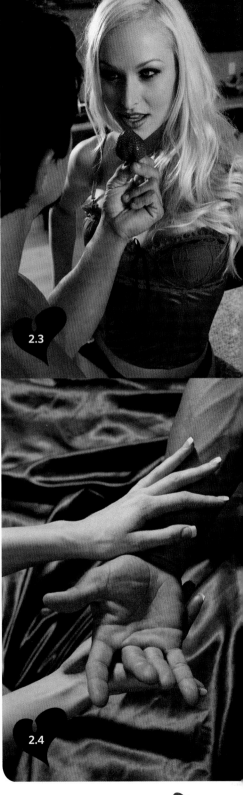

2.3

2.4

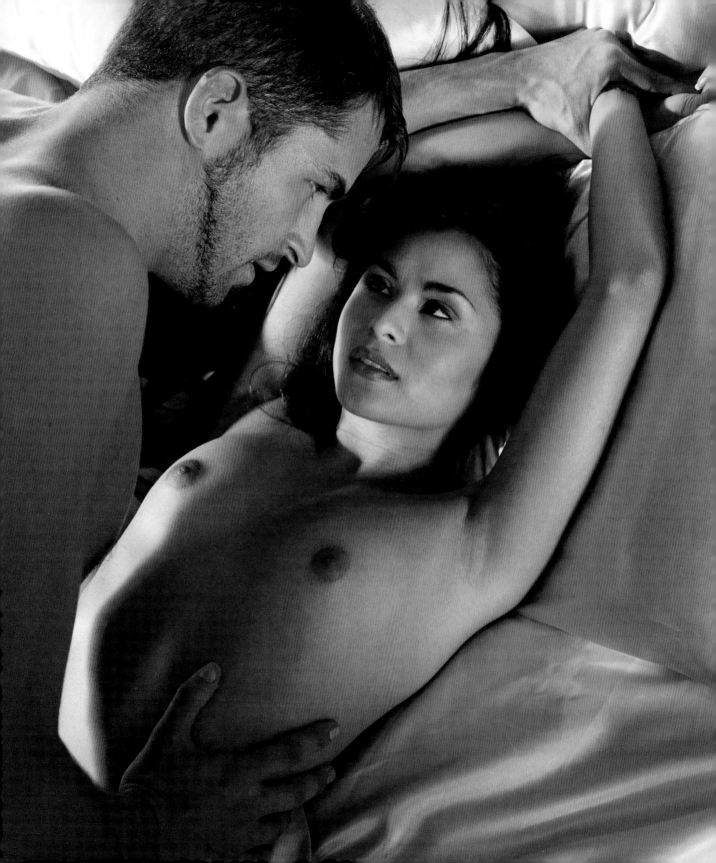

SEX TASK 2: Take turns showing each other what your favorite way of touching somebody is when it comes to touch that is . . .

- Healing
- Affectionate
- Sensual
- Erotic
- Sexual

Get as creative and daring as you want to. A lover may want to hug for five full minutes or make out for an hour or suck on your nipples . . . . Let your lover know how it felt to be touched in "that" way and if you'd like to do it again sometime.

Exercise 2.5: Have Sex

As explained earlier, sex fuels the desire for more sex. It is also significant in its ability to act as a vehicle to emotional intimacy.

SEX TASK 1: Have sex—any kind of sex. Even if you're not in the mood, have it. Let yourself slip back into that time and place when you really loved being sexually intimate. Discover what kind of amorous feelings it awakens.

Exercise 2.6: Live Sensually

Having a sensual environment and doing things that continually keep you tuned in to yourself and the sensuous can keep you primed for love. In taking steps to feel "delicious" as much as possible, you'll work up a sexual hunger as well.

SEX TASK 1: Focus on your self-care practices, things such as regularly applying moisturizer, for instance. Consider how you eat and drink. Do you wolf things down or allow yourself to luxuriate in every sip and bite? Observe how you carry your naked form. Do your gait and stance exude your sexual energy to the fullest? What are the loving gestures you carry out daily that make people fall in love with you? How can your place of work, home, and bedroom all be revamped so that they invite more pleasure energy?

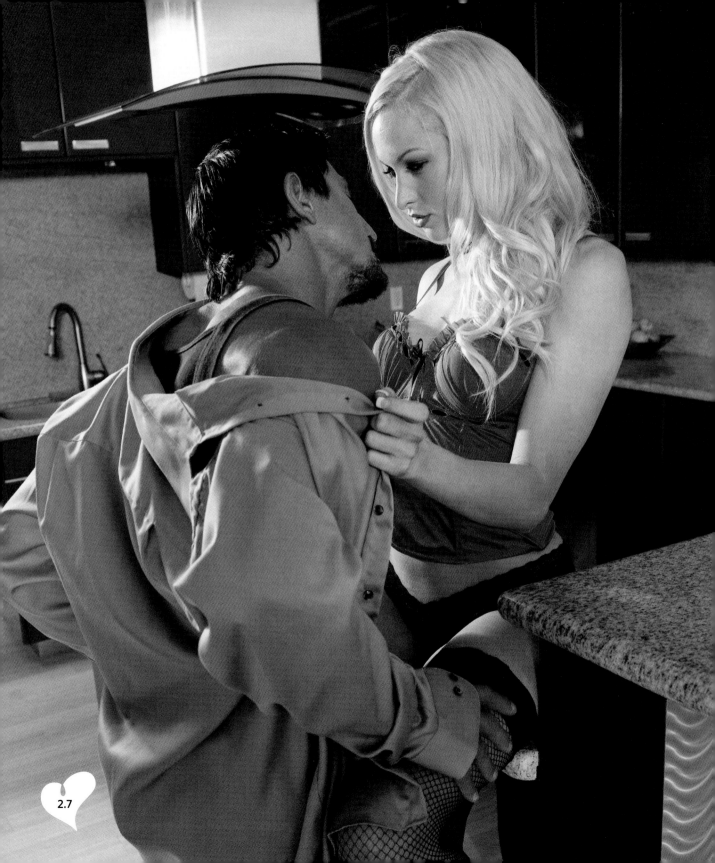

SEX RX

Don't be afraid to express your love and desire and to create an atmosphere
full of smells and sounds, welcoming in the erotic. This includes, most importantly, getting rid of anything electronic or work-related in your bedroom.
Your boudoir should be for two things only: sex and sleep.

Exercise 2.7: Incorporate Risk

Any activity involving an element of danger can increase your sense of bonding.
Many couples thrive off of pushing the envelope in a variety of settings during
a number of different activities, sexual and not.

SEX TASK 1: Brainstorm scenarios that will get your heart rate going. Go
indoor sky diving, take a trapeze class, or go bungee jumping. Consider sex in a
public place. Are you not so bold or afraid of getting arrested? Some people do
better with a little less danger, such as having sex in the great outdoors or under a blanket at a seemingly secluded beach. Even mild anxiety has been found
to facilitate sexual arousal, as published in the Journal of Abnormal Psychology.

Exercise 2.8: Aim for the Novel

Keeping things new and fresh are a must in having a hotter sex life. After all,
the exotic is erotic. This is in large part because dopamine, which is increased
with new experiences, can trigger lust in humans. So make sexual exploration a
goal when it comes to lovemaking, getting out of any routine that can kill your
sex drive. When your sex life becomes predictable, you run the risk of becoming bored and dissatisfied as your sexual excitement and motivation plummet.

SEX TASK 1: Try something new, whether it's as tame as reading an erotic
book together or as freewheeling as sex in the great outdoors—couples who
play together stay together. And this can include doing nonsexual new things,
such as exploring a never-trekked hiking trail or learning how to parasail.

$S\mathscr{e}\mathcal{x}$ercise 2.9: Practice Kegel Exercises

Learning how to strengthen your pubococcygeus (PC) muscle, the collective term for your pelvic-floor muscles, results in amazing sex. Also known as Kegel exercises—named after Dr. Arnold Kegel, who developed these exercises as a way to help women who suffered from urinary incontinence—such practices can increase your enjoyment, orgasmic response, sensations, ejaculatory control, and sex duration.

SEX TASK 1: Identify the same muscles you use to stop your urine flow. That's your PC muscle. Now, if you're a female, squeeze those muscles inward and upward, doing three sets of 10 to 20 repetitions three times per day, gradually increasing your reps. You can also use a Kegel "barbell," such as the Natural Contours Energie, to help isolate this muscle. Men, you want to initially aim for 15 reps twice a day, working your way up to 75 reps for each session, over the course of four to six weeks.

Note that you can do these exercises anytime, anywhere and no one will ever know! Given the importance and benefits of having a strong PC muscle, we will definitely be hitting on this topic again in the Orgasm section.

TALK ABOUT SEX

Perhaps you have a sexual desire you'd like to share. Or maybe you're a bit concerned about something going on in the bedroom. Or there's something a little "kinky" you'd like to try. Or you're so angry at your partner about a non-sex-related issue that even makeup sex is out of the question . . . .

When it comes to sexual intimacy, couples have plenty of issues to talk about. To maintain open and healthy sex communication, you need to assess your needs, desires, and issues on a regular basis. This allows you to stay in tune with each other. It helps you to get a handle on a problem earlier versus later.

So learning how to express yourself whenever necessary—and not in a way that is driven by anger, fear, intimidation or pain—is critical to maintaining sexual intimacy. Holding back only makes for regret, so don't be afraid to ask for your needs and wants. Take the time to address your feelings and concerns. And equally important, encourage your partner to do the same. Take turns in voicing your wishes, grievances, or feelings, and don't interrupt one another. Just listen. When it is your turn, stay positive, be specific, and be behavioral. You do this by not complaining and by making a specific request, such as, "I would really appreciate it if you could help me put the kids to bed so that we have more time to be intimate." Stick with what you want, taking care not to focus on what you don't want.

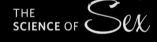

THE SCIENCE OF $S\mathscr{e}\mathcal{x}$

In general, the ways men and women communicate are different. According to clinical neuroscientist and brain-imaging expert Daniel Amen, M.D., men are hardwired to be more detail-oriented and to the point while women are more fluent. So you and your lover may process information differently. If that's the case, make a conscientious effort to make sure that you hear and understand one another; make sure that you're listening!

SEXUAL FANTASIES TO FUEL DESIRE

A sexual fantasy is a deliberate or unexpected pattern of thoughts used to create or enhance sexual feelings and arousal. Ranging from the tame to the bizarre, such erotic mental imagery may involve a quick "flash" or an entire story. You can use sexual fantasy to pass time, to get turned on, or to consider and explore sexual behaviors, scenarios, and desires you may or may not actually want to enact. The frequency and content of sexual fantasies vary from person to person and time to time. Famed sex researcher Alfred C. Kinsey found that 64 percent of females and almost all men used fantasy during self-stimulation.

The appeal of sexual fantasy is this: You can imagine anything, unconstrained by social convention, fears of embarrassment, rejection, criticism, or practical and legal barriers. In many ways, the more we learn about fantasies, the more we come to know about what we find erotic.

In many respects, sexual fantasies are the great sexual equalizer, since most people engage in them at least occasionally, with romantic fantasy (daydreaming about kissing a crush, for instance) nearly universal. Anybody can have them. Very much self-defined, fantasies are generally recognized as part of a healthy sexuality. They can be experienced as positive or negative, though few are regarded as unwanted.

THE RANGE OF SEXUAL FANTASIES

No study to date has investigated our erotic imagination using a complete list of most human sexual fantasies. That said, there are themes that run through the most common sexual fantasies, including:

1. Having sex with your current partner
2. Having sex with an imaginary lover or stranger
3. Being forced or overpowering another
4. Group sex
5. Reliving a previous sexual experience
6. Having sex in different positions or locations
7. Doing things that you would never do in reality

Typically, people the world over love sexual fantasies involving power dynamics (having control or being controlled), doing the taboo, breaking the law, being sexual in front of others or in public, being a voyeur or being watched, threesomes, orgies, "innocence," romance, danger, feeling desired, being naughty or deviant, or fetishes. In many cases, more than one theme can be found in fantasy scenarios.

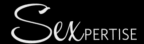

S*ex*PERTISE

"The Sex in America: A Definitive Survey," published in *The New England Journal of Medicine,* found that 54 percent of men and 19 percent of women think about sex daily or several times per day. Research has found anywhere from 47 to 92 percent of males report sexual fantasy while having sexual intercourse, while women range from 37 to 94 percent in doing such. Fantasy is also regarded as one mechanism monogamous couples use to stay faithful and together for the long-term. Those who are daydreamers are likelier to have fantasies.

Sexual fantasies can help you to:

- Get aroused
- Attain orgasm
- To get turned on anytime, anywhere
- Introduce new ideas for sexual exploration
- Boost your sexual self-image

ONCE UPON A SEXUAL ENCOUNTER

The types of sexual fantasies people have are practically innumerable, involving story lines such as these:

- Sex with an authority figure
- Sex in a public place
- People around me being naked
- Being sexually victimized
- Sex acts against one's religion
- Indecently exposing one's self
- Masturbating in a public place
- Joining the "Mile High Club" (sex in an airplane)
- Elevator sex
- Watching two men or two women have sex
- Having sex with another couple
- Watching men and women masturbate
- French kissing after a blow job
- Sex with a call girl/stripper
- Having same-sex interactions
- Double penetration
- Anonymous stranger sex
- Dressing up in leather
- Playing cowboy
- Wearing boots/heels
- Being videotaped
- Dressing up in plastic, rubber, and women's clothes

WHEN SEXUAL FANTASIES ARE REPRESSED

Sexual fantasies aren't welcomed by all. Some people repress their fantasies. A considerable number feel guilty, shameful, anxiety-ridden, or uneasy for having sexual fantasies, especially during intercourse. According to research in *The Journal of Sex Research*, more than 15 percent of males and females try to repress feelings of arousal when having a sexual fantasy or thought. Seen by many as forbidden, uncommon, abnormal, socially unacceptable, and sinful, not surprisingly, an article in this same journal reported that almost half of a conservative Christian group surveyed said that sexual fantasy was "morally flawed or unacceptable."

WHAT MEN FANTASIZE ABOUT

Males have sexual fantasies more frequently than females. They also report a significantly higher number of fantasies per month than women. Men tend to engage in fantasy more often than women when it comes to masturbation and when they're not engaged in sexual activity. A 2004 study in *The Journal of Sex Research* found that, overall, male fantasies tend to involve more visual imagery and explicit anatomical detail than those of females. They tend to lack any romantic or emotional context yet more frequently involve a partner's sexual desire and pleasure than do women's fantasies. They are also more active than passive in "doing" a sex act rather than receiving it.

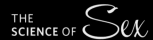

THE
SCIENCE OF *Sex*

Most surveys that depend on adult recall have found that the majority of people start having sexual fantasies somewhere between the ages of eleven and thirteen. While males tend to fantasize more in adolescence, they fantasize less with age, whereas women begin fantasizing more as they enter their twenties. There has not been any notable change in the number of people reporting fantasizing about sex since Kinsey's research from the 1950s.

SEXUAL Q&A: RAPE FANTASY

Despite being a feminist, I still have the occasional rape fantasy where I'm being overpowered by a faceless lover. I feel guilty that it's so thrilling. Is there something wrong with me?

Fantasies involving force, being overpowered, or forcing someone to engage in a sex act are quite common in both men and women. A 1997 study on American women, published in the book *Making Sense of Sex*, found that they were nearly two times as likely as men to actively fantasize about being "done to" as opposed to "doing." Yet a national U.S.-based study in 1994 by Edward Laumann, Ph.D., and colleagues found that less than half of 1 percent of women actually want to be forced. They also found that less than 1 percent of men enjoy forcing women to have coitus.

Given that the reality of this type of fantasy would be horrific and illegal, people—feminists or not—can become distressed and anxious in having them. Research in the *Journal of Sex Education and Therapy* on rape fantasies has found that females who visualize being forced into sex by a male often feel more guilty, unhappy, frightened, and disgusted than those women who do not imagine such force story lines.

Know that there is nothing wrong with you or this fantasy. It does not mean that you want this behavior to happen or support it in real life. Many people love the idea of being so irresistible and attractive that a lover can't help but do anything to "have" them, even if it involves nonconsent.

WHAT WOMEN FANTASIZE ABOUT

Female sexual fantasies, on the other hand, involve more affection, emotion, romance, and story line, such as sex after a walk on the beach. Their fantasies, which contain more detailed descriptions of the setting, tend to involve more of an emotional connection with a particular lover, where they are the passive receiver of the sexual interaction. Academics have speculated that this preference for familiar lovers may be due to the fact that females are raised to be chaste and selective when it comes to sexual partners.

Both men and women fantasize about having sex with other people besides their current partner. In fact, one study in *The Journal of Sex Research* found that 98 percent of men and 80 percent of women had fantasized about someone other than their current partner in the last two months. For both genders, these fantasies are quite common, despite any social ideas about it not being "proper." Men are also likelier to fantasize about someone other than their current partner in most of their fantasies (54 percent of all fantasies), whereas women are likelier to fantasize about the current partner (64 percent of all fantasies) over someone else. Women were also likelier to fantasize about past partners than were men, as well as have fewer externally generated sexual thoughts.

WHAT DO YOUR SEXUAL FANTASIES REALLY MEAN?

Much like dreams, people are often curious about whether their fantasies have any meaning, especially if they're recurring. Yet there is no point in overinterpreting your sexual fantasies. After all, everyone has favorite fantasy scenarios—namely the ones that deliver satisfying results. Still, the following fantasy story lines may reveal certain sexual desires you may possibly want to eventually act out.

Engaging in a threesome or group sex

Sex with at least one other person is sexy, especially if you're being worshipped by both lovers at the same time. You like the idea of being stimulated in many areas of the body all at once, as well as breaking taboos. Such fantasy scenarios may also give an individual the opportunity to have sexual relations that test their sexual orientation.

THE SCIENCE OF *Sex*

A 2006 study in *The Journal of Sex Research,* which involved participants writing their favorite or most frequent sexual desires, found that women who have more unrestricted sexuality have more fantasies involving dominance (exerting power over a partner).

Being tied up

You want someone to take charge and control the sex session, teasing you and telling you what to do. In not having a say in what you do, and in simply being receptive to sexual commands, you can relinquish yourself of any sex guilt— and that, in and of itself, can feel sexually satiating.

Sex in public

The thought of getting caught thrills you, and you like the idea of being the center of attention when people spot you. You also like the idea of nonconformity and free sexual expression.

Anal sex

You want to break social convention and do something that's often considered wrong, dirty, and taboo. You're also curious about the great pleasures this erogenous zone can hold, especially given that it can result in a different and even more powerful orgasm, for many.

Being unfaithful

Your sex life possibly lacks excitement and/or you need to feel desired by another. You need to recharge your sex life and evaluate what can be improved in your current relationship. Your sexual desires are likely going unfulfilled.

$\mathcal{S}$ex ercise 2.10: Fantasy, Please

Review the list of fantasy story lines on page 64 and reflect on the following:

- Which sexual fantasies have you had?
- Which ones turn you on?
- Which ones have you acted out?
- Which ones would you consider acting out?
- Which ones can help you to expand your own fantasizing?
- How could the enhanced fantasizing boost your own sex life and sexual repertoire?

EROTIC DREAMS TO FUEL DESIRE

Erotic dreams give us further insight into our sexual desires and sexual potential. More than simply stimulating ideas, these dreams involve much more unexpected twists and turns, often giving the dreamer some of the best sex and orgasms!

More symbolic and abstract than anything, erotic dreams are enjoyed by many simply for the lack of responsibility. Since you didn't intentionally imagine that, then you can enjoy or dismiss even the most "disturbing" or "crazy" sexual imagery guilt-free. Erotic dreams are also fancied in that they:

- Give us ideas for fun and pleasuring, possibly increasing our sexual response
- Help us to feel closer to our sexual selves and sense of ourselves as lovers
- Can make for titillating stories and role-playing ideas when shared with a partner
- Enable us to understand our sexual desires and passions even more
- Offer resolutions to our dilemmas when focusing on a current real-life situation
- Help us to make better sexual and relationship decisions, helping us to feel better and more confident in our sexual relationships

DREAM A LITTLE DREAM OF ME

According to dream researcher Dr. Gillian Holloway, the most common erotic dreams can be explained as follows:

The Faceless Lover

Impossible to identify, your sexual partner may be a stranger or not. This anonymity is exciting and the sex is so stellar that you don't need to see a face. Seeing a face makes for obligations. Faceless means that you have no requirements beyond this sexual liaison. All you need to do is get lost in this moment, the qualities you love in this sexual partner, and the naughty stranger element.

Celebrity Sex

Sex with a famous person such as Brad Pitt or Marilyn Monroe is a quite common fantasy, especially among young people who daydream about being stars themselves. These dreams are relished in that you are being erotically recognized by someone you admire so much. You are thrilled to have been "chosen" as the worthy recipient of the famous one's sexual attention.

Sex with Your Ex

Having dreams about sex with an ex or former lover can have multiple interpretations. If you had a wonderful sex life, it's only natural to get caught up in such moments again, especially if that lover represented a significant first for you or was a recent love affair. Such dreams may also be the mind's attempt to assess your current relationship and life in general. They may be a calling for getting in touch with your life passions again.

Group Sex

Despite being quite sexual, dreams involving multiple partners are mostly about power and passions—and a person's need to feel supported. They also symbolize the need to clarify your feelings, to sort through choices, to reprioritize desires and options and to basically step back and reevaluate your life and sex life.

$\mathcal{S}$exercise 2.11: Keeping a Sex-Dream Journal

Look for any patterns or greater insight as to what your dreams may be telling you about your sex life, relationship, or life in general. Go ahead and share your nonthreatening erotic dreams with your partner. If you're shy in doing so, remember that you can be held "blameless" for your nocturnal visions. Given the private nature of your dreams, sharing them can be a meaningful and quite stimulating bonding experience for lovers.

APHRODISIACS TO FUEL DESIRE

Named after the Greek goddess of love, Aphrodite, an aphrodisiac is any substance thought to arouse sexual desire and/or enhance sexual response. For centuries, humans have tried to identify a safe and effective aphrodisiac, experimenting with substances such as elephant tusks, rhinoceros horns, and bull testicles without much luck. So great is the desire for heightened desire that humans have even ingested toxic substances in hopes of boosting their libidos and response.

Amyl nitrate, also known as "poppers," which is meant to reduce chest pain in heart patients, is a classic example. While the medication can facilitate erection, possibly prolong orgasm, and facilitate anal intercourse by relaxing the anal sphincter muscle, it's also associated with disturbing side effects. These include headaches, fainting, dizziness, and even death in extreme cases.

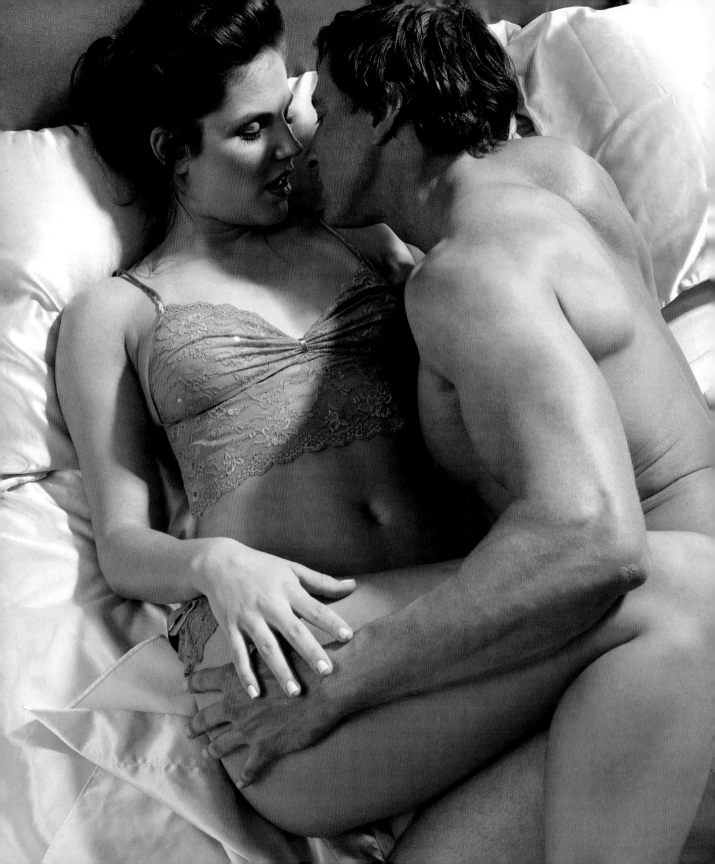

Alcohol and drugs such as marijuana have also been regarded as aphrodisiacs over the years, yet their drawback is that they can diminish judgment, resulting in high-risk sexual behaviors. Alcohol is also a central nervous system depressant, which can actually interfere with sexual arousal rather than enhance it. While a drink or two may help lovers feel more relaxed, anything more than that actually hampers their sexual response more than boost it.

That's not to say, however, that all aphrodisiacs are ineffective. One substance that may be an actual aphrodisiac is yohimbine hydrochloride, which is from the sap of a West African tree called the yohimbine tree. This substance, as reported in *The Journal of Urology*, has enabled some men with erectile dysfunction to attain and maintain an erection long enough for sexual intercourse. It does not, however, work for all men with this sexual disorder.

LIGHT HIS FIRE: USE MALE SEXUAL PSYCHOLOGY TO PLEASE YOUR MAN

As we learned in Chapter 1, male sex drive and desire are said to be synonymous and more testosterone-based than that of the female. Many academics hold that a man's sex drive is governed by nature, thus he turns inward when tuning in to his sexual desire. In recognizing his sexual needs, a man's partner needs to focus her attentions on certain areas, primarily:

- Flirting. A man sometimes needs blatant signs that you're interested in him, especially considering that he must respect women by being hands-off.
- Direct genital contact. While the rest of his body feels good, teasing his privates is an ultimate pleasure.
- Giving up control. Many men love playing with a woman's body—exploring it, titillating it, watching it react. Making yourself his "plaything" brings him a great deal of gratification.
- Recognizing his efforts. He needs praise and affirmation throughout a lovemaking session.

Beyond these key components, much of what lights his fire is in the world around him. That is, males are aroused by the visual, since they are typically more spatially adept than women. In short, men like to look. They are visually stimulated and are known to focus heavily on body parts and copulation during fantasy.

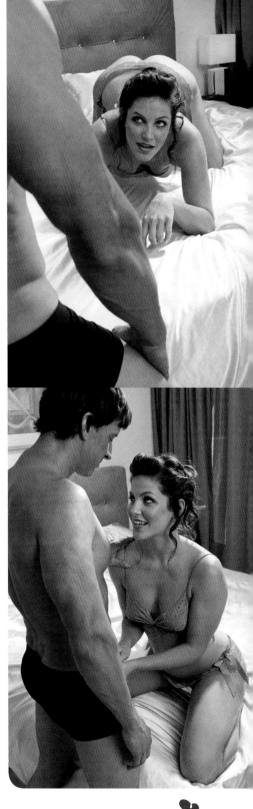

According to love and brain researcher Helen Fisher, Ph.D., men show more activity in brain regions associated with visual processing, especially the face. Research appraising gender differences in focusing on different parts of the same photographs has found that men looked at the faces much more than women did, while both genders looked comparably at the genitals. This may be because men look for cues in a woman's face as to her sexual arousal since her body doesn't give it away as easily as does a man's body.

Research out the University of Nevada published in 2007 has further confirmed sex differences in the processing of erotic material. Twenty heterosexual men and twenty heterosexual women were presented with erotic and nonerotic images of heterosexual couples. In tracking participants' eye movements, researchers found that men looked at opposite-sex figures much longer than women did. The women looked at same-sex figures significantly longer than the males in both erotic and nonerotic images.

SO LET HIM LOOK

To turn him on, play to his visual acuity.

Wear sexy clothes

Wear whatever complements your figure best: a pair of jeans that hug your hips, a form-fitted tee to show off your breasts, a low-cut dress revealing a glimpse of your cleavage, thigh-highs, a G-string. While many think the racier the garment or lingerie, the better, go for articles of clothing that show off your assets and that allow you to be the most confident in your skin and in being sexual. If you feel good about your form in a particular style of clothing, your sexual energy will radiate even more. Remember, too, that much of what is left to the imagination is often seen as sexier.

Maintain an attractive face

Given a male will look to your face for cues concerning your arousal, you want to look your best, going the extra mile to be special. No matter what your age, strive for a clear, healthy complexion, and play up your attributes when applying makeup. More than anything, always wear a smile, flashing pearly whites. Furthermore, make the extra effort to dress the way your partner likes you best; for example, if you usually wear pants and he loves you in a dress, humor him every now and then.

*Sex*PERTISE

Don't assume that a man is always ready for sex. Men want to be seduced, too.

Adjust your communication style

Be clear about your desires, presenting facts and feelings. Make direct statements by saying things such as, "I need to feel your pulsating penis in me" instead of, "I hope that we can be sexually intimate." You don't want him to feel like he needs to be a mind reader. Finally, to top things off, soften the level of your voice. This will also force him to get closer to you.

Incorporate erotic visuals into your sex play

There are a number of different types of visual images available for every couple's pleasure, from the tame to the soft-core to the hard-core, depending upon their tastes. Get to know his tastes, focusing on erotica that features some of his favorite fantasies, whether that be woman-on-woman action or oral sex. Ask him what he'd like to re-create from the scenario, and tell him what aroused you, too.

Put on a strip show

Once again, here, you want to show off your assets and talents. If you're flexible, then work those splits and backbends. If you're a good dancer, shake those hips and swivel around him. If you feel more confident giving him a close-up and letting him provide some assistance, give him an erection-inducing lap dance. And when you get to areas of your body that you're a bit self-conscious about, have a special surprise waiting that will actually help to divert his attention and make you feel more at ease. If you don't care for your chest, for example, realize that many men love cleavage for the mere fact that it's something they don't have. So sport a sexy brassiere or wear titty tassels, if only to help you feel sexier. If, ultimately, you find yourself unable to put on your own performance, you could consider inviting him to a high-class strip club.

Re-create voyeurism/exhibitionism scenarios

Tell him you want him but that he can't have you right away. Tell him that you were hoping, instead, that he might be willing to watch you for the next hour or so while you get ready for sex. Then take to the shower and let him watch you wash yourself, allowing yourself to forget that he's even there as the water washes all over you. Let him watch you walk around the house naked as you do a couple of things that you normally wouldn't do in the nude. Let him gaze at you as you put on the crotchless underwear you've bought just for him and "forget" to put on a bra before retreating to your bed for some self-pleasuring. All the while, don't be afraid to talk out loud, playing up the act of innocence in "thinking" you're alone to further play up the story you're developing.

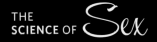

THE SCIENCE OF *Sex*

Research in *Personal Relationships* has found that both men and women think that male and female sexual desires have different causes. Male sexual desire is thought to be caused by intra-individual and erotic environmental factors whereas interpersonal and romantic environmental factors are thought to cause female sexual desire. Both sexes see physical attractiveness and overall personality as sexually desirable characteristics for both genders.

Capture your sex life

Make use of your digital camera (including the fact that you can easily delete photos) by snapping shots of yourselves during sex. While stopping may not initially hold appeal, taking even a brief bit of time to look at your sexual response, such as hardened nipples, or to take a shot of his hard penis penetrating your vagina could make for some true "capture the moment" good times. Plus, such snapshots will slow down your sexual response, making your pleasure last longer.

THINK LIKE A MAN . . . IN BED

You can use male sexual psychology to erotically exploit his sense of intimacy in other ways as well by:

- Simply having sex. Men are four times more likely than women to equate sexual activity with emotional closeness.
- Working or playing side by side. Men don't like to be engaged as directly as do women, in general. So in being intimate, pursue activities that involve being more physically by each other's side than face-to-face, such as hiking, driving, or going to a movie.
- Doing or talking about things that men, stereotypically, enjoy. He's going to be more drawn to a partner who joins him in skiing, tennis, chess, rock climbing, for example, and who enjoys talking about sports, business, world affairs, and politics.

LIGHT HER FIRE: USE FEMALE SEXUAL PSYCHOLOGY TO PLEASE YOUR WOMAN

A woman's sexual desire is less influenced by the visual and more governed by other factors, primarily cultural norms, when it comes to sexuality. A number of external issues and messages come into play, including her perception of her role as a woman and sexual being, relationship issues, and how she feels about her physical appearance.

THE
SCIENCE OF *Sex*

Your personality appears to play a role in your sexual desire experiences. A 1992 study in the *Journal of Sex and Marital Therapy* found that women who scored higher on sensation-seeking had higher levels of sexual desire and arousability. (Note: This is not to say that they necessarily had sex more frequently than women who didn't score as high.)

Thus, perhaps most important to lighting her fire is helping her feel safe enough to surrender to desire. You can do this by:

- Giving her permission to take the time for intimacy. Let her know that she deserves a break. She sometimes needs a reminder that she can do things such as take off her work and/or "mommy" hat.
- Reaching emotional and cognitive levels of relaxation; for example, describe the lovely bath you're about to draw for her before lusciously drying her off to make love to her.
- Giving her emotional reminders of how much she means to you; you can do this by leaving her small notes or gifts.
- Using touch to "check in" with her. She craves physical affirmation that she's emotionally and physically desired, so do things such as coming up from behind to kiss her on the neck.

Tell Me a Sexy Story

Women are more turned on by romantic words, images, and themes in stories. That's not to say that women do not like visual imagery, which they do, indeed, respond to—a fact that is often understated given that being visually stimulated is typically unfairly relegated to being a "male thing." One 2007 study at Emory University found that it was the female participants who lingered longer and took greater pleasure in looking at photos of men performing oral sex on women.

The Mystery of Female Desire

For women, being aroused and knowing that they are aroused are often two different things. Many women may show genital signs of arousal but not feel aroused. They may not even be aware of physical changes taking place, such as becoming lubricated.

Yet women's genitals appear to respond to all types of sex. Research at the Centre for Addiction and Mental Health in Canada found that females' genitals became engorged with blood and lubricated when participants were shown scenes of a man and woman having sex, two women having sex, two men having sex, as well as two chimps having sex—despite, in many cases, the women being unaware of their response. Researchers found a discrepancy, too, between a woman's stated preference for certain visuals and her physiological arousal. That is, women were turned on by same-sex scenarios despite thinking otherwise.

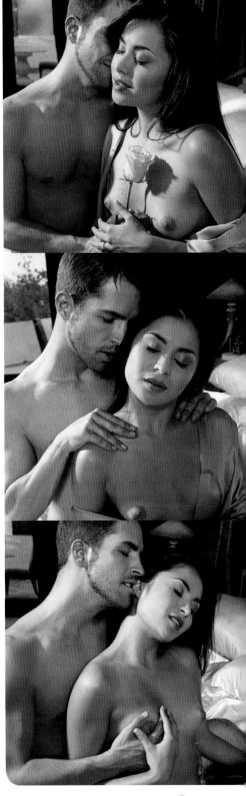

Talk to Her

All in all, a woman's sexual desire is more driven by affection, commitment, and sex with familiar partners. Women in new relationships are likelier to experience spontaneous sexual desire, namely sexual thoughts and fantasies, than are women in established relationships, who may find themselves thinking about sex less frequently.

So to turn her on, be sure to:

1. Court her with words. Women are more linguistically gifted; they tend to enjoy talking about emotional and personal issues. Not surprisingly, women report more intimacy if they talk with their partner before sex. So keep your language sexy, self-revealing, and meaningful—a combination likelier to win her interest.

2. Play upon her fondness for stories. Send her love letters, full of scenarios of what you want to do to her later, of the naughty fantasies you've been having, or recapturing a recent hot sex session that still causes a stir in you.

3. Talk face-to-face. Return her gaze so she doesn't feel as though she's being ignored.

4. Pay attention to her. Connection, trust, and a willingness to risk all are incredibly sexy to women. The more you can be engaging, the more she'll feel sexually drawn to you.

5. Notice her in sexual touch. Don't just dive in for her erogenous zones. Take the time to play with all of her, getting her body warmed up. For women, sex is not as much of a genitally-focused experience as it is a whole-body experience.

6. Exercise with her. Studies out of the University of British Columbia have demonstrated that moderate exercise boosts genital response/arousal to erotic stimuli in women. This boost may be due to changes in mood, neurotransmitter and/or hormone levels, and autonomic nervous system activity. Plus, with increased endorphins and much of your arousal mechanisms already fired up, both of you will be in the mood for amour, if even in the shower.

THE SCIENCE OF *Sex*

Female sexual desire does not necessarily cease with age. A longitudinal study in Gothenburg, Sweden, on the changes in sexual desire in midlife, which was published in the *Archives of Sexual Behavior*, found that two-thirds of women do not experience a decline in libido. Another study found that 40 percent of middle-aged women actually complained of not having enough sex!

7. Speak her love language. Ask for her opinion. Practice active listening. Use adjectives. In the very least, look interested in what she's saying.

8. Do something for her that alleviates her workload. Women respond emotionally when their partners do something for them such as washing the dishes or mopping the floor, as found by relationship researcher John Gottman, Ph.D. Such nonsexual acts are considered an act of emotional intimacy for women, with many motivated to seek out a sexual response.

Sexual Homework

Given our appetite for sexual stimulation, the means we have to fuel our desire is, thankfully, practically endless. While this chapter just equipped you with a number of ways to enhance your desire, we've got even more assignments for increasing your amorous efforts with the following:

Allure Yourselves with Aphrodisiacs. Plan a quiet evening that involves no more than feeding each other well-known oral delights. Arrange assorted plates of foods such as:

- **Chocolate.** The chemicals, primarily caffeine, anandamide, and phenylethylamine, in this sweet are thought to make you feel randier!
- **Fruits.** Given their texture, aromas, soft flesh, and sensual nature, apricots, bananas, peaches, pears, and oranges can be erotically inspiring.
- **Vegetables.** Their texture and long, firm phallic shapes make veggies such as cucumbers, carrots, and asparagus pique the imagination.
- **Seafood.** The slippery texture and likeness to the female genitals has made foods such as oysters, scallops, and clams the delight of lovers for centuries.

Go with the Flow. Lie on your back as your lover caresses your genitals. As you receive this loving touch, say whatever comes to mind without censoring or editing it. Let your sexual thoughts spontaneously arise. Allow any emotional reactions to happen. As the giving partner, focus on how your caress affects your lover. Kindly encourage your partner to keep talking if there is a lengthy silence. After twenty minutes, switch roles. When you are finished, talk about the feelings that came up. Or have sex if you're feeling sexually aroused.

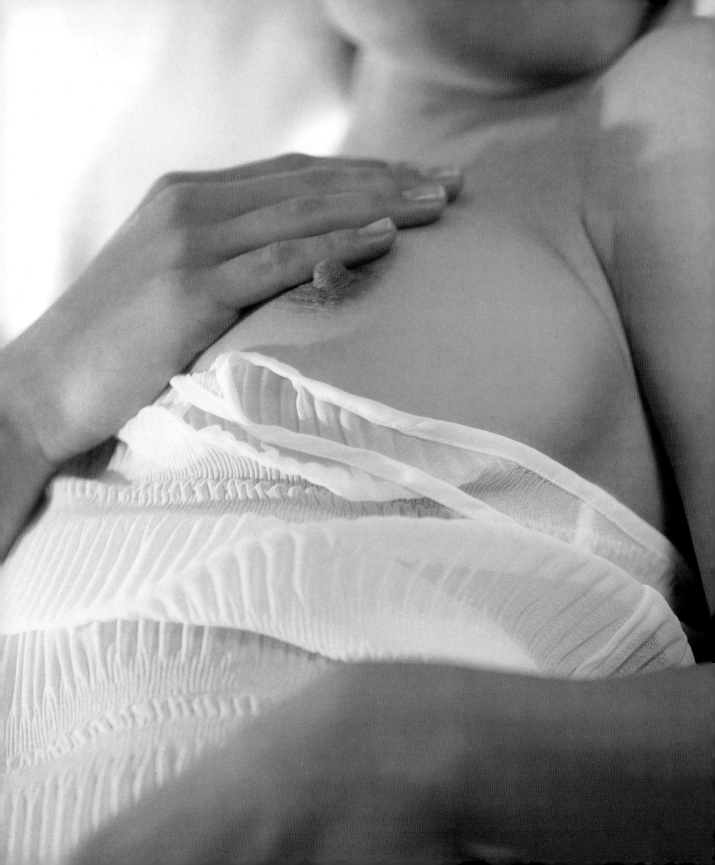

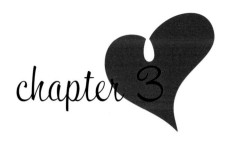

chapter 3

Know Your Terrain: Sexual Knowledge Is Sexual Power

IT IS IN OUR FIRST critical years that our parents and caretakers teach us about our body parts. We're asked to find our nose, or we're asked what "this" is called. Yet in this process of discovering the body, few parents are good at highlighting our private parts. In many cases, they refer to the child's genitals using slang terms instead of the proper medical ones. Between a lack of adequate sex education in the home and in the school system, many people grow up not knowing a whole lot about their sexual anatomy and sexual response. This is unfortunate since it's important to know your body and response in order to understand both you and your lover's capacity for sexual arousal and pleasure.

Your body is a work of art, including your sexual anatomy. Realizing that his penis and her vulva house many erogenous zones themselves helps us to see genitals in a whole new light. Such knowledge also enables us to expand our sexual repertoire and sexual response as we work toward enhanced sex.

"You know what happens when we touch! You laugh like the sun coming up laughs at a star that disappears into it. Love opens my chest, and thought returns to its confines."

—RUMI

KNOW HIS BODY TO RAVISH HIS BODY: MAPPING OUT HIS SEXUAL PLEASURE

Fairly or not, most regard the penis as the centerpiece of a man's sexuality. Yet few know that this male reproductive and sex organ offers both him and his lover so much more in having individual, highly erotic hot spots. The penis consists of the following structural divisions:

Foreskin—The foreskin, or prepuce, is present in males who are uncircumcised, meaning this retractable, double-layered fold of skin is in tact (men who are circumcised have had this erogenous tissue removed). Full of rich blood vessels, nerve endings, and muscle fibers, the foreskin is an extension of the shaft, covering and often extending beyond the glans. It contains sebaceous glands that secrete emollients, lubricants, and protective antibodies that help to keep the surface of the glans soft and moist.

Glans—This is the smooth, incredibly sensitive helmet-shaped knob, full of nerve endings, at the tip, or head, of the penis.

Shaft—Filled with blood vessels, the body, or shaft, of the penis contains spongy cylinders, a pair of corpora cavernosa, and a corpus spongiosum, which have the potential to fill and expand for an erection. The corpora cavernosa extend back into his body, its roots, or crura, attaching to the surface of the ischiopubic rami, the branches of the pelvis. This prevents his penis from sinking into his perineum during thrusting. (Note: While covered with muscles, the penis itself is not a muscle.)

Root—The base that attaches the penis to the body.

Penises come in all shapes and sizes, varying in length and girth. It is the larger nonerect (flaccid) penises that tend not to increase as much in size when erect (as do penises that are smaller when flaccid).

Corona—Also known as the coronal ridge, the corona is the sexually excitable raised ridge at the bottom of the glans, which separates the shaft from the head of the penis.

Frenulum—Also referred to as the fraenum, this hot spot is the small bump of loose skin at the indentation on the underside of the penis, where the shaft and head of the penis meet. On men who are circumcised, the frenulum can appear as an area of scar tissue, which can be more sensitive than regular skin. It is an extremely sensitive part of the penis that reacts quickly to stimulation.

Scrotum—The scrotum is the dark thick-skinned sack of flesh under the penis that hangs between a male's legs, housing the testicles. In maintaining an ideal temperature for the production of sperm, the scrotum contracts muscles when cold, drawing the testicles closer to the body, and relaxes the muscles when hot, lowering the testicles away from the body. Highly sensitive, it contains a number of sebaceous glands and is covered with hair. This area should be handled with care, since every man is different in the amount of scrotal stimulation he can bear.

Testicles—Protected by the scrotal sack, the testicles, also called testes or gonads, are the oval glands that produce sperm and sex hormones, primarily testosterone, the hormone that controls a male's sex drive. Each testicle contains seminiferous tubules, tiny coiled tubules that produce about three hundred thousand sperm for every ejaculate. They vary in size and shape from male to male, with the left testicle typically hanging down farther than the right. It may also be slightly larger than the other.

Prostate—Sometimes known as the "P-spot," this golfball-sized wonder surrounds the urethra like a donut, sitting just below the bladder above the perineum. When a man is sexually aroused, this firm gland, made of smooth muscle fibers, connective tissues, small tubes, clusters of glands, and tiny blood vessels, begins to throb, sending sensations throughout his groin as it swells with prostatic fluid. This fluid is meant to protect the sperm from the vagina's acidity by increasing the pH of their environment, facilitating sperm movement and the chance of fertilization.

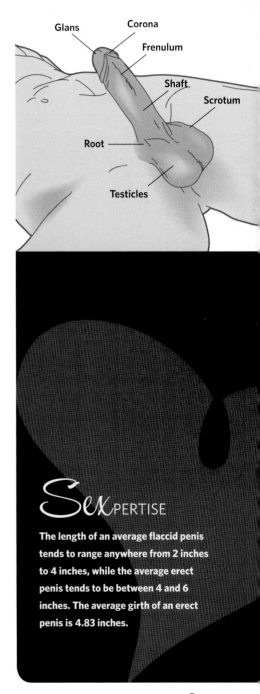

$\mathcal{S}$e𝓧PERTISE

The length of an average flaccid penis tends to range anywhere from 2 inches to 4 inches, while the average erect penis tends to be between 4 and 6 inches. The average girth of an erect penis is 4.83 inches.

KNOW HER BODY TO RAVISH HER BODY: MAPPING OUT HER SEXUAL PLEASURE

Beyond her supple curves, soft skin, and scintillating sensuality, the female form is rich with erogenous zones meant to bring her inner goddess to life . . .

Vulva—The vulva, or pudendum, is the collective term for a female's external genitals. This area consists of her mons pubis, inner and outer lips, clitoris, the clitoral hood, two Bartholin's glands (which produce lubrication), the vaginal opening, and the urethral opening. Vulvas vary greatly from female to female, presenting themselves in a variety of shapes, sizes, and colors.

Mons Pubis—The mons pubis, also called *mons veneris* (Latin for "hill of Venus," Venus being the Roman goddess of love), is the fatty pad of tissue, covered with pubic hair, that sits on a woman's pubic bone. It is thought that the pubic hair is meant to protect the vulval area, while the fatty tissue is meant to protect a female's pubic bone from the impact of sexual intercourse.

Urethral Opening—This is the protrusion between a female's clitoris and her vaginal opening through which urine passes.

Clitoris—Packed with eight thousand nerve endings, the clitoris is, for most females, the primary source of sexual pleasuring and orgasm. This incredibly sensitive sexual organ, ranging in external length from two to four centimeters, is nestled between the labia and actually extends back into the body. Every female is different when it comes to the size and look of her clitoris. This hot spot can be as small as a seed pearl to seemingly "enlarged" in protruding a bit.

The clitoris is protected by a sheath of tissue called the clitoral hood, or prepuce, and an area of skin called the commissure (which can be seen in gently pulling back the outer lips and hood). The clitoral hood protects this hot button from overstimulation. It is composed of a clitoral glans, or "head," which sits at the top of the vulva, where the inner and outer lips meet. Its clitoral shaft, or corpus (body), contains spongy erectile tissue known as a pair of corpora cavernosa, which wrap around the vaginal opening, urethra, urethral sponge, and vagina. The two clitoral shafts, also referred to as "legs" or "crura," extend inward, straddling each side of the vaginal canal, for a total clitoral length of up to nine centimeters.

When stimulated, the clitoris swells with blood, its erectile tissue becoming erect and possibly doubling in size. Some clitorises swell more than others with sexual arousal, with those that extend beyond the clitoral hood and lips more visible and firm.

$\mathcal{S}ex$PERTISE

Every woman is different when it comes to the amount of pressure and touch she likes on her clitoris during manual or oral stimulation. Every woman is unique in preferring indirect versus direct stimulation, and this can vary from one lovemaking experience to the next, especially given that the clitoris is sensitive to temperature. The vast majority of women need clitoral stimulation in order to reach orgasm, no matter what the sexual activity.

Labia—A collective term for the inner and outer lips, or labia majora and labia minora, the labia encompasses the rounded, sensitive skin folds that create the vulva's outermost area. Consisting of fatty tissue, they protect the inner vulva. The outer lips, or labia majora, are covered with pubic hair and contain fatty and sweat glands that produce every woman's unique perspiration and scent.

The inner lips, or labia minora, are the oftentimes thinner (though sometimes more pronounced in some females) and smoother parallel folds of skin housed between the outer lips and vaginal entrance. Typically damp, they are filled with nerve endings, and may appear pink, bright red, or deep brown to black. In containing sebaceous glands that produce sebum, they also serve to lubricate the skin, forming a waterproof, protective covering when combined with secretions from the vagina and sweat glands. The two inner lips join at the top of the clitoris, forming the clitoral hood. Both the inner and outer lips fill with blood when a woman is aroused. Most are not as symmetrical as is typically depicted in medical drawings or erotic materials.

Vaginal Opening and Vagina—Also known as the "introitus," the vaginal opening leads to the female's vaginal canal, which is, on average, about one inch in diameter. Sitting at a forty-five-degree angle, the vaginal canal runs four inches deep in a woman's unaroused state. When a woman is aroused, this elastic canal can double in depth and width. The vagina is a highly muscular organ that connects the vaginal opening with the cervix. The greatest concentration of its nerve supply is in its lower one-third.

Cervix—The cervix is the small, fleshy dome-like opening to the uterus. It contains few nerve endings and is as small as a cherry in some nulliparous women (those who have not had a child). It is surrounded by the cervical fornix. While an erogenous zone for some, many women find pressure or thrusting against the cervix rather uncomfortable if not downright painful.

G spot—Also referred to as the Gräfenberg spot, female prostate, or urethral sponge, the G spot is located about two inches up the front (stomach side) wall of the vaginal canal. This small mass of erectile tissue, made up of paraurethral glands, ducts, blood vessels, and tissue, surrounds the urethra. The size of the spongy tissue, which swells during sexual arousal, and glands found in the urethral sponge differ from woman to woman.

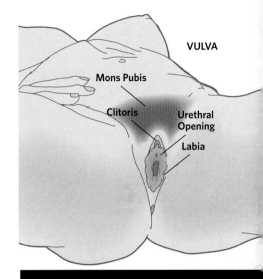

VULVA

Mons Pubis

Clitoris

Urethral Opening

Labia

$\mathcal{S}ex$PERTISE

One major reason the G spot is such a noted erogenous zone is that this area is turned on by the pelvic nerve, one of the body's most powerful nerves, which is also connected to her bladder, uterus, urethra, PC muscle, and uterine muscles. The G spot can be found only once a female is aroused, when the urethral sponge is bulging, becoming firmer. It is an erogenous zone that is not necessarily on the vaginal wall; rather it can be felt through it. (Note: Not all women can locate a G spot, and even some who do may not notice any difference in sensation.)

KNOW YOUR MUTUAL PLEASURE ZONES

Breasts and Nipples—Regarded as secondary sex organs, the breasts and nipples are important sources of pleasure. Full of pleasure-receptive nerve endings, each breast consists of fatty fibrous tissues and fifteen to twenty clusters of mammary glands. Stimulating this area often results in perkier breasts and hardened nipples for some. This is in large part because the area becomes engorged with blood during sexual stimulation, thereby becoming more sensitive to touch for some.

Perineum—The perineum is the area located between the scrotum and anus of a male and between the vagina and anus of a female. This incredibly soft, sensitive area, full of nerve endings and spongy erectile tissue, is made of tissue similar to that of the vaginal lips. It is here where the pelvic-floor muscles crisscross one another, making it a big hot spot. Thus, lightly or firmly stroking or tickling the area can activate this pleasure zone, particularly by triggering the pudendal nerve. The pudendal nerve runs through the PC muscle and lets your brain know that you're experiencing sexual arousal.

Anal Opening and Anus—Packed with densely concentrated nerve endings, the anus is the area of soft tissue folds, the opening of which may be covered with hair. During sexual arousal, the anal opening and anal canal are engorged with blood, heightening sensitivity and arousal potential when directly stimulated. The area is quite sensitive to touch for most people, sometimes resulting in orgasm when stimulated.

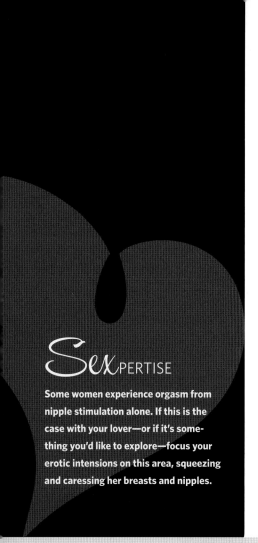

$\mathcal{S}ex$PERTISE

Some women experience orgasm from nipple stimulation alone. If this is the case with your lover—or if it's something you'd like to explore—focus your erotic intensions on this area, squeezing and caressing her breasts and nipples.

SEXUAL Q&A: MALE NIPPLE STIMULATION

My husband threw me off the other day by asking me to stimulate his nipples during sex. He says that it feels good. I'm willing to oblige, but I thought that only women could have sensitive nipples. Is he the odd man out or is this fairly normal?

Despite the prevailing notion that breasts are a female-only hot spot, plenty of men get turned on from having their own breasts and nipples stimulated. Many thrive off of chest and nipple play. In fact, 60 percent of men's nipples harden when they're turned on. Whether direct or indirect stimulation, men thoroughly enjoy having their nipples stroked, kneaded, rubbed, pinched, pulled, stretched, flicked . . . gently, firmly, or vigorously. So have fun finding out what he likes, being sure to ask him what feels good and when he would like more or less stimulation or pressure.

KNOW YOUR SEXUAL-RESPONSE CYCLE

As mentioned in the introduction, this book's sex program approach is based on three major stages of the sexual-response cycle, the sequence of physiological and psychological changes that take place with sexual stimulation. So before going any further, working our way to the Arousal section, let's examine the stages of the sexual-response cycle: Excitement, Plateau, Orgasm, Resolution.

EXCITEMENT

The arousal stage of the sexual-response cycle, which the next section will explore in much greater depth, is also known as the excitement phase. Fueled by desire and an increased sensitivity to stimulation, it is heavily defined by vasocongestion, the accumulation of blood in a body part's blood vessels, particularly the genitals and breasts. Both sexes can experience what's known as a "sex flush" as your muscles tense and the body's pulse rate and blood pressure steadily rise.

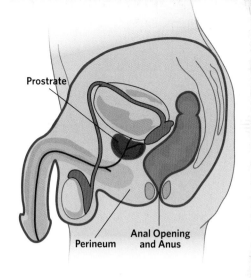

Prostrate

Perineum

Anal Opening and Anus

What Happens When He's Aroused

During the excitement phase, the male's penis fills with blood, becoming erect, with the foreskin of those who are uncircumcised pulling back. His scrotal skin will thicken as the scrotal sac tenses, pulling itself up closer to the body. The testes it houses become slightly elevated, as well.

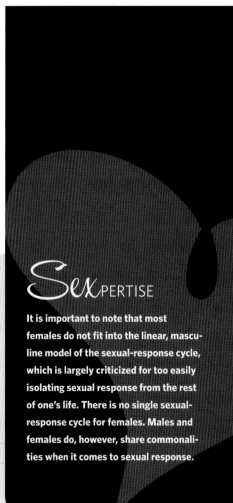

𝒮𝑒𝑥PERTISE

It is important to note that most females do not fit into the linear, masculine model of the sexual-response cycle, which is largely criticized for too easily isolating sexual response from the rest of one's life. There is no single sexual-response cycle for females. Males and females do, however, share commonalities when it comes to sexual response.

In the Bedroom:
Your Own Personal Anatomy Lesson

IN A RELAXED SPACE, take turns stripping down for your own personal anatomy lesson, making an effort to actually make it as nonarousing as possible. Instead, armed with the diagrams in this book, allow your partner to take his or her time looking for and/or looking at these spots. Allow her to touch. Allow him to prod. Let your lover get up close and personal to truly understand where these areas are exactly and to assess how they might be best stimulated.

What Happens When She's Aroused

With arousal, a woman or her lover will notice vaginal swelling and natural lubrication of the vaginal walls. This is due to blood flow to the muscular middle layer of her vagina, during which lubrication is actually pushed through her vaginal walls, for an effect known as "vaginal sweating," or transudation. At this point, her entire clitoris—external and internal—fills with blood, increasing in size as it becomes erect. The part of the clitoris surrounding the urethra, called the vaginal sponge or paraurethral sponge, swells with the vasocongestion of its tiny blood vessels. Her inner and outer lips also increase in size, with the inner labia spreading apart as they thicken and deepen in their hue. Internally, a female's vagina is experiencing a "ballooning" effect, expanding dramatically as her cervix and uterus are pulled upward.

The excitement phase can be short or may last for several hours. During longer sex sessions, the penis may occasionally become less erect and vaginal lubrication may decrease periodically, as well.

PLATEAU

As an individual becomes increasingly aroused, s/he enters the plateau phase, with the amount of blood in the genitals reaching its maximum level. One's breathing, pulse rate, and blood pressure are at their highest. Some individuals may experience short muscle spasms in their face, hands, or feet.

When He Plateaus

The healthy male has a total erection at this point. His penis may appear darker in color, its head possibly a shade of purple. His testes and scrotum, engorged with blood and pulled ever closer to the body, may be swelling up to 50 percent larger than its regular unaroused size. As his glans swells, a few drops of pre-ejaculatory fluid, containing active sperm, may appear at the tip of his penis thanks to his Cowper's glands, located at the base of the penis. This preseminal fluid appears meant for neutralizing and cleansing the urethra after urination.

When She Plateaus

A female in the plateau phase is equally charged, with her clitoris practically numb with excitement as it's drawn up into the body. Her labia may be very dark, a state known as what Kaplan and other sexologists have referred to as "sex skin." Her body is preparing itself for climactic release with an "orgasmic platform," which namely involves the thickening of the outer third of her

As many as 75 percent of women and 25 percent of men will exhibit a sex flush, a reddening of the face, throat, chest, and abdomen. A female's chest may swell and enlarge by up to 20 percent, with the nipples becoming erect in some individuals, thanks to muscle contractions of the nipples' muscle fibers. Both sexes feel alive in this state of heightened physiological activity, their bodies alive, radiant, and full of well-being and a sense of euphoria as they anticipate what will happen next.

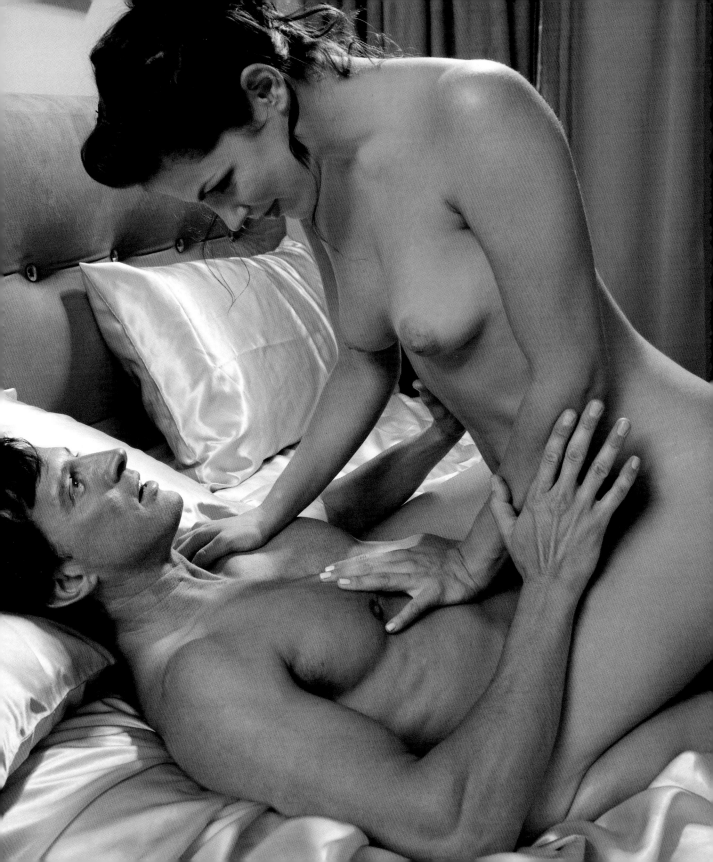

vagina. Her uterus is also becoming fully elevated. Any fingers or penis that have penetrated her may notice that there is a tightening of the vaginal opening here as well. Her Bartholin's glands, located under the skin of the inner lips, about partway between the bottom and top of the vagina, may secrete a couple of drops of clear fluid. The glans folds into the hood just prior to orgasm, a reaction caused when a suspensory ligament that is attached to both glans and ovaries becomes stretched at peak arousal as the woman's internal reproductive system braces for climax.

During the plateau phase, a female may also experience a tightening and lifting of the vaginal canal as the muscles and ligaments tighten for a uterine "tenting" effect. Researchers speculate that the "tenting" effect of the uterus during the plateau phase may have two purposes:

1. It reduces friction on the penis, delaying ejaculation.

2. It lifts the cervix away from the semen pool following ejaculation. This creates a "reservoir" for the semen, allowing time for decoagulation so that the sperm are no longer clotted.

Research featured in The G spot: And Other Discoveries About Human Sexuality has found that no tenting takes place if the G spot (located on the anterior vaginal wall) area is stimulated and the female experiences orgasm.

ORGASM

Often chalked up as "indescribable," physiologically speaking, the orgasm phase of the sexual-response cycle consists of a temporal succession of pelvic, including uterine and anal, rhythmic contractions, spaced at 0.8-second intervals. It is the peak of sexual arousal, with vasocongestion, myotonia, breathing, blood pressure, and pulse rates at their highest, unable to go any higher. During orgasm, blood that has collected in the genital area is actually forced out.

While the shortest phase of the cycle, psychologically you can feel temporarily suspended in time as warm, tingly sensations course through your body. It is also during the orgasm phase that lovers may feel closer to each other. With the release of the "bonding hormone" oxytocin at climax, the level of which can impact an orgasm's intensity, lovers can feel increased emotional attachment and intimacy. Some may also have atypical reactions postorgasm, such as feeling slightly melancholy or depressed.

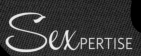

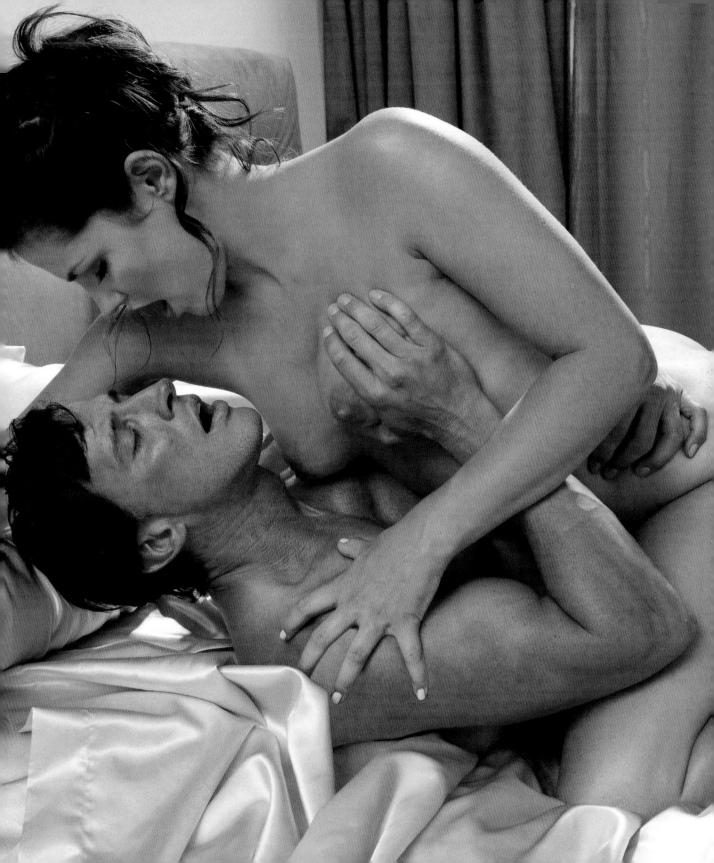

For either sex, the experience of orgasm can involve multiple orgasms. Every person has the potential to experience multiple orgasms. Every person has the potential to experience different types of multiple orgasms, since humans can have a number of different climactic reactions. Multiple orgasms can happen successively within a few seconds of one another or may be a minute or two apart. They are generally described as any of the following:

Compound single orgasms: Each orgasm occurs individually and is distinct. You return to a partially aroused state in between each peak during a lovemaking session; for instance, a woman experiences an orgasm during foreplay and then another one thirty minutes later during intercourse.

Sequential multiple orgasms: A series of orgasms, each climax happening two to ten minutes apart. You experience minimal reduced arousal between orgasms, as though you're riding a roller coaster. Such may occur, for example, when a woman has an orgasm from cunnilingus, after which her partner enters her, with thrusting bringing her to another orgasm. Orgasms are regarded as more "sequential" if restimulation is needed.

Serial multiple orgasms: Each orgasm happens one right after the other, possibly separated by seconds. For some, this may feel like one long orgasm, with spasms of varied intensity. For others, these are experienced more as wave after wave of pleasure.

RESOLUTION

As the final stage of sexual response, the resolution phase involves the body returning to its previous, unaroused state. Both sexes lose any sex flush, with pulse, blood pressure, and breathing rates returning to their normal levels.

When He Comes Down

For men, the loss of erection, or detumescence, defines the resolution phase for him. As blood leaves the penis, a refractory period settles in, where a male cannot experience sexual arousal, an erection, or orgasm again. The length of time experienced in the refractory period varies from man to man, with younger males having the ability to bounce back sooner than their older counterparts.

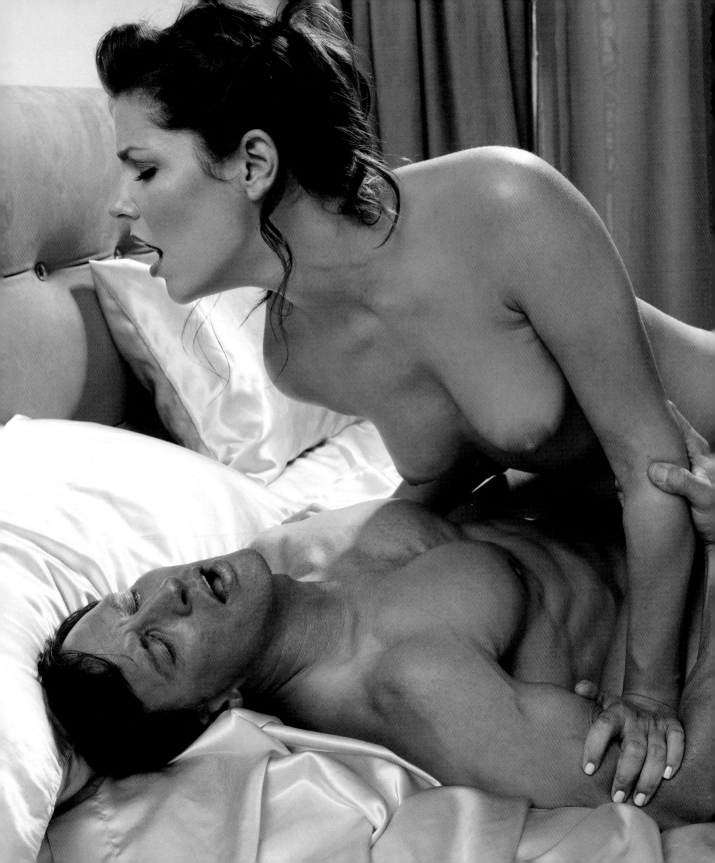

THE SCIENCE OF *Sex*

A woman who is breastfeeding may experience unexpected sexual desire. This is because the suckling/nipple stimulation results in a release of oxytocin into the bloodstream. This hormone, then, acts on the mammary myoepithelium, causing the milk to eject out the nipple. As it does this, it also causes a contraction of the uterine muscles. Breastfeeding further results in the release of prolactin, which ultimately decreases sexual desire in lactating women.

When She Comes Down

A female's cleavage is the first to "come down," followed by the clitoris returning to its normal size and position. As her orgasmic platform relaxes, her uterus shrinks back to its previous state and her vaginal canal shortens in length. All of this can take up to a half an hour total, though with more arousal, a female can be thrown back into an earlier phase of the cycle, in some cases experiencing orgasm all over again!

SEXUAL CHEMISTRY: THE ULTIMATE APHRODISIAC

It would not be fair to leave this section without mentioning the role of sexual chemistry in lovers' desire for one another. This mysterious, unknowable, and undefinable condition is often used to assess the quality of one's sexual relationship and ability to feel sexual desire and response. Based on a combination of traits, this physical, emotional, and sexual state is what drives us toward sexual intimacy and mutual pleasure.

SEXUAL Q&A: MALE EJACULATION VS. ORGASM

What happens when a man ejaculates? How is this different from his orgasm, if at all?

For men, orgasm is almost always accompanied by ejaculation, which occurs in two stages. Yet these are two distinct experiences. When it comes to ejaculation, in the preliminary stage, or emission phase, semen moves from the testes, receiving fluid from the prostate gland before being driven to the urethral bulb at the urethra's base. His reproductive system's smooth muscles are also contracting, causing his semen to move into the widening of the urethra found at the base of the penis. Together, this results in the sensation known as "ejaculatory inevitability." It is at this point that a male knows that he is about to ejaculate and that this reaction cannot be stopped, leading to the expulsion phase.

During the expulsion phase, a male's urethral bulb and the pelvic muscles at the base of his penis are contracting rhythmically, pumping the seminal fluid through his urethra and out of the head of the penis. This can happen because his internal urethral sphincter remains contracted so that urine and semen do not mix. At the same time, his external urethral sphincter relaxes as the muscles surrounding the urethra and urethral bulb contract to expel the accumulated semen from the urethral opening.

Yet, while the pelvic contractions are experienced as orgasm, ejaculation doesn't automatically trigger climax. Emission and expulsion are controlled by different nerve groups, making it possible to experience one reaction without the other. So a man can emit semen, typically as more of a dribble, without orgasmic release. His pelvic muscles can also contract for a climactic reaction, but without releasing ejaculate.

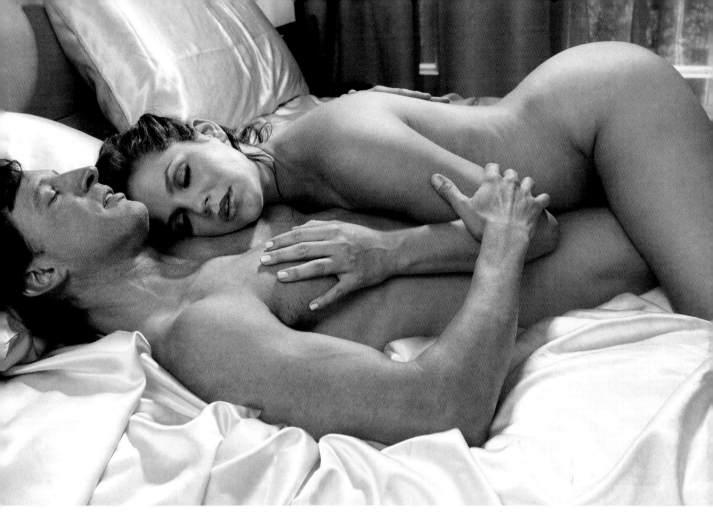

Captured as a state of "magic," sexual chemistry does not necessarily translate into sexual frequency. It is more about the quality of a couple's connection, namely the ease, intensity, and passion in their sexual union. If you've got it, you know it. More than anything, enjoy it! In Arousal, we plan to capitalize on it.

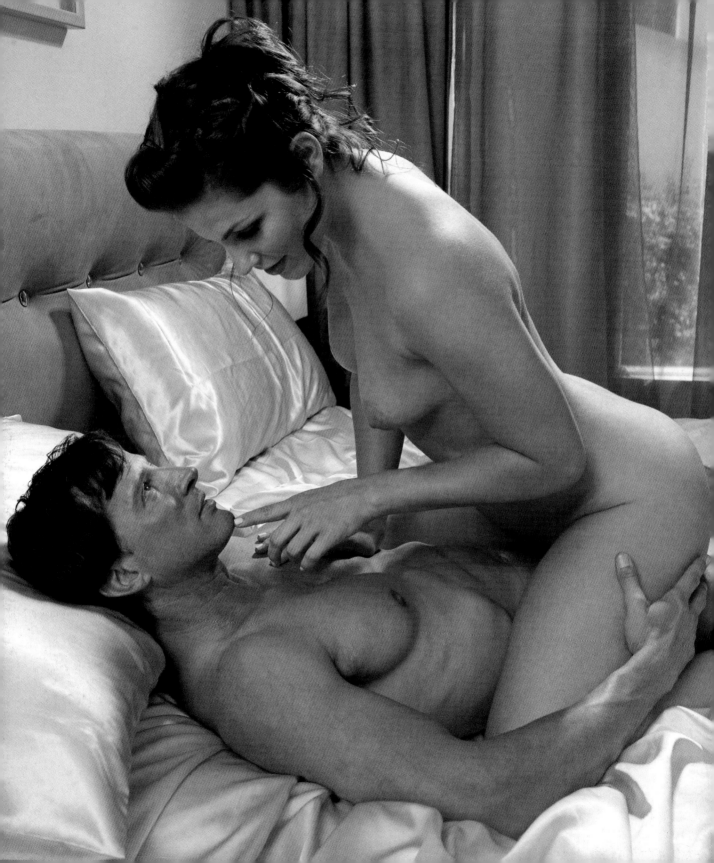

"If only I could walk into your eyes and pull the lids behind me and leave all the world outside."

—SHEILA GRAHAM

Sexual Homework

Now that you know all about your genitals and sexual-response cycle, celebrate your sexual selves!

Take Sexy Pictures! Turn up the heat by snapping a few self-portraits. But be sure to set the mood first. This will depend on the type of photos you want to take. Lighting candles and playing soft music will make for a romantic atmosphere, while colored lighting and tunes with a fast beat will provide a totally different atmosphere. Know, though, that soft lighting will be the most flattering (so start with your camera's flash off). Try shooting just after sunrise or right before sunset. Do yourselves up. To boost your confidence and to feel less intimidated, treat yourself to a nice hairdo, a waxing, and a sexy outfit. Note that red and white colors work well on film. As you pose, be yourself, moving and acting in ways that you feel comfortable and sexy. If you're feeling a bit timid or need some ideas, check out an erotic magazine or pictures,

noting the poses that are most flattering. Looking at these pictures later, especially the close-ups of your genitals, is one way to learn more about your own and each other's most intimate erogenous zones. Plus, it's a divine way to get yourselves aroused for even more!

Merge. The next time you become one, just hold each other, gazing into your lover's eyes as the penis lies still in the vagina. Forget the need to perform. Just enjoy the sensations of this sexual bonding as you look at one another. Express your appreciation for your partner, your lover's body, and your partner's genitals. Feel the energy build from your physical closeness and connection. After five, ten, or fifteen minutes, you may feel the desire to proceed with sexual intercourse. Either lover may fall asleep, which is fine. Or you may just want to keep holding each other. Sexual intimacy takes all types of forms, and this exercise encompasses many of them.

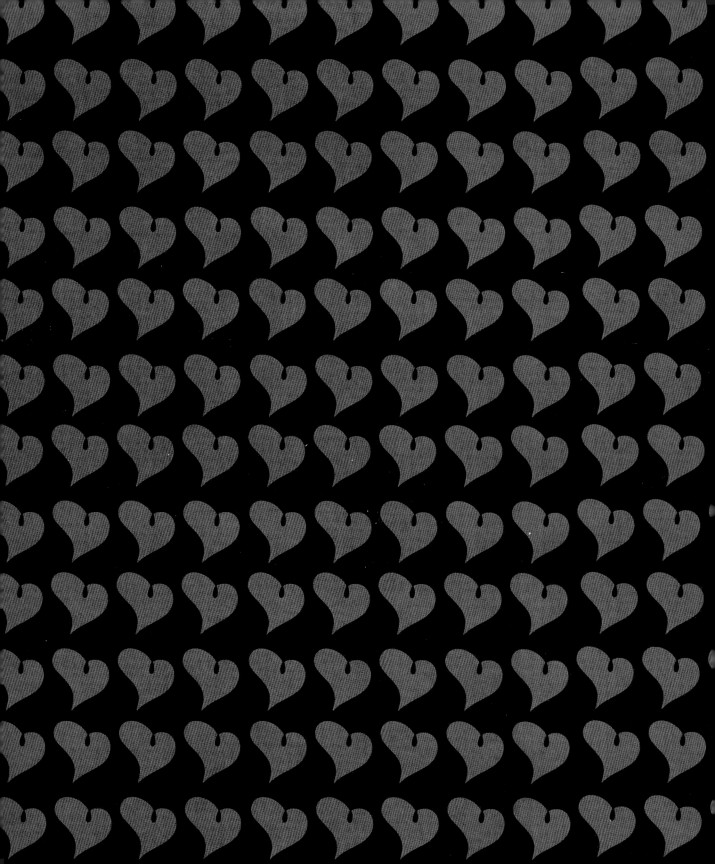

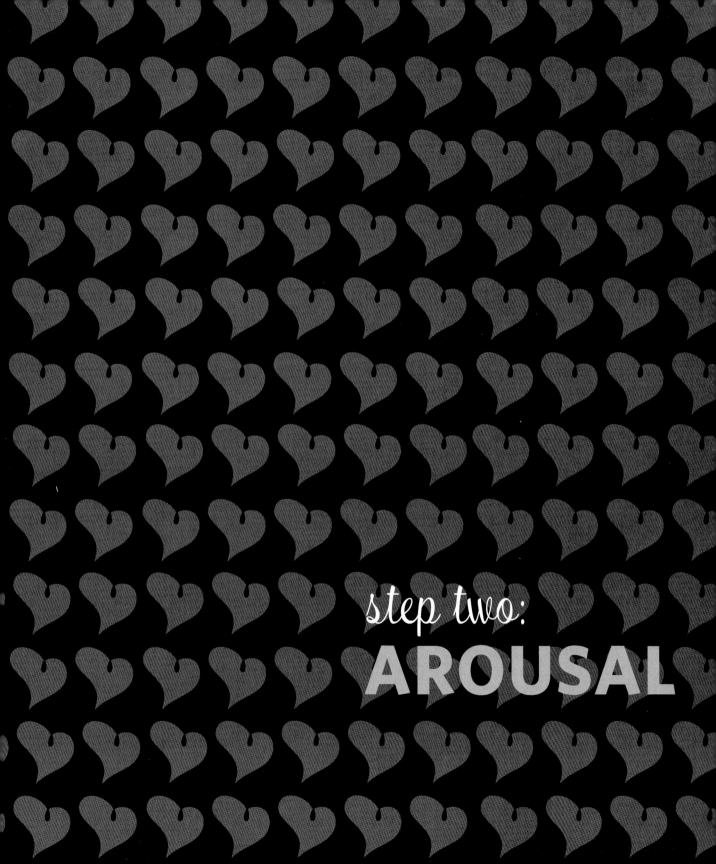

step two:
AROUSAL

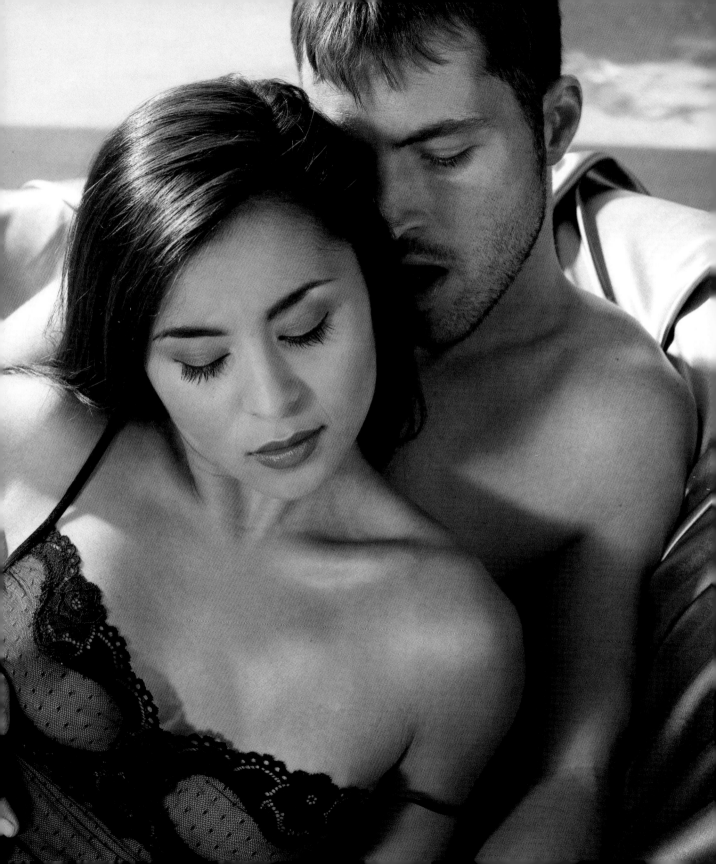

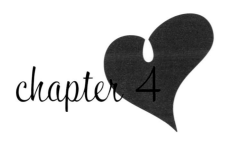

chapter 4

Learn the Nature of Arousal

THERE'S NOTHING LIKE that stirring in your groin, that insatiable sexual energy motivating you to action, urging you to seek more and more. Feeding your sexual appetite will make it grow and grow . . . setting the stage for powerfully satisfying sex.

Quality sex simply isn't possible without adequate arousal. Yet even lovers who are well aware of this fact often fall into relying on some mythical, instantaneous "hot button" reaction to spark their libidos—and then wonder what's gone wrong when the fireworks fail to launch. Sex that is physically, emotionally, and mutually satisfying for both you and your lover requires mastering the art of sexual arousal. The arousal potential itself in both of you must be seduced with sensual playfulness, emotional intimacy, eroticism, and sexual enhancement.

"The mind can make substance, and people planets of its own, with beings brighter than have been, and give a breath to forms which can outlive all flesh."

In this chapter, you'll learn how to achieve the total mind-body focus that you need to maximize arousal for better sex. You'll learn what to do inside and outside of the bedroom to pique your passion-play to its fullest. The more you nurture your basic needs and take care of each other in that process, the more you'll activate your arousal on the physiological, psychological, emotional, and spiritual levels.

There are three major arousal styles when it comes to sexual excitement:

1. **Partner interaction:** You focus on your lover in building your craving, or both lovers play off of one other in increasing sexual tension.

2. **Self-entrancement:** You focus on your body in becoming sexually excited.

3. **Role enactment:** A scenario, something new, or sexual experimentation lends itself to your sexual arousal.

Any of these styles tend to be fueled in one of two ways—physically or mentally—which makes for a more powerful reaction when such efforts are combined. Physical arousal involves tapping into your body's senses: sight, hearing, taste, touch, and smell.

Just consider that your tongue has nine thousand taste buds. Your nose can distinguish ten thousand scents with its 10 million olfactory receptacles. Your eyes can identify 10 million different colors. Your ears hear more than four hundred thousand unique sounds. So you have countless ways to titillate one another!

All of these abilities play into your sexual potency by stimulating and opening your body up to the sensual nourishment that foreplay, which will be covered in Chapter 6, invites. They're made even more intense when you give ample attention to mental factors that play into arousal.

SET THE STAGE . . . MENTALLY

Great sex is all in your mind—as well as in your body. Sexual response is reliant upon getting "in the mood." So make the time to do what you know as a couple has helped you to get in the mood in the past. Think back to the early days of your relationship for clues, or try something new. A few suggestions:

- Take a midnight dip in the ocean or a pool.
- Slow dance in the dark.
- Relax in a bubble bath.
- Playfully undress each other while blindfolded.
- Watch the sunset together.

THE SCIENCE OF *Sex*

In interviewing people about their sex lives, sex researcher Shere Hite, Ph.D., found that not one person interviewed disliked arousal, with most feeling sensations all over the body in becoming aroused. Hite also found that long periods of arousal feel good to many women, with some complaining that their male partners wouldn't wait long enough in making sure they were fully aroused. Lesson learned: Don't shortchange yourselves! Milk the arousal stage for everything it's worth!

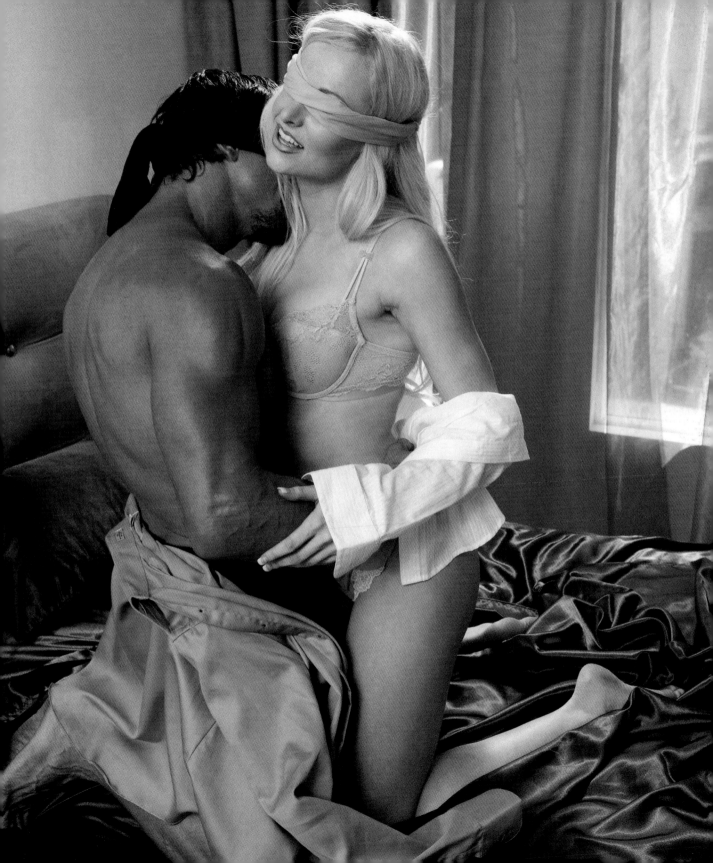

ALL SEXED UP: THE ROLE OF AROUSAL IN SEXUAL RESPONSE

When you come alive with sexual excitement, your body's response is nothing less than orchestral. With the brain as its sexual conductor, your body's electrical, chemical, and mechanical compositions combine in hot-and-heavy harmony. As this master of the body interprets the stimulus you've come across, it strikes up an activation response, turning you into one melodious musical marvel. Several different parts of your body, such as the nervous, circulatory, and reproductive systems, coordinate for some riveting reactions, with psychological feelings of arousal complementing these physiological reactions. When this sexual symphony is on, it can prove orgasmic. But when it's even a little less than fine-tuned, your reactions are in nowhere near as lyrical. So let's first take a look at what makes for an amorous arousal arrangement before exploring why things can get thrown out of key.

WIRED FOR GREAT SEX

Your peripheral nervous system is a major player when it comes to arousal. This system of the body includes all of the nerves from your spinal cord to your internal organs and limbs, including the involuntary autonomic nervous system (ANS). Your ANS is made up of the sympathetic nervous system (SNS), which depletes your energy, and the parasympathetic nervous system (PNS), which conserves your energy. These two "subnervous systems" connect to parts of your body through a network of nerves.

As you become sexually aroused, messages are sent via these nerves to a body part, telling it to react. This is important to know since sexual arousal and orgasm depend on the balance of these two systems and how they interact. The two systems work together during orgasm. This is necessary because, while the SNS causes your heart rate to shoot up, your muscles to tense, and your breathing to become heavy, it also causes blood to flow to your limbs, away from the genitals. So while the SNS revs up the body, much like when you feel danger and suddenly spring into action, the PNS kicks in to slow things down. Evidence indicates that the PNS is stimulated by oxytocin, which acts as a neurotransmitter when released within the central nervous system (CNS), primarily your spinal cord and brain.

Now, you may be wondering why it's necessary to have this short biology lesson in the middle of a better-sex book. Knowing the basics of these very complex responses can help you in your efforts. They help to explain why it is hard for us to get in the mood at times, why our bodies don't respond the way we want them to when we're stressed or anxious. They also help to explain why it's easier to feel erotic and sexually excited when you're in a relaxed state.

Since your SNS cannot be turned off, no matter how much you try, the only way to make sure that you're ready for arousal is to work on activating your parasympathetic system. The healthy-body and relaxation exercises in this chapter seek to do just that, especially in helping you to avoid a couple of the most common issues lovers face at the arousal stage of sexual response.

DEALING WITH ERECTILE DYSFUNCTION (ED)

Erectile dysfunction (ED) is a condition where a man is unable to attain or maintain a penile erection adequate enough for sexual satisfaction. This sexual disorder affects millions of men worldwide and can be due to a single or combination of any of the following reasons:

A. **Organic:** All sorts of physiological issues can hamper a man's erectile response, including cardiovascular and neurological disorders, diabetes, spinal cord injury, infection, Peyronie's disease, high blood pressure, medications, alcohol, drugs, nicotine, toxic exposure, hormonal deficiency, prostate disease, and fatigue, just to name a few. ED becomes much more common as men age and in men with diabetes or with risk factors for heart disease, including high cholesterol. This is because conditions that affect blood flow to the penis are the most common causes for ED in older men.

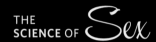

THE SCIENCE OF *Sex*

Endorphins released during sexual excitement create euphoria since they latch onto the same areas that interact with opioid drugs such as heroin.

SEXUAL Q&A: UNDERSTANDING ERECTIONS

What causes an erection? Does the same thing happen to both the penis and the clitoris during sexual response?

As your body becomes more physically and cognitively turned on, it responds by sending more blood to the genitals. Certain arteries, primarily the ones in the penis and clitoris, are opened, which allows more blood to flow through. This dilation of the arteries causes a female's clitoris or a male's penis to become erect as blood rushes into each structure's spongy tissues. Both the clitoris and penis have a pair of spongy erectile tissues, known as corpora cavernosa, which become firm when filled with blood. The penis has a third spongy cylinder, the corpus spongiosum, which also fills and expands with blood in further

causing a male's erection. Nerve and muscle constriction then hold the blood in place for a male's "hard-on" as he becomes increasingly swollen.

Muscles surrounding the reproductive organs of both sexes contract during arousal. In the male, this response causes fluids from the Cowper's gland, seminal vesicles, and prostate gland to be secreted into what we know as semen. In the female, this heightened blood flow to her genitals, known as engorgement, also puts pressure on the walls of her vagina, causing vaginal lubrication.

B. **Psychological:** Emotional and mental matters such as stress, depression, anger, lack of desire, frustration, distraction, unresolved partner conflict, death, and not feeling mentally aroused, can affect a man's game. Even when men take medication to address any organic reasons for ED, the problem often persists since many fail to address any psychological issues at hand.

C. **Partnership:** Problems in the relationship can be at the root of a man's erectile response, like miscommunication, a partner's issues with sex, guilt over infidelity, a lack of attraction for his partner, or being in a sexually demanding, coercive, or intimidating relationship. ED itself can cause a lot of strain between partners, with both individuals taking his lack of reaction very personally.

There are a couple of things to consider about a potential ED situation before you even head to the doctor's. First, as Hite once wrote, we expect men to have "coitus a la James Bond," meaning he should be able to have an erection at will and with no problems. So when things go wrong, from issues as simple as exhaustion, we tend to think that it's unnatural for a man to be reacting in a way that's perfectly normal given certain circumstances. While ED is not inevitable for every man, in many cases, it may just be temporary and situational; for example, he's likelier to become erect two months versus two days after mourning a death. So couples shouldn't jump the gun in assuming that they have a sexual catastrophe on their hands.

Second, don't put so much pressure on the penis when it comes to sexual fulfillment. A penis isn't always necessary for orgasm. And it's okay for you or your lover to receive pleasure in other ways. As plenty of couples will tell you, lovers don't necessarily need to enjoy an erection in order to be sexually satisfied. There's more to a male's sexuality than his penis, and ED situations invite the opportunity, and excuse, for lovers to look into other ways of enjoying each other and experimenting.

If you find yourself dealing with ED, talk to your urologist about the situation in detail. Your physician will then review your medications and psychological history and possibly run some tests in evaluating your vascular, neurological, and hormonal functioning. You and your physician will work together to determine the cause and to decide on a course of treatment. In treating and preventing ED, it is important to remember, as research like that published in the American Journal of Men's Health has confirmed, that simple lifestyle changes, especially ones that target your cardiovascular functioning, can help thwart ED. A Harvard study involving more than thirty-one thousand men found that those who were physically active had a 30 percent lower risk for erectile dysfunction than those men who engaged in little or no physical activity. So make sure that, in addition to any treatments, you're taking care of yourself mind, body, and soul. Make sure that you're integrating the treatment with your relationship's style of pleasuring and intimacy.

Since medications with the active ingredient sildenafil citrate are often used to treat ED, it's wise to be aware of the following: Your erection can last from four to thirty-six hours, depending on the brand. The brand also determines how quickly you'll get an erection, which can be anywhere from fifteen minutes to four hours. (Note: This reaction is highly dependent upon whether or not you're feeling desire.) If you're not feeling stimulated in any way, the drug is not going to be of much help in your arousal efforts. Effects of certain brands are also slowed when taken in combination with a high-fat meal, and each comes with its own side effects, such as diarrhea or increased frequency of urination, neither of which is sexy. Ultimately, the decision is yours to make after consulting with your doctor.

It's important to realize, too, that erection drugs aren't magic pills and they do not work for everyone. ED medications are likely to provide you with an erection sufficient for intercourse given you have adequate penile stimulation 60 to 85 percent of the time. So you may need to combine treatments. In addition to or in place of an erection drug, you may want to try using a vacuum device, penile brace, vacuum constriction device, surgical penile prostheses, intracavernous drugs, erection-enhancing Medicated Urethral Suppository for Erection (MUSE) (alprostadil), or having penile vascular surgery. Yohimbine and phentolamine mesylate can also be used.

DEALING WITH FEMALE SEXUAL AROUSAL DISORDER

When it comes to female sexual arousal disorder (FSAD), a woman can psychologically feel all the passion in the world but have absolutely no genital response. Conversely, she may experience "ravish me" sexual responses that do absolutely nothing for her emotionally. FSAD occurs when a woman cannot attain or maintain physical and/or psychological sexual arousal, including lubrication, for sex. It is the second most common sexual disorder after sexual desire disorder and is typically classified as one of four types:

1. **Genital arousal disorder:** A woman is aware of psychological pleasures yet experiences decreased or a lack of vaginal lubrication, swelling, or genital tingling that comes with arousal.

2. **Subjective arousal disorder:** This is a condition where a female does not feel subjective sexual arousal, despite physical congestion in the genitals. There is no mental awareness of sexual pleasure. In many cases, a woman will avoid direct genital stimulation, feeling less physically during intercourse.

3. **Anhedonic sexual arousal:** Genital congestive response has occurred, yet despite being aware of her genital response, the woman is not joyous or satisfied.

4. **Combined arousal disorder:** Both genital and psychological responses to sexual stimulation are absent.

Reasons for FSAD are often overlapping, including prolonged illnesses (especially ones such as diabetes that can eventually decrease genital sensation), reproductive system conditions or surgeries, depression, stress, exhaustion, lack of sleep, alcohol/drug use, hormonal/endocrine system imbalances, menopause, childbirth, medications (including the birth control pill), history of sexual trauma, or relationship problems. The pain from lack of lubrication during intercourse can also impact a woman's arousal factor.

If you suspect that you have this condition, be sure to get physically and psychosocially examined by a specialist in female-sexual medicine. Treatment options may include the discontinuation of certain medications, sex and relationship therapy, the use of erotic materials, sensual massage, Zestra (a botanical female-stimulation oil that's good for up to twenty-four hours in relieving vaginal dryness), position changes, pelvic floor muscle exercises, a vibrator, a vacuum pump such as the EROS clitoral therapy device, herbal treatments, lubricant use, or hormone therapy.

AROUSING YOURSELF OUTSIDE OF THE BEDROOM

It would be nice if that "do not disturb" sign kept out all life matters that can affect your sexual response. Unfortunately, there's no way to compartmentalize sex. Everything that happens in the bigger world comes into the bedroom and vice versa. That's why it's so important for you to practice prevention in attending to the many physical, emotional, and relational factors that can affect your sex life. You need to be proactive!

Aim for a Well-Balanced Diet

You want to eat sensibly since fatty foods can limit testosterone production, possibly decreasing your sex drive. Sticking with healthful foods will help you to keep weight off. And reducing weight increases testosterone, which increases sexual function, particularly in men. At the same time, realize that you need fat to produce hormones, so stick with foods rich in monounsaturated and polyunsaturated fats—the "good" fats—such as salmon, nuts, and olive oil. You also want to include antioxidant-rich foods such as red peppers, garlic, spinach, and berries, which keep your cells healthy.

$\mathcal{S}\text{e}\mathcal{X}$PERTISE

Remember, arousal issues affect both of you—and resolving them requires a team approach. Healthy sexuality plays a major role in a couple's satisfaction. Dissatisfaction can stem from not valuing your lover, the relationship, or your sex life, which can be interpreted, or misinterpreted, in how you react to a sexual disorder. In preventing and dealing with issues, you need to cultivate a strong couple identity. You need to be able to recognize and address conflicts and differences before they become a bigger a problem. You can do this by learning to communicate effectively, by admiring each other's strengths, by recognizing your vulnerabilities, and by being respectful and loving despite any difficulties.

Foods that help to lower your cholesterol will keep your cardiovascular system in better shape, helping to avoid any sex issues involving blocked blood supply. Chili peppers and ginger are also thought to improve circulation and stimulate nerve endings, which could ultimately improve sexual sensations. Soy, which binds estrogen receptors, can keep the vagina more lubricated and combat hot flashes, among other menopause symptoms, as reported in the European journal *Maturitas*. Soy, in moderation, is also beneficial to the prostate, as studies, such as a 2004 Australian investigation published in *Urology*, have indicated.

Limit Toxins

A number of legal and illegal stimulants, sedatives, and antihistamines can hurt your sexual response. So keep your alcohol to a minimum, don't smoke, and stay away from drugs, including supplements that can have negative sexual side effects.

Evaluate Your Meds

Work with your healthcare provider to determine which medications, such as antidepressants and cholesterol-lowering drugs, may be affecting your sexual response. Then consider whether you should switch brands or change your dosage to meet both your sexual and medical needs.

Get Your Rest

While "Honey, I'm tired" gets old, you do want to sleep for sex since being fatigued does affect your sex drive. To stay healthy and manage stress, be sure to get an adequate amount of rest (the Centers for Disease Control recommends seven to nine hours of sleep a night for adults).

Take Care of Your Psychological Health

Keep issues such as anxiety, depression, fear, and tension out of the bedroom by addressing whatever is causing you distress. If you need therapy, get some. If you need a vacation, book one. If you need to reduce your hours at work, do so. Consider taking up holistic activities such as Reiki, yoga, Ayurvedic cooking, acupressure, and meditation, which help you to recharge and stay mentally healthy.

Do a Relationship Read

Take the "temperature" of your relationship on occasion. Is there anything going on—such as poor communication or not making enough time for one another—that is adversely affecting your sexuality and/or relationship? If necessary, work with a certified sex therapist on any past or present personal and/or relationship matters you need to iron out to improve your sex life.

Stay Fit

Be sure to pursue a moderate amount of exercise to keep toned, maintain a healthful weight, and to help you get a good night's sleep, all of which will help you in the bedroom. Exercise has been linked to a better sex life, helping to maintain or revitalize your sexual performance and making for greater satisfaction. Research, such as that in the Electronic Journal of Human Sexuality, has found that those who exercise feel better about themselves, feel more sexually desirable, and report higher levels of sexual satisfaction. In getting physically active, you'll alleviate stress, feel energized, and feel better in your body.

So get active together, making the time for skiing, walking, aerobics, gardening, horseback riding, canoeing, golfing, tennis, swimming, running, etc. In taking care of yourself, you take care of your sex life, increasing your stamina, coordination, and strength—all of which can boost your bedroom performance and endurance. Better muscle tone will also increase your sexual responsiveness. You will be able to engage in a greater variety of sex positions for greater pleasure. Exercising regularly also combats cardiovascular disease, stress, and high cholesterol, all of which can lead to sexual disorders. Best yet, you'll look sexier, something that is sure to fire up your sex life.

Court One Another

Don't make the mistake of thinking that just because you're in the mood your lover will be, too—and at the drop of a hat. If you want action, especially better sex, you need to seduce your lover on a regular basis—and throughout the day, not just after the late-night monologue. Let your partner know hours earlier that you want to make slow, luscious love or go for a heart-pounding quickie later. Remind your lover that your heart still skips a beat when you remember your first kiss, first touch, first time . . . slip a sticky note in his lunch, or send her a sexy text message with some ravenous rendezvous ideas. Place a card on his dashboard, or send her an erotic email, with all the dirty details of what's to come later. Leave a rose by her briefcase, or slip a pair of satin panties in his coat pocket. Your lover will get the hint.

$\mathcal{S}ex$ercise 4.1 Becoming Sexually Fit

Sit down with a notebook and plan for a healthier sex life. As not to overwhelm yourselves, think about what you can start to do in the next couple of weeks to get yourselves sexually primed for lovemaking. Evaluate and strategize the following:

- **Your Diet:** What foods do you need to eliminate or cut back on? What foods should be incorporated into your diet for sensuous sex? With cookbooks, online recipes, or food-oriented TV shows, map out your meals for the next week. Decide how you will purchase the food, cook it, and, most important, stick to your nutritional commitment for the week. Don't look at this as a weight-loss plan; rather see this as eating for better lovemaking.

- **Substances**: Decide if either of you needs to quit smoking or decrease your alcohol consumption for more invigorating sex and sexual response. What other medications and drugs, legal or not, need to be reconsidered in your amazing sex efforts? Ridding yourself of toxins will make for a new high in the bedroom!

- **Exercise:** Map out an exercise plan for the week, aiming for at least thirty minutes of walking or a more vigorous physical activity daily. What activities do you enjoy that can whip you into shape? What exercises can the two of you do together? With or without the help of a personal trainer, map out an exercise routine. More important, make sure you stick to it!

- **Sleep:** First, consider how many hours of sleep you're getting a night and if that is adequate. If not, figure out how you can go to bed earlier or sleep in later. Also know that physical activity should make for a better night's sleep as long as you're not exercising right before bedtime.

- **Mental Recharge:** Think about ways you can take care of your psychological well-being. You may want to take a couple's yoga class, learn to meditate at home together, spend time luxuriating in a hot tub, listen to classical music, or give each other sensual massages.

- **Seduce:** Talk about ways to sexually tempt one another. Don't put pressure on each other; after all, part of the pleasure in being seduced is the surprise factor. At the same time, don't be afraid to let your lover know what could put a smile on your face or what has the potential to arouse you.

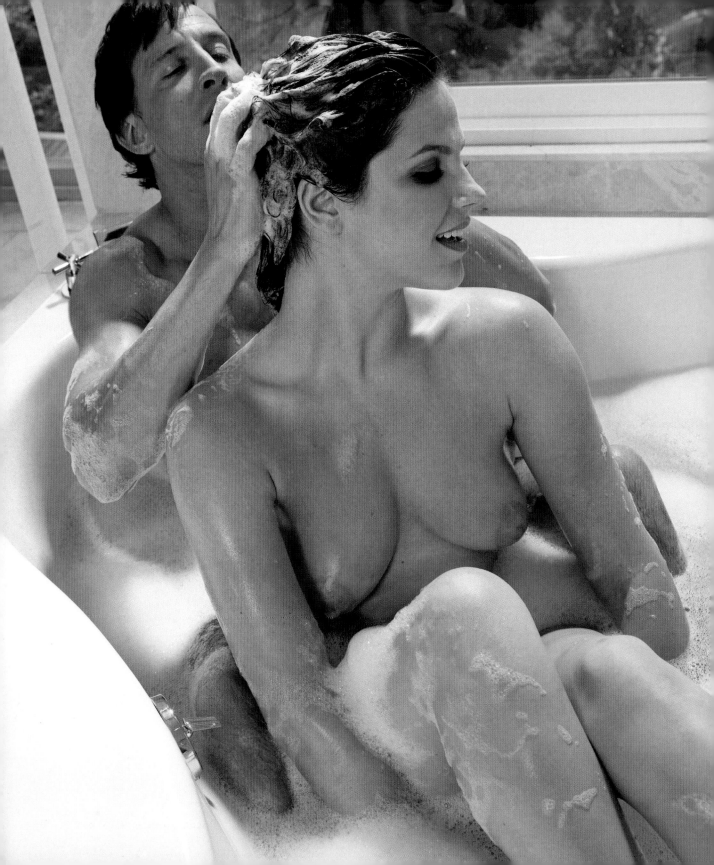

PREPARE FOR A SATISFYING SEX SESSION

True, there are times you can hardly make it to the bedroom fast enough to ravish one another. But since getting caught up in such whirlwind sexual energy is the exception to the rule, you can spend the time between such breathtaking sex sessions planning for your next round of lovemaking:

Clean Up

A clean lover is a sexy lover. Don't get lazy when it comes to hygiene. Taking pride in your appearance and good health helps to maintain lust. So even though it should go without saying, be sure to shower, use deodorant, brush your teeth, rinse with mouthwash, clean and file your fingernails, and groom yourself.

Eliminate Distraction

Identify and address anything that might destroy the mood. For instance, be sure to ensure privacy, attend to any lighting issues, make sure that pets and kids are somewhere safe and happy, and forget about that to-do list (it will be there tomorrow). Distraction-free, you can better focus on sexual intimacy.

Avoid Sleep Triggers

Don't foil your own efforts last minute by consuming too much alcohol, eating a heavy meal, or sitting down in front of the television set. You want to get sexy, not sleepy! Energize yourselves for what's to come.

Feel out Foreplay

Lovers, especially new ones, will often assume that if they're in the mood then their lover will be, too, or will at least oblige. Be courteous to your lover, and ask if it's okay to be intimate. This shows respect for your partner and that you are committed to a mutually pleasing sex life.

Attitude Check

Do what you need to do to get in the mood. This might be as easy as how you carry yourself or dressing to feel sexy. Also, don't let any body-image issues get in the way. You are a sexual being and that alone is sexy. You're about to have sex with your lover, a form of intimacy many would want to experience. So give yourself permission to feel sensual, to be sexy, and to experience one of life's greatest gifts with your special someone.

Clear the Air

Eliminate any anger or resentment you feel toward your partner. Being hurt or resentful or feeling disconnected isn't going to enhance sex. If anything, it will decrease desire and emotional intimacy. Try to sort through any issues that will prevent you from feeling relaxed and connected with your lover, letting go of any anger to let love in. Clear any negative energy by letting your partner know what "I need," "I feel," "I hope," "I notice." Make requests that are behavioral rather than complaint-oriented. Don't blame or complain. Stay calm, focusing on what you want, not on what you don't want. Express appreciation, and stay positive. Validate your partner's feelings. This "weather report" sharing can even be done during pillow talk.

Talk about Sex

Even if you're uncomfortable and embarrassed, having the best sex for you starts with talking about sex. You and your lover need to communicate your likes, dislikes, needs, and desires. Doing so can help you to feel more connected to your partner while increasing your pleasure.

RELAX YOUR WAY TO ORGASM

While it sounds rather ironic, sweaty, heart-pounding sex starts with relaxation. Sexual arousal and orgasm are both greatly dependent upon your relaxation response. In relaxing, you activate your parasympathetic nervous system. To do this, you may need some downtime before you are ready to receive sexual pleasure. Studies, such as that out of University of Groningen in the Netherlands, have shown that in order for a woman to have an orgasm, the part of her brain associated with stress, emotion, and anxiety has to shut down. Relaxation techniques as simple as giving each other a footbath, reading a romantic book, or having a picnic on the beach can give you that relaxation time you need. Lovers who have frequent sex often report handling stress better—and thus are more relaxed and ready for great sex.

Relaxation Breathing

When we're stressed, we often hold tension in our bellies. This tightness greatly affects our energy, overall health, and, of course, the breath we need to keep us pumped during sex. Relaxation breathing helps release this tension and also heightens your sexual sensitivity. By channeling fresh oxygen throughout your body using the breath, your improved circulation enhances your sexual responsiveness and sensations.

In the Bedroom:
Ask Away

IN BUILDING EFFECTIVE sex communication, set aside time to ask for what you want. Nothing can happen in the bedroom until a lover has asked for it. Each of you is to take a turn requesting what you want the other to do. You can ask for anything you care for, being specific. If your partner chooses to honor your request, but doesn't do it exactly as you desire, give further instructions until your lover is doing exactly what you want. Each partner has the right to refuse a request. If your request is met with a "no," do not use this time to process the why. Save that for another time, and simply move on and ask for something else.

In the Bedroom:
Belly Breathing

PRACTICE THE FOLLOWING relaxation exercise to ultimately help arouse you and your lover for sex: With belly breathing, also called diaphragmatic breathing, lovers are able to open up the abdominal area so that the diaphragm moves more deeply with inhalations. These exercises train your diaphragm, the sheet of muscle at the bottom of the lungs, to "unwind" the chest muscles, using the entire abdomen to boost energy and stamina—namely sexual stamina.

Belly breathing is best done anywhere you can lie on your back comfortably: a mat, carpet, or firm bed, though you can sit in a chair as well. To begin a belly breathing practice, do the following:

1. Lie on your back, knees bent upward and feet flat on the floor; calm your mind. (Or if sitting, sit up straight, lengthening your abdomen as though a string is being pulled up through your spine through the head.) Let go of any thought that enters your mind. Mentally envision the thought rolling down your back and out of your attention.

2. Begin breathing in through your nose and out through your mouth, then tune into your regular inhales and exhales for a minute. Note where your breath goes in the body.

3. Begin rubbing your hands together as you continue noticing your breath, until your hands are quite warm. Place one of your hands on your belly so that the center of it is touching your navel. Place the other hand on top, noticing any change in your breath; for instance, notice if your abdomen wants to expand with your inhalation.

4. Rub your hands to get them warm again, and then massage your belly when you touch it, noticing any softening effects.

5. Repeat steps two and three again, this time observing your belly's greater expansion and retraction. Press down on your belly as you exhale if the breath is still tight. Release this press with the next inhale, repeating this process several times.

6. Now, work to make your exhalations twice as long as your inhalation; for example, if your inhale is three counts, then make your exhale six counts, without forcing it. Take care not to breathe too quickly or you may get light-headed.

7. Bask in the sensations you've created for yourself—the warm relaxing feelings and cleansing energy. Try to breathe this way most of the time.

Belly breathing is just one of many relaxation breathing exercises at your disposal for joyous sex. Doing this exercise, or any breathing practice, on a regular basis will help you to breathe more fully, lowering your blood pressure, stress, and anxiety levels. Research out of Harvard Medical School has found that such breathing in the context of meditation, prayer, or yoga can improve your health. These activities actually change patterns of gene activity that affect your body's stress response. Your mind actually counters the effect of genes that are "switched" on or off by stress. All of this stress management helps you in the bedroom.

"This is a place for the exercises that will bring me to where I want to be."

—JOSEPH CAMPBELL

Sexual Homework

In recapping the nature of arousal and what can influence your sexual response at this stage, this chapter has focused heavily on relaxation and better lifestyle techniques. So for your sexual homework, we're going to stay in line with that in practicing the following . . .

Savasana: Known as "corpse pose," this yoga pose is a great way to soothe your sense organs.

1. Lie in a neutral position by lifting your pelvis and pushing the back of it toward your tailbone with your hands.

2. Return the pelvis to the floor, making sure that your legs are extended, with your feet turned out equally. (Note: as your groin softens, you do not want your lower back to flatten.)

3. Lengthen your head away from the body, slipping a folded blanket under the back of the head and neck for support, if necessary.

4. Place your arms at your side, rocking your body to broaden the back ribs and to rest the shoulder blades away from the spine. Turn your arms so that they rest outward, backs of the hands on the floor.

5. Stay in this "dead man" pose for at least five minutes, letting your body sink into the floor as you breathe deeply. If your mind starts to wander, focus on your breath.

Deep Muscle Relaxation: Progressive muscle relaxation is a tension-reducing technique where you contract and release specific muscle groups. Start with the muscles in your face, tensing them for ten seconds; then completely relax your facial muscles for ten seconds. Now, repeat the process with the muscles in your neck. You want to slowly work your way down the body, attending to every muscle group, until your entire body is relaxed. Over time, with practice, you'll be able to relax your entire body within seconds, getting rid of toxins that get stored up in a tense, stressed body.

Unwinding Together: While it is good to spend some time relaxing on your own, you can also bond with your lover doing relaxation exercises together. The following exercises can improve your sex life by relieving tension, stimulating your energy flow, improving your flexibility, and increasing your sexual capabilities and pleasures. These positions will act as an aphrodisiac in and of themselves by loosening your thighs, groins, and hips. You may also feel more connected to each other in new ways, realizing that you're able to engage in public displays of affection, such as holding hands and giving hugs, more easily.

So take turns attending to each other, with the receiving partner lying on his or her back as the giver takes his or her time doing the following:

1. Take your lover's foot and pound lightly on the sole with loose fists; change feet.

2. Shake each of your lover's legs before bending each knee and pushing the thigh into the lower abdominals. For a good hip and lower-back stretch, slowly push the thigh across the body so that the knee (almost) touches the floor. Repeat on the other side.

3. Cover your partner's body with light love taps using your fists, being sensitive to bony areas or ones that are not so muscular.

4. Sit at your lover's head, place your feet on your love's shoulder's, and gently pull her head.

5. Gently and slowly help your lover to sit up. Staying behind your partner, rest your feet on his back as you pull his arms back.

6. Slip your arms under your lover's armpits, and bend your arms back so that you can cup the back of her head with your hands as you stretch her upper arms back.

7. Have your lover move into butterfly position, where he sits with his knees bent, soles of the feet touching one another, back straight. As your lover holds his ankles, he should gently press his knees toward the floor for an inner-thigh stretch; then take your lover's shoulders and gently stretch them back.

8. Ask your lover to roll forward into "child's pose." To get into this yoga pose, also called balasana, your lover needs to kneel on the floor, bringing her big toes together so that she can sit on her heels, before separating her knees hip-distance apart. As she exhales, she will lean forward so that her head touches the floor, arms back beside her torso, palms up. As she is in this resting pose, gently press on her lower back with one palm and on the area between her shoulder blades with the other palm. Check in with her as to whether or not more pressure is desired.

Note: Be sure to breathe fully during these exercises, communicating with each other. You need to make sure that everything feels good, and if it does, don't hold back in giving generous thanks with oohs, aahs, and moans!

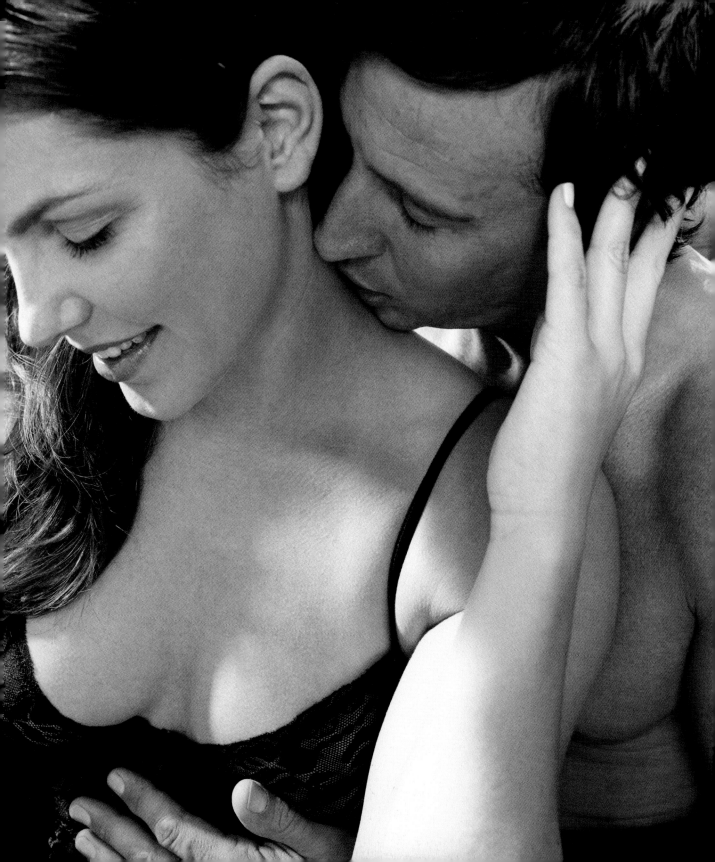

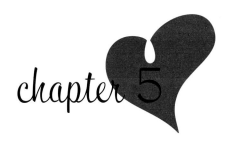

chapter 5

The Right Touch: The Secrets to Touching Yourself and Your Partner in Powerful, Unprecedented Ways

UNLESS YOU'RE TOUCH-PHOBIC, chances are, you love touch. Whether titillating or tender, you know that it can do wonders for you, especially when it involves your partner. Even if you're not consciously thinking "I want touch" or "I need touch," a simple pat on the back, squeeze of the hand, or a warm hug can suddenly make you want to immerse yourself in more feel-good head-to-toe touch. People thrive on it! We literally live on it. Craving all kinds of positive touch is in our nature.

As our most innate need, touch is one of the first senses we develop the moment we come out of the womb. Unable to see clearly or differentiate various sounds, we rely on our skin to navigate our new world. Through it, we feel safe and "valued" by how we are touched. Research, such as that published in *AORN Journal*, has found that infants who are regularly, lovingly touched are less stressed. This, in turn, enables them to gain weight, sleep better, and cry less. Babies and children who receive healthful touch throughout childhood grow up to be competent, well-adjusted adults. Infants who are deprived of touch, on the other hand, fail to flourish, suffering

"*Seduce my mind, and you can have my body; Find my soul, and I'm yours forever.*"

—ANONYMOUS

from abnormal physical development and behavior as adults. Humans deprived of physical contact also have higher death rates. So you can see, we do need touch for our survival. And who better to reach out and touch than your sweetheart, especially in unprecedented ways?

DIFFERENT TYPES OF TOUCH

When it comes to the role of touch for better sex, many lovers—and sex writers, for that matter—tend to focus on sexual touch, namely sex acts. They think that this makes for what they frame as "mind-blowing" sex. And while we certainly can't snub the value of learning a few sex maneuvers, technique alone doesn't make for satisfying sex. You need to incorporate other types of touch in and out of the bedroom for the best of sex.

These other touches are what fuel your libido when you're not in the bedroom, making you all the more eager to rush back to bed for more lascivious loving. Vibrant sexual relationships include healthy doses of sexual, erotic touch, plus all of the other types of positive touch at your disposal, primarily:

- **Healing touch.** Often given when you're sick, tired, or in pain, healing touches such as massage can do wonders to lift your spirits and help you to restore yourself and your sexual desire.
- **Affectionate touch.** These gestures of caring, nurturance, and friendship (think an arm around the shoulder) can offer a lover much support and encouragement. Some touches, such as a pat on the buttocks, can also add a playful dynamic to your relationship, making for more successful sexual relations.
- **Sensual touch.** Suggestive, lingering touches focusing on pleasure bring lovers closer together and invite more erotic touches.

In giving and receiving scintillating sexual touch, lovers often need to go back to the basics. This is because a person's quest for sexual liaisons is often based more on the need for human contact than all-out sex. Phrased differently, our desire for sex is often more of a desire for healing, affectionate, sensual touch than physical, sexual gratification alone. So to isolate your touch exchanges to primarily erotic ones deprives you and your lover of rewarding sex in so many ways. Simply touching your partner, including hugging regularly or cuddling, can boost your sense of belonging and sense of support. You and your lover will feel more connected, invested in each other, and happier. You'll also be much more relaxed.

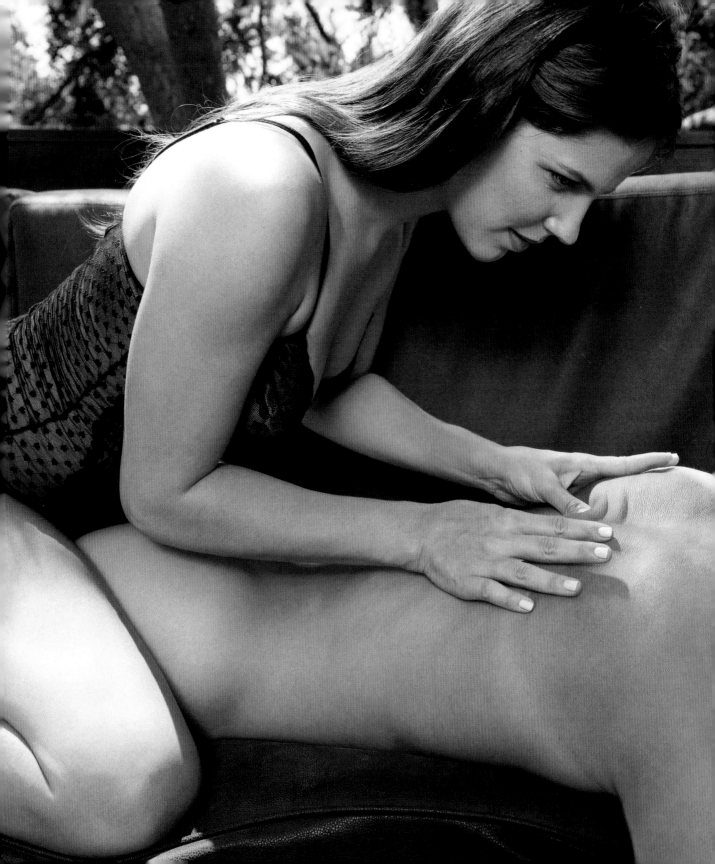

In feeling safe, pleasured, soothed, and just plain good through different types of touch, your body will feel at ease and healthier. Stroking, massaging, and holding another person leads to oxytocin production and the release of endorphins, both of which result in feelings of attachment. With the release of oxytocin, you'll feel calm and reap health benefits such as lower blood pressure and heart rate (plus lowered risk of heart attack). Your overall sense of well-being will also improve as cortisol (the hormone linked to stress) is reduced in the body. Touch also acts as an antidepressant, lowering anxiety, reducing cravings (even resulting in weight loss for some), and promoting a sense of healing and connection.

Why is all of this so important to better sex? Happy lovers make for more pleasant partners, which makes for better-functioning relationships. As mentioned in Chapter 4, relaxed, healthy lovers also get in the mood for sex more readily. They're more receptive to touch and able to get turned on with relative ease. Being in a healthier place both physically and mentally makes them more turned on to sexual intimacy. Being in such a positive space fuels their longing for more loving touch, helping to keep their sex life alive and well.

FEEDING YOUR "SKIN HUNGER"

Gender stereotypes have it that men do not like to cuddle, while women do. And while females are much more sensitive to touch than males from the time they are infants, people of both sexes love to share affection and comfort in snuggling. While we're all different when it comes to touch, in general, people's bodies yearn to be touched beyond their erogenous zones. In fact, many people will describe a "skin hunger," where they're completely ravenous in wanting to be wrapped around or enveloped by a lover. When this appetite goes unfed, lovers can become dissatisfied with their sex lives and with each other. That's why it's so important for you to explore the unexpected pleasures that can be realized in different forms of touch and deeper sexual intimacy.

So how do we start satiating this skin hunger? Our first task focuses on activities that can help you to discover "right" touches for connecting, pleasure, and sharing. We're going to then look into how solo pleasuring can aid you in your "perfect" touch exploration. Before you can have gratifying sex with your lover, you have to have it with yourself. Solo-touch time, including sex, allows you to build a foundation for amazing sex, enabling you to get connected with your own body, touch needs, and where and how you like to be physically touched. It is this private touch time that complements your together time, especially as you share your discoveries.

Hand Exploration: Our hands are one of the most intimate parts of our body, yet how much attention do they get in your love life? Take the time to study nothing but your partner's hands. Be affectionate as you:

1. Close your eyes, and without talking, take one of your partner's hands.

2. Get to know the hand. Feel the texture, the shape. Explore the fingers.

3. As though you're reading Braille, trace your fingertips over the length of each finger, starting at the wrist.

4. Massage the palm, pressing your thumb up to the pad of each fingertip.

5. Do the same exploration with the other hand, this time with your eyes open.

When you're done, share what you both liked about the experience. What made you uncomfortable? What do your lover's hands mean to you? What do they tend to communicate to you in and out of the bedroom? How would you like to be more connected with them on a regular basis?

In the Bedroom:
Body Bonding

THE EXERCISES IN THIS SECTION are about connecting to the body and to your core as a couple. Their aim is to help you to understand how we move in our bodies, allowing yourselves to relax and breathe deeply. As you practice these pleasure exchanges, focus on letting go of tension, being vocal, and trusting your lover. Not only are these vital steps in bettering sex, but doing so fills you with a sense of sensuality that grows only more vibrant as you get in touch with your sexual self. All of these touches are ways lovers can feel closer, express love, relax, and relish physical and emotional pleasures.

In body bonding, there are several things you need to keep in mind. More than anything, make sure that you are allowing yourself adequate time for these body bonding dates. These intimate activities should not be rushed.

Furthermore, ensure the privacy to pursue them. You need moments free from distractions.

Before engaging in any of the activities, you may also want to ground and calm yourself. You'll get a lot more out of these exercises in doing this. Clearing your mind via meditation, for example, can help you to more readily connect with the exercise and your partner. You may find that it's more effective to pursue these activities after you've exercised, had a nice walk or a hot bath, or done some yoga. In further getting yourself in the mood for body bonding, consider what's going to make you and your lover comfortable and more sensually seduced. You may want to lay a mat, pillows, or blankets on the floor. It may help to have the room at a warm temperature, enhanced by soft lighting and scented candles.

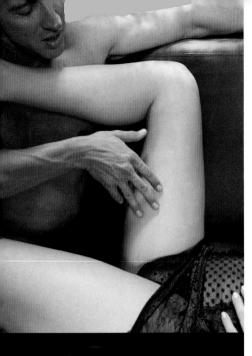

Face Caress: Before beginning the face caress, thoroughly wash your hands with warm soap and water. Now, get in a comfortable seated position, and ask your partner to lie on his or her back, eyes closed, head in your lap. Study your partner's face as though you've just met, as you do the following:

1. Cupping your hands around your lover's head, place your thumbs on the forehead and fingertips at the temples.

2. Press the thumbs between the eyebrows before firmly running them along the eyebrows, working toward the hairline.

3. Move the thumbs up the hairline to the center of the forehead, and massage the temples.

4. Continue that massaging action as your fingers move down the jawbone to the chin.

5. Using the pads of your index and middle fingers, work your way back up the face, massaging the "moustache" area, moving to each cheekbone, then up each side of the nose and around the upper bone of the eye sockets and under each eye.

6. Finally, massage each ear between your thumb and fingers, starting at the earlobe and working your way up around the top of the ear.

Tell your partner what you love about his or her face. Share how much it means to you every time you see it.

Spider's Legs: This exercise can be done anywhere, depending on how much body you want to cover. A French love game, spider's legs, or pattes d'aragnee, involves the lightest possible touch, going for tiny skin hairs on sensitive zones such as the stomach, armpits, chest, and thighs. Using your fingertips and the pads of your fingers, play on and tickle your partner's hair and skin with lightest touches. This action brings your lover's skin to life, enticing them to want more and more touch.

Full-Body Press: Lie either on your sides or with one lover on top of the other. Either way, your goal is to press every inch of your self up against each other. Submerge yourself in this full-body press, letting your bodies melt into one another in silence for ten minutes or so. As you bask in this safe space, think about how it feels. Note the heat, your connectedness, and your energy in this relaxed, merged space. How does your partner's body feel? Share your thoughts with your partner.

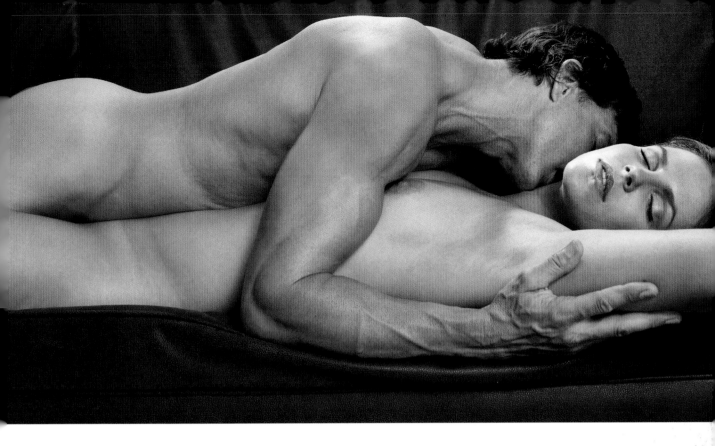

Complements to the full-body press include synchronizing your breaths. Loosely connect your lips so that your breaths move in and out together. You can also alternate between keeping your eyes closed or open. Observe how that is different for you. Why is it important for lovers to engage in the occasional full-body press? How can it benefit you?

Cuddle Parties: Have your own private cuddle party. Modeled after the social, nonsexual workshops coined "Cuddle Party," set aside one evening or an afternoon where you and your partner lounge around in your pajamas and focus on nonsexual touch and affection. Start slowly and with tenderness, much like you would if initiating lovemaking. Ask for hugs and massages when you feel like it. Take a nice long nap, or catch up with intimate conversation, including why it's good for you to have this kind of quality time.

DISCOVER YOUR PHYSICAL PLEASURE ZONES ALONE TO ENHANCE SEX WITH YOUR PARTNER

Masturbation is self-stimulation of the genitals for sexual arousal, gratification, and pleasure, often to the point of climax. Such self-pleasuring is a very common behavior (and not just among humans—other animals, including dogs, cats, horses, bulls, rats, hamsters, deer, and whales, practice it as well). It is the foundation of sexual health in many ways, enabling lovers to have more satisfying sex. Couples who masturbate individually or together often have better sex lives, since such practices offer a plethora of rewards, such as:

- **Sexual empowerment and confidence**. Lovers feel better about themselves, their bodies, their genitals, and their sexual desires, arousal, and response.
- **More powerful orgasms.** Masturbators often experience more intense orgasms during masturbation, in part, because they aren't distracted by a lover's body, movements, and response. They eventually learn how to re-create these intense reactions with their lovers.
- **Greater sexual awareness**. Lovers know what physically and mentally fuels their desire and arousal, and what feels good, for the ultimate in sexual satisfaction.
- **An enhanced sex life.** More sexually informed, lovers can teach each other about what feels wonderful, equipping each other with vital information for longer arousal, better orgasms, and a richer sex life.

COMBATING ISSUES WITH MASTURBATION

Often the first sexual act experienced by many males and females, masturbation has been consistently reported by people in studies over the years. Research since Kinsey has consistently found that about 90 percent of males and 60 percent of females report having masturbated. Among couples living together, both Laumann's *The Social Organization of Sexuality: Sexual Practices in the United States* and Robert Michael's *Sex in America: A Definitive Survey* found that 85 percent of men and 45 percent of women had masturbated within the past year. Yet despite being extremely common and delivering a number of health and relationship benefits, people have a lot of reservations about self-pleasuring.

With religion, law, medicine, and even the media having all worked at some point to keep masturbation a dirty secret, ménage à moi, as it has been coined, has historically been cast as a sinful perversion, mental problem, or medical or ethical issue. Self-pleasuring was thought to lead to disease, jaundice, epilepsy, and a whole host of other negative health conditions. Unfortunately, the major consequence for these misconceptions is sex guilt: Many men and women have been unable to fully enjoy their masturbation experiences because they feel guilty for touching themselves.

In interviewing thousands of women, Hite found that many masturbators felt lonely, guilty, unwanted, selfish, bad, silly, uncomfortable, cheap, dirty, self-centered, ashamed, pathetic, and disgusted with themselves. Almost all of these women were brought up not to masturbate. Some had trouble enjoying their self-pleasuring but were eventually able to get over it and enjoy it, though more physically than psychologically. Most felt the main importance of masturbation was to substitute for sex or orgasm with a partner, feeling that sex with another is better. Some simply saw it as a learning experience and a means of independence and self-reliance.

If you or your partner has an issue with self-pleasuring, be rest assured that masturbation is a perfectly natural, safe, acceptable form of sex play at any age. It is a harmless type of sexual expression for both males and females. In fact, in 1972, the American Medical Association (AMA) declared masturbation a "normal" sexual activity. And research since has confirmed that self-pleasuring offers one a number of physical and emotional health benefits. Both sexes reap rewards such as:

- Stress relief
- Decreased risk for depression
- Increased self-esteem
- Safe sex
- Improved mood
- Better sleep
- Stronger pelvic floor muscles
- More energy
- Improved heart health in being a cardiovascular workout

According to brain researcher Daniel Amen, sexual gratification and release through masturbation may be helpful for your brain. It can also be used as a form of treatment in working through a sexual dysfunction such as lack of orgasm or early ejaculation.

When it comes to males specifically, research summarized in a 2007 article in "Sexual and Relationship Therapy" found that taking matters into one's own hands boosts a man's immune system functioning, bolsters his resistance to prostate gland infection, and makes for a healthier prostate. One study out of Australia's Cancer Council Victoria found that a man who ejaculates from masturbating more than fives times per week is one-third less likely to develop prostate cancer than one who does not.

As summarized in a review of the literature published in Praeger Perspectives Sexual Health series, when it comes to a woman's health, self-pleasuring delivers health benefits for her, as well, by keeping her vagina lubricated and building her resistance to yeast infections. Masturbating also relieves chronic back pain and increases a woman's threshold for pain. Finally, it provides much relief in matters related to a woman's menstrual cycle: Self-pleasuring alleviates premenstrual tension and other physical conditions, such as cramps. It also provides relief for those suffering from dysmenorrhea (painful menstruation) by increasing blood flow to the pelvic region. This reduces pelvic cramping and related backaches. For women who are menopausal, masturbating to orgasm can reduce symptoms including hot flashes by increasing estrogen production. Self-pleasuring can also protect the health of her urinary tract and vaginal tissue.

The only time masturbation is considered a problem by mental health professionals for either sex is when it is done in public, when it causes an individual a significant amount of distress, or when it inhibits sexual activity with a partner.

In realizing pleasing sex, lovers need to take responsibility for their sexual enjoyment, practicing self-acceptance and openness. Masturbating is one way to do this, and a great starting point, all while keeping you primed for sex with your partner. You can do it by yourself and on your own terms. In many ways, it's the best way to learn what works for you. It is a means to discovering and fulfilling your sexual needs and desires—the perfect way to experiment with new sexual practices, to develop your orgasmic abilities, to learn to prolong sexual pleasures, and to expand your sexual potential. For women in general, masturbation and the fantasy that often accompanies it results in more orgasms, including multiple orgasms, during partnered sex. It also makes her more sexually receptive and responsive when she's making love, with married women who masturbate reporting more relationship satisfaction, according to a study published in the *Journal of Sex Education and Therapy*.

MASTURBATION FEARS ONLY HURT YOUR EFFORTS

People have a lot of unfounded concerns when it comes to masturbation. Here, some of the most common fears are alleviated:

FEAR: Masturbating will reduce the quality of my lovemaking.

Masturbating will definitely not reduce the quality of sex. If anything, it will improve your sexual intimacy. This is not only because of shared body knowledge equipping partners with the information they need to turn each other on, but also because it serves you well in bringing you back to your sexual core. The more connected you are with your self, the more connected you can be with your lover.

FEAR: Masturbation desensitizes the clitoris.

Masturbation does not desensitize or numb the clitoris, ultimately preventing a female from reaching climax during intercourse. In fact, self-pleasuring, with or without a sex toy, can help women to increase their clitoral sensations, making for a better orgasm.

FEAR: Masturbating is like cheating on my partner.

People tend to think that masturbation is only for those who don't have partners or for those whose lovers are ill or disabled. As with everything in life, you can depend only on yourself when it comes to meeting your needs. You have to watch that you don't become sexually codependent, meaning that you expect your partner to fulfill your every sexual need. When this happens, you become empty, losing touch with the self and being able to fulfill your own desires. This kills the sexual empowerment that lovers find to be a turn-on, both when it's experienced from within and emanating off of your partner. Ultimately, having a close sexual relationship with yourself puts you in charge of your sex life. Your partner shouldn't be your only source of sexual relief or pleasure. It is unfair to expect such. In making it "okay" to masturbate while in a relationship, solo sex also decreases the tension around one lover wanting to engage in sex more frequently than the other.

FEAR: Masturbating indicates that I'm not sexually fulfilled.

While elderly men have reported, in the Journal of Aging and Health, masturbating more when less physically satisfied with their partners, this isn't necessarily the rule. People can have very fulfilling sex with a partner and still want solo time. That's in part because you're fulfilling a different set of needs; for instance, you may want to be alone to view erotica or to focus only on your own pleasuring. You may want to consider, however, whether you're using masturbation as a way to avoid sex with your partner. If so, that's a pretty good indicator that something is wrong.

FEAR: There is a point where one can masturbate too much.

People will often ask sexologists if there is a certain number of times per day or week that's considered "normal" versus "abnormal" when it comes to masturbating—and there is not. How much a person masturbates in his or her lifetime is very individual and can vary significantly at different points in a person's life. It is considered problematic only if it replaces your interest in other forms of pleasure, such as your hobbies or hanging out with friends. As long as your solo sex isn't interfering with your daily life and activities, then you can masturbate as often as privacy, and chafing, allows.

FEAR: Masturbation trains my body to respond a certain way.

In order to avoid patterns that transfer to partner sex, keep your masturbation practices varied. This includes how you seduce yourself, what you fantasize about, and how you stimulate yourself. Also, don't go for quickies, as is often the case for males, who may then go on to suffer from premature ejaculation with a lover. Treat yourself to slower, gentler solo sex, and you'll realize greater benefits.

S*ex*PERTISE

People like to experiment with all sorts of objects when it comes to masturbation. Don't take a chance with any unsafe objects, such as a glass bottle or pine needles, lest you land yourself in the emergency room. Be smart and play it safe, with enhancements from reputable sex toy companies such as the Sinclair Institute.

PREPARING FOR YOUR SOLO PLEASURE SESSION

Before embarking upon the preparation needed for self-pleasuring, it's important to highlight the fact that there is no wrong way to pleasure yourself. Everyone is different. Everyone has his or her own preferences. So the following tips may not work for you, and that's all right. That said, let's look at some primary preparation strategies for sex with yourself.

KNOW YOUR LUBRICANTS

Lubricants can enhance any sex session, whether partnered or solo, making for greater pleasure and sensitivity for many (though this is not the rule). Even if lube isn't something you like to use, or you don't see a need for it, know that it can come in useful at different points in your sex life. A woman, for example, may feel "dry" from new motherhood, her oral contraceptive, medications, alcohol consumption, or menopause. She may be completely aroused and simply need a little assistance in getting wet (which is why wetness should never be used as a gauge of arousal). So it's always useful to know about the different types of lubricants at your disposal, and the pros and cons of each.

Water-Based Lubes: Considered the most user-friendly and all-purpose of the four major types of lubricant, water-based lubes are great in that they:

- Wash easily off of the body or clothing
- Involve no pore-clogging oil
- Are non-irritating for most users
- Take just a few drops of water or saliva to become "rejuvenated" when dry
- Are latex-friendly, and thus are safe to use with condoms, dental dams, diaphragms, and other safer sex products
- Can be used with all sex toys
- Don't stain the sheets
- Can be used with all types of sex
- Are odorless and tasteless

Primary drawbacks to water-based lubricants include that they dry faster than other types and that some women may be sensitive to its use during vaginal penetration. A number of water-based lubes also contain glycerin, which can contribute to irritation and yeast infections.

Silicone-Based Lubes: Providing a slicker feel for some lovers, silicone-based lubes are great in that they:

- Last
- Are latex-safe
- Can be used in water without washing off
- Don't irritate the skin
- Can be used for all types of sex

Drawbacks to silicone-based lubes are that they can leave an oily stain (that may not come out in the wash), can be cleaned only with soap and water, can cause upset stomach if ingested, should not be used on silicone or "real-feel" toys since the lube can gradually break down the silicone in the toy. Also, be careful not to use silicone with electrical devices, as the risk of electric shock is real. Using a condom over the toy can help you to keep your toys clean.

Oil-Based Lubes: Oil-based lubricants, and petroleum jellies or lotion, have the primary advantage of not drying out and are primarily used for male masturbation. They are, however, known for their drawbacks, primarily in that they:

- Are not latex-safe (they should never be used with a condom or latex toy since the oil breaks down these materials)
- Will stain the sheets
- Can be used only externally (never use oil-based lube vaginally or anally since it can leave a coating that can lead to infection)
- Are hard to clean and require you to shower after use

Flavored Lubes: Originally developed to mask the scent and taste of condoms, they are ideal and primarily used for oral sex. They awaken more of the senses in providing smell and taste. The fragrance alone can be a turn-on. Flavored varieties are good in that they are:

- Latex-safe
- Fine to use with sex toys
- Great for oral sex

Drawbacks to flavored lubes are the same as any water-based lube. They can dry more quickly (though they can become slick again with water or saliva), certain colors can stain the sheets or make washing off difficult, and can be too sticky for masturbation or anal sex. Some are not recommended for vaginal use in sensitive women, as they can irritate the skin, depending on the ingredients.

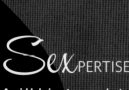

SEXPERTISE

Avoid lubricants or products with nonoxynol-9. This spermicide is highly irritating and may increase one's chance of contracting HIV.

Everybody has his or her own preferences when it comes to lubricants, and there are certainly plenty to choose from. Sold at drugstores, through mail order, adult shops both off- and online, and other retail stores that carry sexual health products, some lubricants are better than others. So be sure to try different ones to see which are best for you and your partner. If you have sensitive skin or are prone to allergies, be sure to spot test an area of your inner arm before use to see if you have a reaction.

Plan a date with yourself

While this sounds a bit cliché, planning a date with yourself requires a bit of thought beyond simply setting aside time. You want to consider when it might be the easiest for you to self-pleasure. Most people actually do so right before they go to sleep or take a nap. You may realize, however, that you're more in the mood after a workout or are better able to enjoy it as a study break. You may also find it more practical to do before a date or to relieve yourself from PMS symptoms.

Get in the mood

Do whatever you need to do to get relaxed and to feel ready to touch yourself, treating yourself like royalty. This may involve a rejuvenating shower, a glass of wine or water, turning off the phone, locking your door, lighting candles, running your fingertips over sensitive skin zones, thinking about the last time you had sensational sex . . . . Don't overlook the power in seducing yourself and how this ultimately boosts your sexual self-confidence in knowing that you're worth such erotic efforts!

Get scantily clad or all-out naked

Sometimes being almost naked or totally buff can make you feel naughtier. This is in part because society holds our nakedness as rather taboo. So "misbehaving" with a peekaboo nightie or your birthday suit can be terribly enticing. Plus, being unrestricted feels so good!

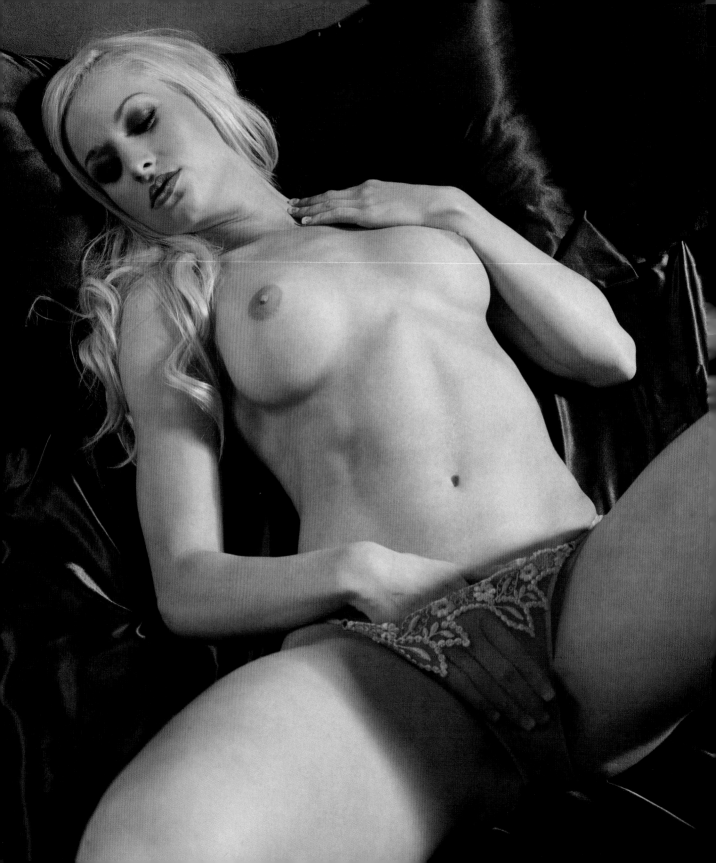

Fantasize

Think about thrilling past sexual encounters. Read an erotic story or flip through a sex magazine for inspiration. Get ideas from an adult movie, imagining yourself in the starring role, being worshipped, being commanded, or feeling sexually insatiable.

Assume the position

People often get in the habit of having solo sex the exact same way every time. While there's comfort in the guarantees that come along with knowing what works for your sexual satisfaction, experimenting with different positions can make for more variety when it comes to sensations. It also enables some lovers to reach climax more easily during partnered sex since they've "trained" their bodies on how to attain orgasm in a certain position while solo. So go ahead and see how masturbation and orgasm feel different from your regular routine with any of these positions:

"Classic" Positions: Many women like to lie comfortably on the back, knees bent, feet flat on the floor, legs open. Many men like to sit at the edge of a chair or bed. But don't let gender preferences confine you. Experiment! As you stimulate yourself, you can grind your hips to mimic thrusting.

"On Your Knees" Position: Whether on a plush carpet or mat, on pillows or on your bed, get on your knees. This position gives you the freedom to swivel your hips, sway, or stretch more easily. Also, as you masturbate, you can lean back on your calves for support.

"Doggie" Position: On one hand and your knees, assume an animalistic approach to sex, stimulating yourself with the other hand.

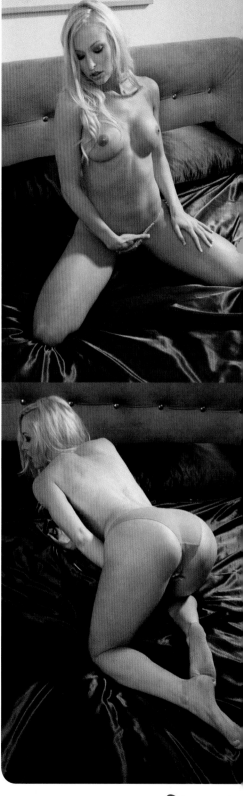

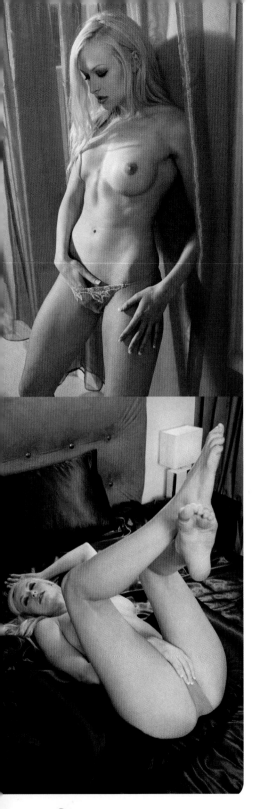

"Standing" Position: Whether in the middle of a room or up against a wall or a support, spread your legs hip-distance apart to give yourself pleasure. You can also prop one leg up on a bed or chair for something different.

"Rocking Chair" Position: Lying on your back, pull your knees into your chest. Open your hips by pulling your knees out gently to either side, and then rock them, creating an energy as you complement your hand's rhythm with your body's beat.

"Head Over Heels" Position: If flexible, you can lie on your back, pulling your legs up over your head. (You can put a pillow under your hips if easier.) From here, you can keep your legs together, spread them apart, or bend your knees. Have easy access to your groin, sides, buttocks, legs . . . in going for a total body effect.

"Gravity Defying" Position: Here, aim for a position where half of your body is on a different level than the other half. This may involve, for example, lying on a bed or floor with your legs up the wall, or laying on your stomach, legs hanging off of the bed.

Touch yourself all over

Part of building excitement is saving the best for last. So run your hands slowly and seductively all over your body, letting them linger at your favorite non-genital erogenous zones. Caress yourself. Make this a total body experience. Gradually work your way to your genitals, employing any of the moves we'll get to in the next two sections to bring yourself to the heights of sexual ecstasy.

Build your excitement

Don't go for the gold all at once. Tease yourself. Build up to a certain point, then back off—reducing or temporarily ceasing all stimulation. Observe how your body responds. Resume by either slowing down the tempo or picking up the pace. Remember, unless you're in need of pulling off a quickie, there's no need to rush. Enjoy yourself!

My weight has always played into my ability to let go during lovemaking. As a result, my husband says that he's sick of my body-image issues and how they're affecting our sex life. He's offering to pay for me to see a therapist. Will doing such really help our sex life?

Before you can have better sex with someone else, you have to be happy with yourself first. This includes having a healthy sense of your body image. Body image is the mental image we have of our own physical appearance. It is impacted by a number of factors, including weight, body shape, values, ethnicity, the media, family, misguided idealized images of the human body, warped self-views, uneven sexual desire in a relationship, being single, and/or sexually inexperienced. Whether it's the pressure to be thinner, to be well-endowed, or have bigger breasts, body image influences much of our sexual behavior and self-esteem, impacting our choice of sex partners and our sex lives.

The better our body image, the more confident we are, and the more sexually confident we are. With this better sexual self-image, we're likelier to pursue a potential partner and become more open to sexual expression that involves exposing the body. Research, including that published in the International Journal of Eating Disorders, confirms that body image significantly predicts the frequency of sexual behaviors for both men and women. People with poor body image, on the other hand, may fear revealing themselves, ultimately shutting down their ability to experience sexual pleasure, intimacy, and even sexual encounters.

With self-acceptance a major means to better sex, lovers need to actively counter their negative self-thinking around body image, especially as it relates to their sexuality. Therapy or counseling is definitely one way to do this. Your sessions, solo or with your partner, will include education,

reframing work, and homework assignments, among other efforts. Even if you choose the therapy route, you may also want to do any of the following in boosting your body image woes:

- Masturbate—make love to your body!
- Focus on what's beautiful about your body as you stand in front of a mirror.
- Become more educated about sexuality and sexual skills in order to boost that aspect of your bedroom confidence.
- Come to terms with the fact that erotica and most media portrayals of "beauty" are not realistic, if that's part of what makes you so hard on yourself.
- Pursue activities that promote self-acceptance, such as yoga and exercise.
- Pamper yourself with strategies that help you feel good in the skin you're in, including getting manicures, brushing your hair, wearing feel-good clothes and fabrics, using soft sheets with high thread counts, applying silky lotions, etc.
- Employ guided imagery and other self-acceptance techniques.

Use your breath

Make sure that you're not holding your breath. Incorporate a breathing technique, such as the belly breathing we covered in the last chapter. Breathe deeply, since this will help you to release your sexual energy. Complement the breath with a pelvic rocking motion, rhythmically clenching and releasing your pelvic floor muscles. Let the breath and rocking get faster and faster in order to attain orgasm, allowing your mind to flood itself with sweet or "sordid" scenes.

Ride it

As you orgasm, continue stimulation, but perhaps easing up a bit at first. Maintaining the stimulation as you ride your climax will make for a longer orgasm and lovely aftershocks.

ME, MYSELF, AND MASTURBATION—PLEASURE YOURSELF TIPS & TRICKS FOR HER

"Me" time for women is critical when it comes to her orgasmic ability, since women are three times more likely to orgasm from masturbation than from sexual intercourse. In fact, Shere Hite found 95 percent of female masturbators could reach orgasm easily and regularly when pleasuring themselves—and in as easily as four or so minutes (the same as for a male). What's working so well for them?

The most common technique women use when masturbating is manual stimulation of the clitoris and the small lips of the vulva while lying on their backs. Some masturbate on their stomachs, against a soft object, by pressing their thighs rhythmically, by using water massage, or via vaginal entry. Less than one-fifth of women masturbate by inserting objects or fingers into their vaginas—and nearly all who do still stimulate the clitoris. Women actually report, however, that clitoral stimulation as more of an "extra" than anything. Many view clitoral stimulation as commonly used for arousal, but not orgasm.

In the Bedroom:
Solo Session for Her Pleasuring

WHETHER MASTURBATING or simply getting to know your sexual self, take the time to get to know your genitalia. Refer back to all of the genital parts we reviewed in Chapter 3, using a mirror to see what your female anatomy looks like. Observe your contours and unique look, taking pride in how sexy you are. Notice the color, size, and shape. Flex your pelvic and sphincter muscles, and observe the reaction. Basically, make friends with your vulva. The vulva can often feel like a foreign being since it is not readily seen, but it's an intricate part of you, benefiting your sex image enormously when attended to lovingly.

With or without your mirror in hand or propped up close by, massage your pubic hair area. When you feel compelled, use one or two fingers to stroke your vulva, tracing every part. (Don't forget lubricant if desired. Alternatively, you can always "dip" into your vaginal juices for some natural lubrication.) Saving the best (your clitoris) for last, increase your arousal by moving your hips as you massage your vulva. You may want to rub your vulva as though it's a figure eight, looping around the vaginal opening and then up around the clitoris and back down again. Use that mirror to see yourself getting turned on. Notice yourself getting wetter and wetter (you may even hear how aroused you're getting). Observe how your genitals become darker in color, fuller, and riper as they're engorged with blood.

As you hone your attention on the clitoris, you will notice that its head will have become more erect and visible. As you stimulate this hot spot, experiment with different moves, seeing what suits you best. You may like to rub your clitoris from up to down, from left to right, or in a circular manner. You may prefer some pressure levels more than others since some females prefer light touch, while others prefer more firm touch. Others are more into direct clitoral stimulation versus indirect, which involves coming at the clitoris more from the side, pulling at the vaginal lips, or massaging the mons pubis.

At any point, experiment with different types of motions and speed, especially in how these complement whatever racy thoughts you're having. Rub and squeeze your thighs together, perhaps by crossing your legs, for added stimulation. Insert one or more fingers into your vagina, either to mimic thrusting or to stimulate the G spot (to learn how to find and stimulate your G spot, turn to page 160). Rub up against an object, such as a pillow or the arm of a couch. Other tricks for enhancing your masturbation experience or adding variety to your solo sex play include:

- Rolling, pinching, tickling, tapping, kneading, pulling, or tugging at any of your hot spots
- Holding your labia apart with two fingers while stimulating your clitoris with your middle finger
- Using one or up to all fingers, your palm, or knuckles
- Paying attention to other body parts that don't want to be ignored; tweak your nipples or cup your breasts
- Contracting your anal muscles
- Pumping your pelvic floor muscles
- Inserting a finger or a sex toy into your rectum (Note: Don't dip either into your vagina without cleaning it first, or else you'll invite infection.)

As you're doing any of these moves, take note of where and how you like to touch yourself. How do you breathe and move? What happens to your energy, sounds, thoughts as you try "this" or transition "here"? What awakens your response? What throws you over the edge? What could you see working with your lover for satisfying sex?

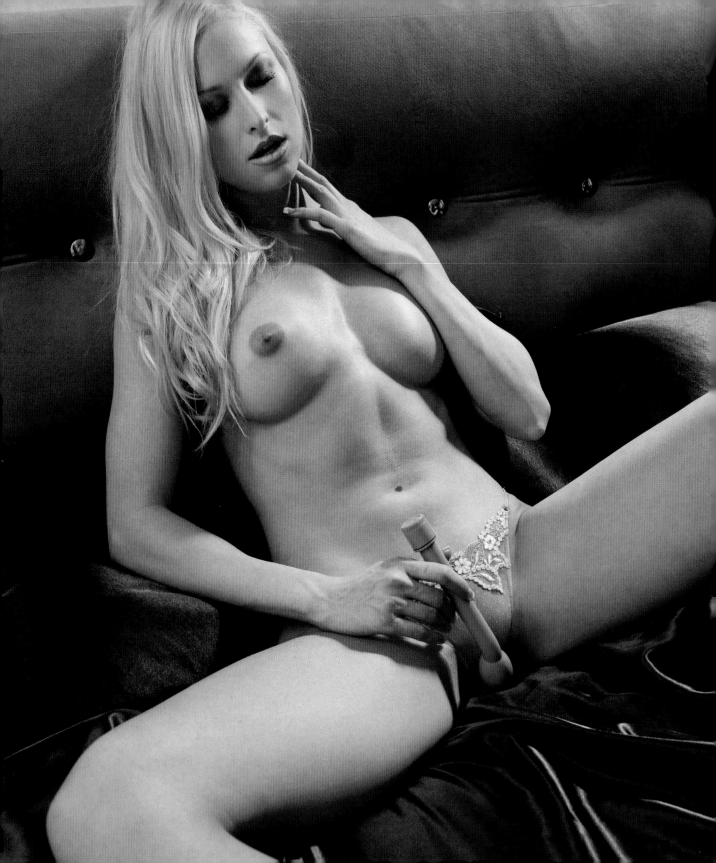

TOYS FOR HER

By far the most popular toy for a woman's self-pleasuring is the vibrator, a handheld device that vibrates to pleasantly stimulate the nerves and enhance sexual responsiveness. It can help a woman to not only become orgasmic, but also multiorgasmic, delivering orgasms consistently and often easily. For use with or without a partner, vibrators are enjoyed by women because the toy alleviates most of the manual labor of sex and focuses on her hot spots for spectacular results. That's not to say, however, that the classic vibrator is a woman's sole means of pleasure. (We do not want to mention specific toys by brand name as there are hundreds, it's better to just stick with types of toys.)

In further adding to your private-time treasure chest, other enhancement products you may want to consider include:

- **External clitoral massagers:** There are a wide range of sizes, shapes and materials from the most basic to the ultra realistic. There are wands which can be used for the entire body.
- **Internal massagers and dual function:** Used internally, and in some cases designed to stimulate both the G spot and the clitoris. There are curved shapes just for the G spot and special shapes to be used for anal play.
- **Attachments:** Some massagers come with attachments. Wand body massagers also have attachments available to stimulate specific areas. Wands can be turned into a clitoral and/or G spot stimulator with attachments that fit snuggly over the head of the wand. Made of soft material, attachments can massage larger surface areas with their hundreds of nubs for unique vibrations, reducing the intense effect of some wand massagers. Some wand attachments are made specifically to stimulate the G spot.
- **Ben Wa balls:** Available in a variety of sizes, these safe, easy-to-clean toys arouse and strengthen your vaginal muscles for more powerful orgasms.
- **Wearable vibrators:** Made of soft material and designed to hit all the hot spots, these vibrators are sometimes wirelessly remote controlled. They fit into panties and can be worn with adjustable straps, similar to a G-string, for self-pleasuring, including on-the-go.

$\mathcal{S}ex$PERTISE

When it comes to a woman's partner, some worry that a vibrator may be more of a foe than a friend. While some may experience mild discomfort after a long vibrator session, especially if the toy is used vigorously, any desensitizing of the clitoris is only temporary—not long-term. The same can happen during long masturbation sessions or during extended oral- or vaginal-sex sessions.

Furthermore, a woman will not prefer her sex toy to partnered sex play. Yes, she may reach orgasm faster with a vibrator, and at times more powerfully. It's important to remember, however, that vibrators are enhancements, as in an addition, not substitutions or replacements for partnered sex. Her toys will never be able to replace human touch and the bond that only emotional human intimacy and sharing can provide.

- **Dildos and dongs:** In offering the fullness of penetration without vibration, dildos and dongs (dongs are typically more realistic) can be pleasurable during clitoral masturbation. Some are curved and used especially in stimulating the G spot. These toys are also used in fantasy role play as a "third partner." Some are used with strap-on harnesses.
- **Love rings (cock rings):** These stretchy rings vibrate stimulation to the clitoris during intercourse. Some have removable bullet-shaped vibrators. These rings can also be used over a dong.

SEXUAL Q&A: BUYING A VIBRATOR

I'm thinking about buying my girlfriend a vibrator for her birthday but don't know where to begin. What sorts of features I should be considering?

There are hundreds, if not thousands, of vibrators available for you to choose from, so here are the major things you should consider in purchasing one:

- **Size and Shape:** Vibrators come in different widths and insertable lengths (mini-vibes can be less than three inches, while others are several inches long). Some slender vibes can easily fit into the vagina alongside a penis or a dildo, providing more stimulation, including for him during partnered sex. Others are thick for the pleasures that come from girth. The size and shape is really going to come down to her personal preference and how she may like to use the toy.
- **Materials:** There are a range of plastics that can be used with any lube, which are frequently inexpensive and easy to clean. Silicone is typically high quality and is nonporous, which means it doesn't absorb odor and is less prone to bacteria; it can be sterilized (usually by boiling); and it's durable and long lasting. Glass has similar qualities to silicone and some glass-based designs can be quite beautiful. "Real-feel" materials are made to feel just like human flesh.
- **Texture:** What will feel good to your lover? Will she like a smooth feel or a vibe with ridges?
- **Color:** Will she like a pretty color, something transparent, a glow-in-the-dark look, or flesh tone, for instance?

- **Stimulation:** There are vibrators for clitoral stimulation, G spot stimulation and stimulation for both at the same time. Some vibrators that deliver G spot stimulation or have a slightly curved head to reach that specific, hidden erogenous zone.
- **Speed control:** Some vibes have a dial to adjust the level of sensation, while others have touch-button controls. Some have variations feature many functions, including a pulsating setting.
- **Noise level.**
- **Rotating feature:** The ubiquitous Rabbit vibrators, for example, are offered with rotating beads.
- **Price.**
- **Power source:** Is it rechargeable, battery-powered, or a corded plug-in model?

Other perks to consider are whether the toy is waterproof, offers a discreet storage/travel case, comes with a designer pouch, or fits in her purse. You may also want to consider if she wants her vibrator to actually look like an erotic device or not. Vibes are now made to be pretty or cute like rubber duckies, penguins, fishes, lipstick (and even comes with a real lipstick case), even blush brushes (with or without sugar-free berry-flavored dusting powder). Many women love that these toys are inconspicuous enough to leave lying around.

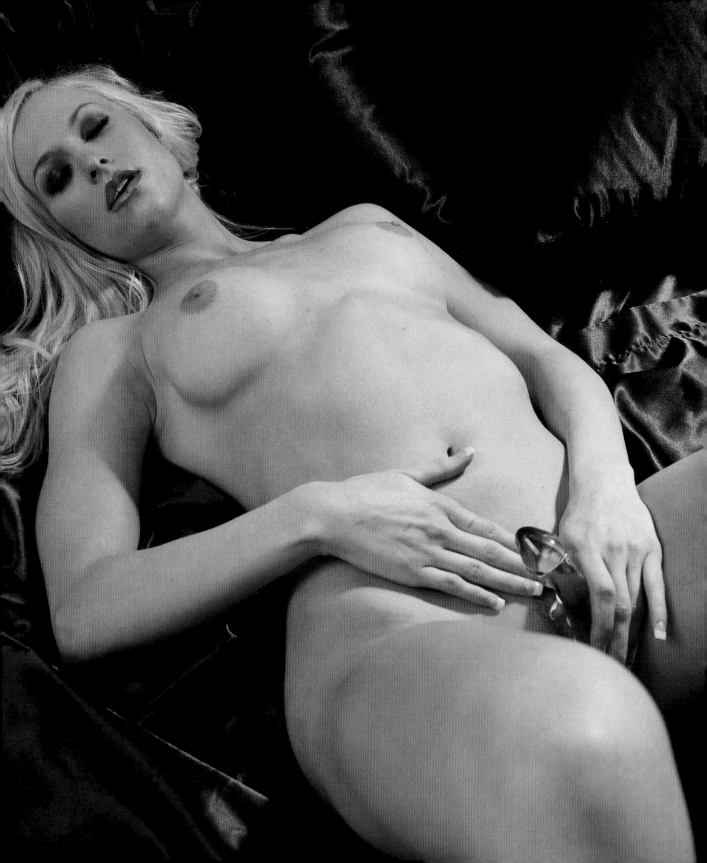

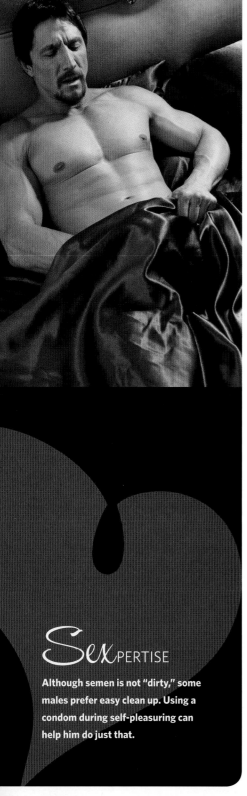

ME, MYSELF, AND MASTURBATION—PLEASURE YOURSELF TIPS & TRICKS FOR HIM

When it comes to male self-pleasuring, most stroke the shaft of the penis with a firm grip in an up-down motion until reaching climax. Sometimes men will concentrate on the head, stroking two of the greatest erogenous zones on his body, the glans and frenulum. This takes, on average, about four minutes, and is often stimulated by erotic literature, films, videos, or the thought of a desired partner. Some men use gadgets to assist them. Many like to lather their penises with soap suds or baby oil beforehand.

Given most men are quite accomplished in being "masters of their own domains," having pleasured themselves a few times since adolescence, providing tips and tricks for them can be a bit more challenging. Yet, in approaching their masturbation practice in terms of great sex, there are quite a few things men can do to vary their routines:

Take time to look at your body

Despite the fact that you see your penis several times daily, do you truly know it? Get to know yourself—and not just the shaft, but all of your pelvic features. Explore your penis, paying attention to its various hot spots, such as the corona. Examine your perineum, the patch of skin between the anus and scrotum. Notice the raphe, the visible line along the center and underside of the scrotum.

Don't rush

Most males are used to pulling off quickies when it comes to self-pleasuring. Afraid of being caught or overly eager for sexual release, many have not given any attention to the full potential of their sexual arousal. So make sure that you're setting aside adequate private time for solo sex and that you're enjoying the journey as much as the destination.

Forget about erotica

Every now and then, focus on yourself instead of on erotica. This is important because some men complain that they are so dependent upon erotica for arousal that they have trouble getting excited or reaching climax with a partner. Abandoning such for a bit can help you to retrain your body to not respond only to such stimuli. Putting erotica aside also benefits you in coming into your body. Paying attention to your sexual response can be incredibly sexy and exciting. In feeling more in tune with yourself instead of a visual, you can pay attention to your breathing, tension in the body, your heart rate . . . and your orgasmic response.

Use the other hand

Most men get into a routine when they masturbate, doing what they know will be the most effective way to reach orgasm, and quite vigorously at that. Diversify your routine. Try the other hand. See what a different rhythm is like. Satiate the newness.

Switch things up

While the standard up-down stroke works well, experiment with different hand moves for different pressures, movements, and speeds. The end result: new sensations, experiences, and orgasms. Use long, twisting strokes. Put one hand at the base of your penis, pressing up toward your body while stroking the shaft of the penis with the other. Roll your penis between your hands, perhaps working your way up and down.

Simulate thrusting

Men have been criticized by men themselves for staying too stiff during solo sex. Don't stay rigid during masturbation. Pretend that you're having sex with someone else. Move your hips, and see how that affects your orgasmic response.

In the Bedroom:
Solo Session for His Pleasuring

YOU CAN AWAKEN the sensitivity of your penis by practicing a slower stroke. While masturbating, use your typical stroke (and lubricant, if that's your norm). Then engage in the following:

1. Slow down your stroke so that it is half as fast as your regular rhythm.

2. After a couple of minutes, reduce your speed by one-half, again.

3. Continue to halve your speed until you find yourself doing more of a genital caress than masturbating.

4. Note which parts of your penis are the most sensitive.

5. Continue with the slow stroke, recognizing that incorporating this practice as a regular part of your masturbating routine will lend itself to greater penile sensitivity.

Note: If you have trouble staying erect, revert to your normal form of stimulation, going back to this newer stroke on occasion.

Hold off

Using your thumb and forefinger as a circle around the top of your scrotum, gently tug on your sac while pleasuring yourself. This will help you to postpone ejaculation, plus spread sensations throughout the body.

Explore your prostate's potential

The prostate can bring your bliss to another level. So go ahead and press on your perineum as you masturbate. Massaging this area rhythmically indirectly stimulates your prostate for more sensations. For more direct stimulation, use a well-lubricated finger or sex toy to stroke your prostate via the anal canal (for more information on prostate stimulation, turn to page 163).

Add accessories

A stereotype of male masturbation is that it never needs to involve more than a dirty magazine. Yet plenty of men like to use sexual enhancements. They know that using different toys can add new kinds of stimulation, increase the intensity, and complement their efforts. Plus, these toys can give your hands a bit of a break. So get creative! Artificial vaginas, fur-like clothes, and inflatable dolls have been reported as masturbatory aids by some men. Penis sleeves, such as the Ribbed Stroker and the Fleshlight, are also becoming more popular, with their firm, comfortable grip and soft ribbed texture, realistic feel, and ability to stretch to accommodate any size. Such penis sleeves provide even more stimulation when accompanied by a vibrator. Male vibrators typically involve a tunnel with a tight grip, natural skin-like feel, and different speeds and pulsation for custom-fit vibration and intensity. Lastly, prostate massagers can be incredible in playing with the P-spot, with some models simultaneously stimulating both the prostate and perineum.

In doing any of the aforementioned, tips for enhancing your efforts include:

- Use light touches on the tip of the penis.
- Pull at the skin of the scrotal sac.
- Vary the degrees of pressure on the shaft.
- Insert a finger into the rectum.
- Roll the penis against your body.
- Massage the anus, scrotum, testicles, nipples, or any point on the body as you stimulate the penis.
- Play with your scrotum. Tickle, scratch, rub, or gently pull at it for more pleasure.

In considering how any of these efforts can help you to have more invigorating sex, consider where and how you like to touch yourself. How do you breathe and move? What happens to your energy, sounds, thoughts at different points and with different tactics? What rituals or patterns awaken you? What would you like to re-create with a partner?

EXPLORE YOUR PLEASURE ZONES TOGETHER TO ENHANCE YOUR MUTUAL GRATIFICATION

A pleasure shared is doubled. And nowhere is that adage truer than when it comes to sharing solo sex. Mutual masturbation is where you both indulge in self-pleasuring at the same time. This type of shared intimacy is a wonderful way to expose your sexual secrets and to teach your lover a few tricks of your own, especially in what garners the greatest reactions in you. You also get to learn where your sweetheart likes to be touched and what you may have to re-create sometime. Given, too, that few get to see us climax while masturbating ourselves, doing so in your partner's presence can be an incredible way of connecting. Mutual masturbation can take you to a different level of intimacy, with some lovers describing these erotic exchanges along the lines of a shared spiritual energy. For many, that in and of itself is better sex. Others end up realizing better sex from first being the mindful masturbation pupils when it comes to this most private kind of show-and-tell.

$\mathcal{S}\!ell$ercise 5.1 Preparing for Mutual Masturbation

As with any successful amorous adventure, lovers do best when they're able to provide each other with a sense of safety. And while mutual masturbation is often cast in sex manuals as a simple form of foreplay, lovers are putting on some of their most passionate performances. Being in the spotlight is a little more than intimidating for many. So before partaking in such sex play, be sure to abide by the following:

A. Make sure that you're comfortable with masturbating on your own first. To be truly comfortable and enjoy your partner's presence, you're going to want to be at ease with your own performance.

B. Talk to each other about masturbation. Talk about self-pleasuring both in general and in the context of mutual masturbation, and the role self-pleasure plays in a relationship. Voice your apprehensions, fears, hopes, and desires. Be sure to acknowledge your lover's thoughts, providing any

$\mathcal{S}\!ell$PERTISE

For those who feel threatened by a partner's sexual solo time, mutual masturbation is an ideal way of letting them into your private world. Showing your lover how you pleasure yourself—and making that a shared experience—can make the time you normally take to self-pleasure feel less threatening. It will also help to diffuse a partner feeling left out or unattractive over the fact that you enjoy private pleasuring.

reassurances needed. You may also want to share stories about moments of self-discovery, such as the first time you truly touched yourself or how you learned to masturbate.

C. Share on your own accord. Don't give into pressure, either your own or your partner's, to mutually masturbate.

THE SEXUAL SHOW-AND-TELL THAT CAN TRANSFORM YOUR SEX LIFE

Mutual masturbation can be the main act of a sexual moment or a form of foreplay. Lovers can stimulate themselves to climax or arouse themselves for other types of sex. Mutual masturbation is ideal for muggy weather when lovers aren't up for full-body contact but long to have sex. This type of sharing is also ideal for those moments you're feeling mellow (versus fatigued or completely energized). For our learning purposes, we're going to focus on lovers playing with themselves at the same time.

If you're feeling shy, go ahead and close your eyes, or wear a blindfold if that makes you feel more at ease. This is especially effective for those who will be distracted by intense eye contact or talking. (Even if both lovers are doing this, hearing each other's movements and breathing can be a major turn-on!) For some people, giving yourself the sense that you're alone may make you feel more comfortable.

THE
SCIENCE OF *Sex*

If masturbating with a female, see if you can note her pupil dilation. This is an indicator of strong sexual arousal and interest. While the function of this response is not understood, it is a distinct response in the female, published in research in the *Archives of Sexual Behavior*, involving vaginal self-stimulation leading to orgasm. It is due to oxytocin acting as a neurotransmitter in the spinal cord.

In the Bedroom: Mutual Masturbation

IN MOVING FORWARD, there are two ways to approach mutual masturbation. Both lovers can masturbate themselves at the same time, since simply engaging in such can be extremely exciting. Lovers who are in sync may even realize simultaneous orgasm. Yet in focusing on your lover and what you can learn from each other, taking turns can work to your advantage. Becoming the focus of attention is what will allow each of you to truly observe the other, noting technique and response. While it may feel awkward at first, and you may become easily distracted, all of this will get easier with time.

As you masturbate, stay present and relaxed, remembering to breathe. Focus on your sensations. Don't put any pressure on yourself by analyzing your technique, being critical, or in focusing on expectations. Take your time, especially as you start your genital caress. Act as though you've got all of the time in the world, since this attitude enhances one's sex appeal.

As you watch your lover masturbate, take everything in—the entire body, the position they're in, the rhythm they're delighting in, the reactions, changes in the skin, the noises being made . . . Notice any wetness, tensing,

throbbing, breathing. Give compliments, such as, "You look so sexy right now," "I've never seen you look so beautiful," "I love the way you . . ." ". . . is so arousing." As your lover masturbates, you can add to the arousal quotient by nibbling at her neck, tracing his nipples with your tongue, or running your fingers up and down the back of your love's legs. But do all of this carefully, as though afraid to interrupt. You're looking to enhance his or her performance, not steal the show. If desired, go ahead and touch your body as well, but stay focused on your lover's reactions.

Over time, the two of you will be able to gaze into each other's eyes as you masturbate, tantalizing yourselves even more while sharing fantasies. As both of you become more confident in your show-and-tells, you can experiment with different types of touch to intensify your experiences, including tapping, scratching, or tickling with different levels of pressure. Or try using peacock feathers, a silk scarf, a sheepskin rug, rabbit-fur mitts, or bristle gloves (for a friction rub) for different sensations. You can also challenge each other. Suggest different positions and situations for these shared solo sessions, perhaps using different pieces of furniture or rooms in the house.

> *"I have loved to the point of madness;*
> *That which is called madness, That which*
> *to me, is the only sensible way to love."*
>
> —F. SAGAN

SEXUAL Q&A: PERFORMANCE ANXIETY

Since learning that my partner's last lover was quite adept in bed, I've been easily losing my erection. Any tips on how I can reclaim my level of performance?

Performance anxiety is when you worry and obsess over how well you're doing when sexually intimate, including how sexy you look. This type of "spectatoring," as Masters and Johnson coined it, is a self-absorption that ruins your sexual response and performance. In becoming fixated on a body part—what it looks like or what it's doing—you're not fully enmeshed in your body's sensations. To resolve this dilemma, men or women can try a few things:

A. Practice "mind talk" for managing your thoughts, emotions, bodily sensations, and past subconscious mind patterns. In countering anxious thoughts, you need to coach yourself through sex with a great deal of self-discipline, much like an athlete does prior to and during a competition. Part of doing this is having a focused internal awareness of what's happening to your body. This needs to first be practiced when nonsexual parts are being stroked. Scan your body in its relaxed, pre-aroused state, observing any tension. Breathe through any tense areas, mentally opposing the tension's presence. Believe in yourself and know that you are in control as you seek to release the tension with your breath. Continue to do this later, when sexual parts are being stroked, realizing that this will be more difficult and likely to take more time.

B. Share your sexual fears. Speak as though you are your genitals. While it may feel silly at first, some find comfort in their genitals taking on a character and apparent mind of its own. This also adds much-needed humor, allowing you to become more vulnerable. This further helps to offset any insecurity your partner may have about the reactions your body is having to the anxiety. Ultimately this enables both of you to work through this issue as a couple.

C. Engage in mutual masturbation. While you can feel anxious stimulating yourself in front of your partner at first, focusing on yourself during this intimate exchange takes the pressure off of pleasing your partner. It also shows that sexual pleasuring and satisfaction is not reliant upon a specific sex act or certain type of sexual response.

D. Realize that it's a temporary situation. Erection problems are normal at points throughout a person's life. Don't give a lack of an erection more power than it has. Allowing yourself to think that it's the end of the world will only make matters harder for you.

Sexual Homework

In keeping with this chapter's themes of types of touch, body bonding, and getting to know each other's bodies, your sexual homework consists of even more erotic exploration . . .

Sensual Massage—Give each other a massage to remember, only let the Hitachi Magic Wand massager—and any of its attachments—do all of the work for you. This body massager is well-known and lauded for its use as a personal massager. So powerful are its effects that some lovers need to place a towel between this device and their hot spots, so proceed with caution. Give each other an overall relaxing body massage, working on tight areas such as the calves and upper back before eventually honing in on the private parts, for what may prove to be some of your most powerful orgasms yet!

Shower Play—When it comes to her pleasuring, women have been known to get creative with anything involving water pressure. Aiming a hot-tub jet at her clitoris, for example, can definitely result in climax. In exploring what your bathroom has to offer (especially in capitalizing on the privacy this room affords), experiment with your shower's massager or hose. Lifting one leg, direct the water flow, varying the pressure, pulsation, and temperature to what's pleasurable. Remember, the faster the water, the more stimulation experienced. As an alternative, a woman can lie on her back and place her buttocks under the faucet. She should then tilt her pelvis and spread her legs, directing the stream of water at her clitoris. (A waterproof toy is also a great option.)

Note: In pursuing such water play, lovers should avoid spraying the water inside the vagina. The shower stream can rinse away healthy bacteria and other natural organisms, upsetting the vagina's pH, or acidic environment. This increases the risk of developing a yeast infection or bacterial vaginosis. Irritated vaginal tissue can further

make a female more susceptible to a sexually transmitted infection. Plus, a contaminated showerhead can introduce an infection, which, when left untreated, can lead to pelvic inflammatory disease (PID). The worst, but rarest, consequence is that the shower stream could force air inside of the vagina, potentially causing an air embolism. If a pocket of air enters her blood stream and reaches the heart, it can cause permanent damage or even death. Don't let these dangers, however, dampen your showerhead play. Just be sensible about it, experimenting with different water pressures and ways to stimulate the vulva without forcing water into the vaginal canal.

Changing Your Focus—Lovers can connect even more by encouraging each other to focus on the sensations of their bodies, including tastes, textures, and feelings. Doing so will develop their sensate-focused abilities. Learning to change your focus during lovemaking can enhance your experience of mutuality while adding to those sensations. While lovers feel a great deal in their genitals during sex, they can practice focusing on sensations in other parts of the body as well as sights, sounds, and scents, to enhance lovemaking. Concentrating on only one partner, both lovers should stimulate the penis or vulva, noting how it feels. After a few minutes, switch, and note the sensations experienced in stimulating the other partner. With your next switch, instead of focusing on the genitals, pay attention to what's taking place with the hands, breathing fully and staying relaxed. With practice, you can focus on more than one sensation, with partners agreeing which sensations they will both focus on at the same time to expand their arousal. Building your focusing skills can be done during almost any mutual sexual activity, with partners getting even more out of the exercise when they discuss what just took place.

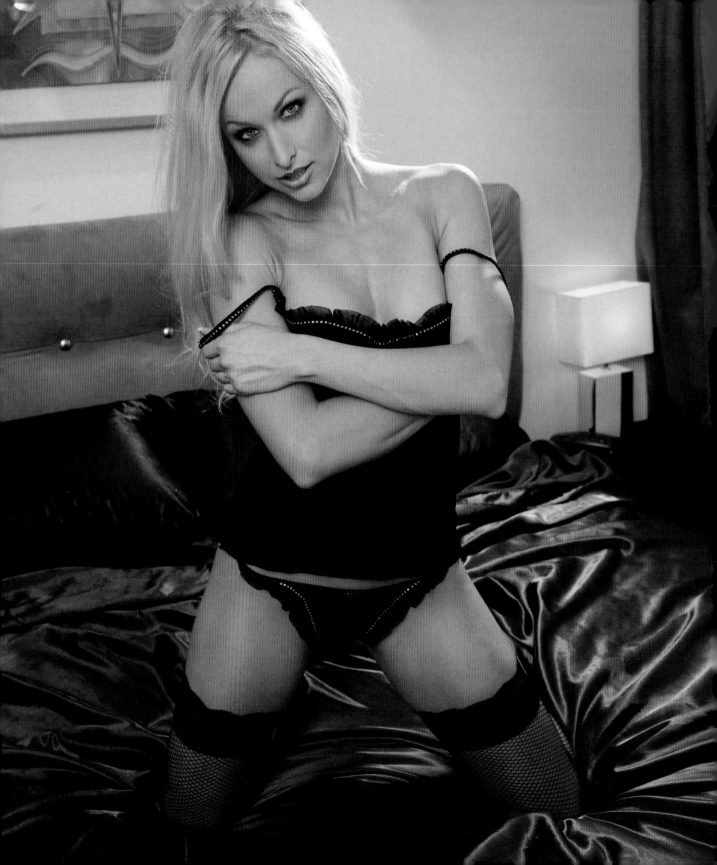

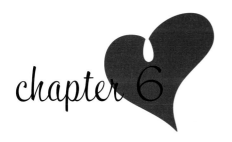

chapter 6

Building Sexual Tension: Fuel Your Foreplay with Red-Hot Touch

IF SEX WERE AN Olympic event, foreplay would be the warm-up. This physical and psychological preparation is the key to the most satisfying sex—and a lot of fun in its own right. Lovers should be mindful not to rush. Foreplay is your opportunity to not only become sufficiently aroused for sex but also to express your love, desire, sensuousness, and feelings—all of which make for better lovemaking. Foreplay is the perfect excuse to show your appreciation for one another, including each other's sexual abilities.

The aim of foreplay is simple: You want to make each other feel good. So indulge yourselves in a sensual warm-up, especially since foreplay is critical when it comes to gratifying sex for women. This is because women need more time to become adequately lubricated for intercourse. They also need this exchange of simultaneous arousal and desire to give their vaginal canal time to lengthen and better receive penetration.

"It is the passion that is in a kiss that gives to it its sweetness; it is the affection in a kiss that sanctifies it."

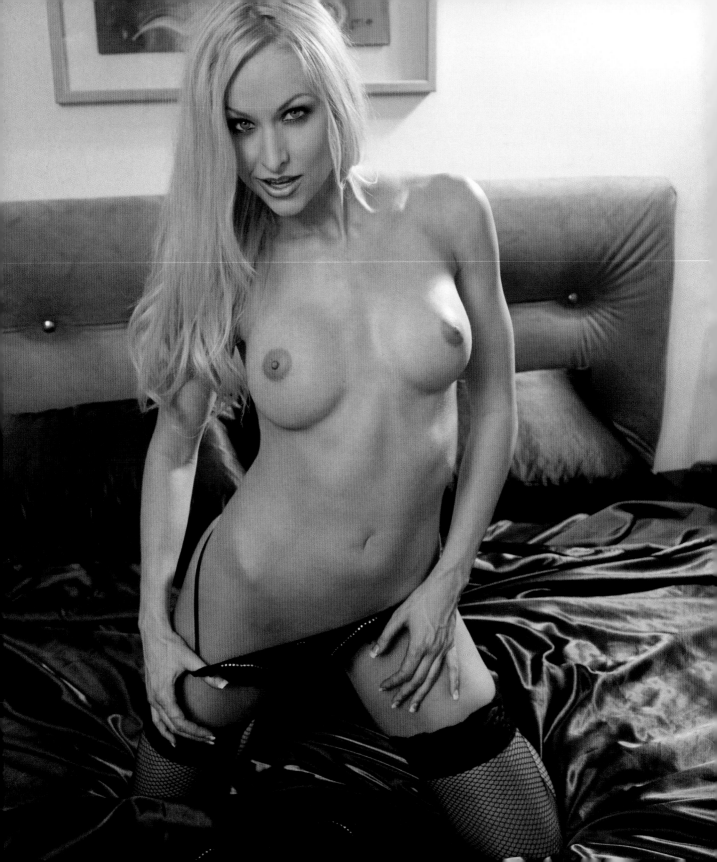

Research out of the University of New Brunswick, Canada, has found, too, that men are as interested in foreplay as women—that they actually want more of it than they're getting. This is in part because they love the extra anticipation and the greater intensity of their eventual orgasm(s).

PIQUING HIS SEXUAL APPETITE

Regardless of their age, men are more frequently sexually aroused and excited by a greater variety of stimuli than women. This includes the sight of an actual or potential sex partner, pictures of nudes and genitals, memories, and the anticipation of new experiences. Males more readily make the association between sexual excitement and stimulus objects. They are better than women at separating the emotional and relational context from physical sex acts. They are more focused on genital stimulation and orgasm, becoming more disturbed than females if they don't take their arousal to orgasm. Not surprisingly, three times as many men as women report masturbating at least one time per week.

Show Him Some Skin

A great way to arouse a man is to show a little skin. According to U.S. News & World Report, Americans—primarily men—spend more money at strip bars than at operas, ballets, Broadway and off-Broadway theaters combined.

The good news: The same impulse that draws men to half-naked women at strip joints draws them to half-naked women at home. In fact, 93 percent of male participants in "Sex in America: A Definitive Survey" reported that it's appealing to watch their partners undress. Luckily for the women who love them, this propensity has not gone unnoticed by the world's lingerie industry, which provides every kind of sexy garment to titillate your partner.

Nearly Naked Lingerie

When it comes to lingerie, sometimes less is more. There's a plethora of choices out there, enough for any woman to find something guaranteed to excite her partner, such as thongs, hipsters, boy shorts, crotchless underwear, body suits, or baby-doll slips.

When it comes to lingerie, it's important to remember that it's not just what you wear. It's how you wear it. Panties take on a whole new look when they're pulled down an inch or two. Breasts in a peekaboo bra become much more hypnotizing. (Hint: Pulling your breasts out of your bra so that it frames your chest can have the same effect.) Sexy heels accented by nylons with a seam that beckons your lover to look up, up, up to your garter belt can make him putty in your hands, practically doing much of the seduction work for you.

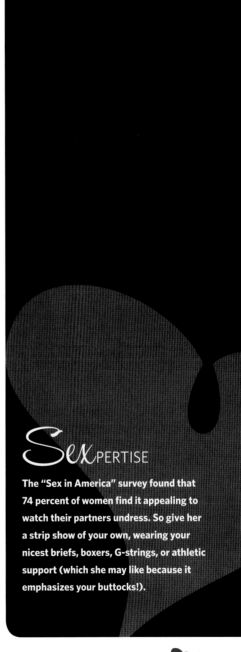

S*EX*PERTISE

The "Sex in America" survey found that 74 percent of women find it appealing to watch their partners undress. So give her a strip show of your own, wearing your nicest briefs, boxers, G-strings, or athletic support (which she may like because it emphasizes your buttocks!).

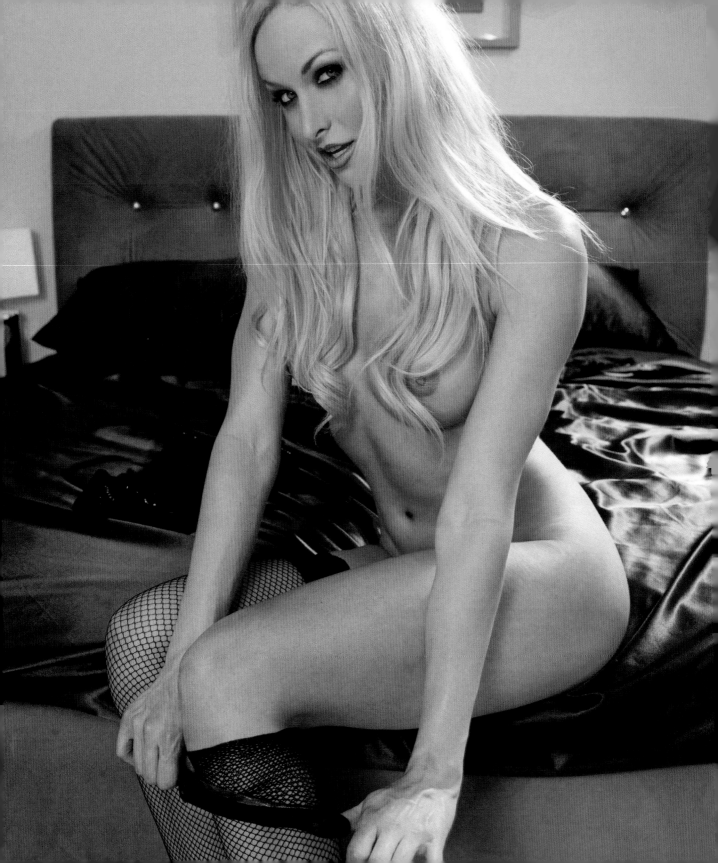

In the Bedroom:
The Sensual Art of Burlesque

THE BEST LINGERIE begs a performance. While you can go the striptease route, some women like to go a more sensual, provocative route, practicing the art of burlesque. In celebrating all body shapes and sizes, slow and seductive burlesque dancing plays upon the power of suggestion in its level of nudity and sensuality. Empowering, glamorous, and elegant, burlesque can keep an entire audience, or one "targeted" viewer, captive. You end up baring more soul than body as you flaunt your wares in a corset, fishnets, garter, matching bra and panties, feather boa, elbow-length gloves, tassels, and glittery powder. Go ahead, unleash your inner sex kitten to bring out the tiger in him.

In exploring the art of burlesque, you can check out a burlesque show, take a class, or rent a video, including Chicago. Look for inspiration in jazz, ballet, or ballroom dancing. Practice dancing in three-inch high heels (feel free to go taller, if you dare). A nice pair of sexy pumps will automatically make you look sexy as they lengthen your legs and straighten your posture. You just need to make sure that you don't look clumsy as you twirl and move with them! To further boost your confidence, practice in front of a mirror to the tune of big band, 1940s show tunes, or something more subtle and provocative—whatever will get you and your lover in the mood and at a tempo that you can keep up with!

As you dance, keep in mind that your aim is fun seduction. You're flirting and giving coy, sweet looks while keeping your movements exaggerated. So arch your back. Stick out your buttocks while placing your hands in your lap or behind your back. Stand on the balls of your feet and do a booty shake, alternately bending each knee. Shimmy your shoulders back and forth, showing off your bosom, and do a cross-step (this is where you cross your left leg over your right leg, then pull your right leg out to a normal stance again). Work your curves, and love that you're in his sexual spotlight! Relish it and take your time, since time is the ultimate tease.

You don't want to rush to strip down since burlesque is more about concealing than revealing, at least at first. You want to torment your audience with little surprises and feminine mystique. For example, as you start stripping down, slide your boa or strand of pearls across your skin, especially all of those places you wish to be touched later. Remove each glove finger by finger, using your teeth. Toss the glove aside when all five fingers have been loosened. Work on removing another article of clothing before revisiting the other glove, perhaps propping your leg on a chair to remove a bow garter. Then return to your shimmy and showing off your form until you feel moved to take off something else . . . .

Men and women can both become aroused by visual materials, often using them as a form of foreplay. While men are often more excited by visual materials, this may be in large part because society gives them more permission to respond so. Academics have also commented that when a man sees a sex film, he may make the actress the target of his lust, fantasizing about having sex with her. Women, on the other hand, are more titillated by identifying with the actress and imagining being the target of a man's wanton desires and attentions. Those women physiologically aroused by erotic films are likelier to respond to scenes of males and females making love than to pictures of a nude male or a genital close-up. Both the Internet and videos offer a wide range of educational, soft-core, hard-core, classic or modern movies, and themed adult-entertainment videos.

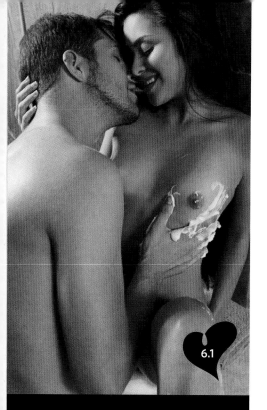

6.1

$\mathcal{S}\!\mathit{ex}$ercise 6.1 Improve Your Nipple Play

Massage the nipples softly, slowly applying more pressure, perhaps using a fabric to vary the sensation. With a bit of lube or massage oil, roll the nipples between your thumbs and index fingers, gradually squeezing them as your lover gets more excited. Ask your partner to breathe deeply as you make love to the entire breast, caressing, squeezing, and kneading it with your fingers and palms. Bring a nipple to your lips and graze it, teasing it with your warm breath before pulling away. Go back and forth between nipples, eventually suckling on each, every time varying the intensity of your tongue stimulation, with your licks hard, then soft, or fast, then slow. Nursing the breasts will bring extra blood to the skin's surface, making the areola area even more easily stimulated, so make sure your lover is feeling nothing but good as the area heaves with sensations.

If your lover can take more intense sensations, you may find that she thrives off of the breasts or nipples being slightly twisted, scratched, tweaked, clenched, pinched, clamped, vibrated, or lightly bitten. Some enjoy having warm wax or drops from ice cubes dripped on their breasts, making their nipples harden and tingle as their body shivers with joy. Nipple clamps (vibrating or not) and nipple rings can make for tingly, and even painful, sensations that lovers enjoy.

Back: On occasion, lovers like to pamper each other with a tender, sensual massage, especially if one needs to be energized for sex. Practically every culture has utilized the use of hot and cold on the body to alter response in the blood and lymph system to bring about healing and rejuvenation. Native American women would place a warm stone on their belly during menses. Roman baths involved hot water followed by the cooling effect of lying on marble tables. So if you find your immune system lagging or energy level low, you will want to consider this wellness practice in particular when giving the back ample attention.

$\mathcal{S}\!\mathit{ex}$ercise 6.2 Activate Hot Spots Using Stone Massage

In activating all of the hot spots on your lover's back simultaneously, consider heating smooth stones for a stone massage. This type of therapeutic bodywork involves hot and cold applications, followed by a massage. Smooth heated stones of various sizes and weights sometimes contrasted with cool ones are used to nurture and enhance your massage. Place them comfortably into the contours of your lover's body that tend to hold tension. Once all the stones are

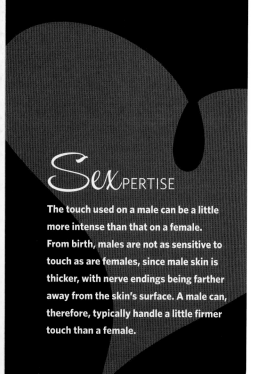

$\mathcal{S}\!\mathit{ex}$PERTISE

The touch used on a male can be a little more intense than that on a female. From birth, males are not as sensitive to touch as are females, since male skin is thicker, with nerve endings being farther away from the skin's surface. A male can, therefore, typically handle a little firmer touch than a female.

placed, slide oiled stones in flowing strokes over your partner's body for greater relaxation. This type of foreplay is excellent for times of mental or physical stress, since it focuses on both body and mind, soothing your lover's entire nervous system, relieving pain, and increasing circulation.

Place the heated stones, available at many holistic wellness stores, on the small of the back, the sacral curve, which is full of nerve endings and where stress often accumulates. Concentrating on this area invites blood flow to the groin, heightening sexual response. Place other stones on the dimple above each buttock cheek. Heating this area, especially with a massaging motion, will spread sensual sensations to the groin.

Hands: Holding hands is often one of the first and most significant exchanges of affection lovers share. Yet beyond this initial hand-holding, lovers often don't give enough attention to their palms and fingers. This is a travesty given that each palm contains forty thousand nerve endings! Instead of using your hands for sexual touch, sexually touch each other's hands. Massage, tease, and tickle palms. Lightly scratch, suck, lick, and kiss the entire hand. Get suggestive with finger play, especially as you feed each other well-known aphrodisiacs such as figs, oysters, or orange slices. Let your lewd intentions be known as you slurp melted chocolate or honey off of each other's fingers, making sure to lick every last drop.

Abdomen: Lovers adore honing in on the navel as the starting point to licking, nibbling, and panting their way down to the genitals. Such loving attention gets things going as blood floods the area, making the hairline treasure trail from the navel to the pubic bone practically stand on end with sensations.

Thighs and Knees: Given their close proximity to the genitals, playing with your lover's inner and upper thighs can leave them longing for more. Leisurely drag your fingernails from the knee to the groin, allowing your fingertips to graze the vulva or penis before going back down to entice the nerve endings at the backs of the knees. Tickle this zone, occasionally letting your fingertips sweep the back of the thigh above the knee. Return to delivering light touches and licks to the inner thigh area as a prelude to oral sex, beating the skin of the inner thigh and groin with your warm breath.

Feet: Packed with pressure sensors, feet are a bona fide erogenous zone. So massage your lover's feet with a generous amount of lotion for a few minutes, relieving the stress between the toes. Firmly press your thumb along your love's arches, working out any tension. Rub, knead, and rap on the ball of the foot. Ask your lover where you should concentrate your efforts.

In the Bedroom Exercises:
Penis Stimulation

THERE ARE A NUMBER of ways to manually stimulate the penis. The following two exercises are among the most effective:

Cylinder Sex

1. While sitting between your lover's legs, warm your palms by rubbing them together.

2. Place one palm on the shaft of the penis with your thumb facing down, palm away from you.

3. Wrap your thumb around his penis, and push your wrist toward his stomach.

4. Form a cylinder with your fingers by gently wrapping them around the base of the penis.

5. Using a firm grip, move your hand up the penis, rotating the palm over the head of the glans, caressing it when you reach the top.

6. Next, keeping your palm against the penis, form a ring with your thumb and first two fingers.

7. Gently glide this ring down to the root of his shaft. Just as you reach the bottom of the shaft of the penis, repeat the process with your other hand.

8. Continue taking turns with each hand, maintaining continuous contact and movement, occasionally focusing on the corona, one of the most excitable spots of a man's penis. Also known as the coronal ridge, the corona is the raised ridge that separates the head of the penis from the shaft of the penis.

Make sure you communicate with your lover as you do this, to learn what feels good and what he would like you to do more or less of.

Glans Delight

The glans, or head of the penis, contains the greatest concentration of nerve endings, so get engrossed with it.

1. Wrap your hand around the glans as though you're about to twist the cap off a bottle of beer.

2. Make the motion like you are twisting off a cap, repeating it several times and asking your lover what pressure and speed feel good. (Note: He may prefer that you do this motion with lubricant.)

3. Then slowly move down the shaft of the penis, using one or two hands, to gently twist it from side to side. Using your palms will provide more pressure.

Know that if your guy has a foreskin, you've got an extra hot spot to work with since this layer of skin is full of nerve endings, muscle fibers, and rich blood vessels. Since this erogenous zone is very sensitive, be sure to communicate with your lover about how much he can handle.

No matter which exercise you choose, whenever possible, don't ignore his testicles. Be sure to avoid being rough, since you're dealing with delicate tissue. To include the testicles, lightly hit them against each thigh. Cup and jiggle his scrotum as you play with his penis, pressing it up against his lower abdominals to indirectly stimulate his prostate. Gently tap them to release his sexual energy. Massage each testicle by placing your fingers under the scrotum, thumbs on top, and rolling 36 times in each direction to build positive energy, increase circulation, and release muscle adhesions. Or have him straddle your thigh so that you can push up against his testicles as you seductively stroke his penis.

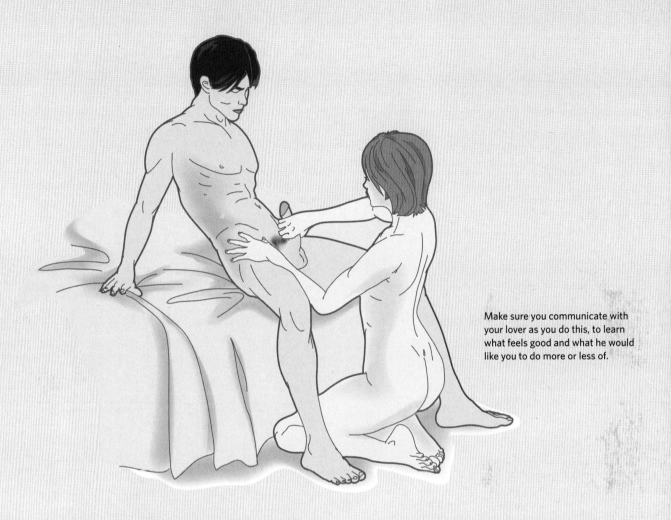

Make sure you communicate with your lover as you do this, to learn what feels good and what he would like you to do more or less of.

Also, consider varying the sensations on his shaft for a whole new experience. Drape panties over your hand, then slide the silky fabric up and down his penis. To create even more sensation, put your panties in the freezer a few hours before sex, or microwave a damp washcloth for about fifteen to twenty seconds; the heat will invite greater blood flow to his groin, increasing his arousal in a most soothing way.

As you're pleasuring your partner, encourage him to invite all of his senses to the party. Encourage him to smell and feel your hair or play with your breasts. Let him feel how wet you are by rubbing your moist vulva against his body. Let him know how badly you want him with your moans and whimpers of desire.

HANDS-ON FOR HIM: EVERY WOMAN'S GUIDE TO HEAD GAMES HE'LL LOVE

When it comes to tantalizing touches, manual stimulation can't be beat in many respects. In bringing him to the brink of bliss, however, you can drive him wild with desire for more than just your hand. But before touching his most private parts, know that there are a few things to keep in mind:

- Trim your fingernails, as jagged nails can hurt.
- Warm your hands.
- Be careful about jewelry snagging his pubic hair.
- Check if he wants you to use lube. Men who are uncircumcised may not find lube as necessary as a man who is circumcised. So find out what his preferences are. If you're planning on using a circular motion, let him know that lube may be preferable since this provides more sensation for the head of his penis.
- Don't be afraid to ask him if he'd like more pressure, a different stroke or massage, or if he'd prefer that you focus on another part of his genitals. Like women, every man is different, and a man's preferences can change with his mood, level of fatigue, and the context of the encounter. So be flexible in playing with his penis, and find out from him what he's in the mood for.
- Make sure that he's breathing. As he gets caught up in the moment, he may unconsciously hold his breath. While flattering, this doesn't do anything for his sexual response. Full, deep breaths will help him to expand the sensations throughout his body.

Like the clitoris, a penis needs to be warmed up. So don't just grab his penis with a firm up-down stroke. While many men like a strong, rhythmic touch and are more responsive to a full-hand hold, begin slowly and gently with light touches and teasing, grazing strokes.

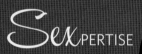

S&X PERTISE

The urethral opening, the orifice through which urine is released from the body, is an erogenous zone for some men and women before, during, or right after orgasm since the area is full of nerve endings. To stimulate this area, use a lubed finger or sex toy to gently rub, press, or circle this area. Confirm that your lover likes the sensations, as some find it unpleasant, nonstimulating, or uncomfortable.

In the Bedroom Exercise: Vulval Stimulation

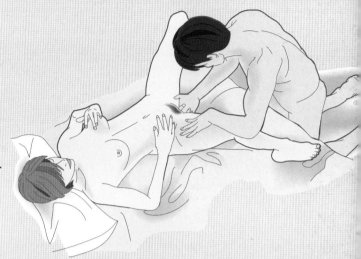

KNEADING, SHAKING, GRASPING, patting, or cupping the mons pubis, the fatty pad of tissue covering her pubic bone, could possibly bring her to orgasm. This is because this area, which is full of nerve endings, ends up indirectly stimulating her clitoris when rubbed, stroked, or massaged. You can also rest the heel of your hand on it while you apply some stimulation with your fingers. With the base of your palm pressed against her pubic mound, drape your fingers against her entire vulva. As you're playing with the mons pubis, you can pursue the following for more intense sensations:

1. Make a rhythmic come-hither motion with your middle finger along her vaginal entrance, allowing it to get wet from her natural lubrication.

2. Lightly stimulate her outer lips with your lubed fingertips, stroking, kneading, fondling, pushing, tickling, or caressing them. Do the same with the inner lips. Feel them swelling and growing slightly larger as they're engorged with blood.

3. Massage the lips against one another before slipping a couple of fingers down to feel her vaginal opening become more inviting, opening, as it prepares for possible penetration.

4. Instead of accepting her invitation, tease her by slipping your fingers a little lower, onto her perineum, the soft tissue between her anus and vaginal opening.

5. Press on this area to stimulate the nerve endings and spongy, erectile tissue it's connected to. (As you do this, use can use your thumb to stimulate her clitoris, which should be getting warmed up now.)

6. Now slowly massage your way up the vulva, caressing the entire area, before honing in on the clitoris.

7. Slowly and softly, apply pressure to her clitoris, checking to see if she prefers direct or indirect stimulation, a different rhythm or touch. If she needs indirect stimulation, approach the clitoris from the side, or pull at or rub the inner lips or mons pubis. If she can handle direct stimulation, tap it, slap it, squeeze it, rock your fingers back and forth across the glans . . . all the while asking her to tell you if it gets to be too much.

For lovers who can handle even more intensity, pull the clitoral hood back as you get faster and faster with your finger play. Make sure that you're still using plenty of lube, as not to make her feel sore, raw, or irritated. Pay attention to her sounds and motion, noting when she's pressing her pelvis into your hand for even more pressure. Be sure to oblige.

Eventually, give your fingers a break by using the tip of your penis against her vulva. Tease her by barely penetrating her before letting the head of your penis linger along her inner and outer lips, occasionally pressing it between the folds of her labia without entering her. Now circle her clitoris with the tip of your penis, occasionally pressing it against her hot spot.

In the Bedroom Exercise: G spot Stimulation

IN FINDING THE G SPOT, a woman must be sexually aroused, her vagina well-lubricated. The urethral sponge will be more prominent when she is sexually excited, making it much easier to find. Her lover's fingers should be well-groomed, preferably lubed, and her bladder should be empty before stimulation, since she may initially experience the urge to urinate, which will soon pass. In assuming a position, the one best suited for finding the G spot involves a woman lying on her stomach, legs apart, hips elevated with a pillow.

1. Once your lover is aroused, insert one, two, or three fingers (whatever is comfortable for her) into her vagina, lightly pressing them down on the front wall.

2. Making sure to stay in the "shallow" end of her vaginal canal, feel for a rough, wrinkled, puckered area along the vaginal wall. Communicate with her, asking if she's comfortable and if she's noting any sexual sensations.

3. Once you feel a raised area, the G spot, continue coaxing it by using the firm, deep pressure rhythmically in a circular, up-down, or side-to-side motion.

4. Increase the rhythm of this steady pressure gradually. Alternatively, you can thrust your fingers in and out of the vagina, hitting against the G spot as you enter.

If you're having trouble locating this spot, place a hand on top of the pubic bone, and gently press on the area where the pubic hairline begins with your hand. Ask her to press against your hand and to give you affirmation when you've stimulated it. You can gently squeeze the area or firmly rock your fingers across it as well.

Don't get frustrated or lose all hope if you haven't found the G spot. Finding it may take multiple attempts, since not all results are instantaneous. The G spot may not be erogenous zone for every woman, and that's okay. Everyone is built differently when it comes to erogenous zones. Be sure to stay relaxed, and don't be too goal-oriented. You're exploring the body, and that can be enthralling fun!

In bettering your chances of finding the G spot, try changing positions and working other erogenous zones, such as the clitoris, with your other hand, mouth, or a sex toy, to increase her arousal and the G spot's chances of becoming more prominent. A woman should also explore her G spot potential on her own during masturbation, which may relieve any performance pressure or anxiety she feels over finding this area with a lover. She also needs to be in a space where she can let go, where she's trying not to be in control, since trying too hard to make things happen can actually shut down her orgasmic response. She needs to stay relaxed, losing herself in the moment, the sensations, or a fantasy. She needs to work on strengthening her pelvic floor muscles, as done in Chapter 14, to heighten this hot spot's sensitivity and responsiveness. Try using a sex toy, specifically a curved G spot vibrator, if you're having trouble finding this area or want even more intense sensation than a finger can provide.

FINGER-PLAY FOR HER: EVERY MAN'S GUIDE TO PUTTING HIS FINGER ON HER PLEASURE

Manual stimulation is one of the most effective ways to build a woman's sexual arousal. Yet, in guaranteeing that such sex play is a pleasant experience for her, be sure to attend to a few things:

- Make sure your nails are trimmed—jagged fingernails can hurt.
- Warm your hands.
- Use lube.
- Communicate. Different parts of her vulva produce different sensations at different times. You may need to adjust your speed and pressure, depending on how she's reacting. So ask her what feels good, what she needs more or less of, and if your stimulation should be continuous, as she could be in need of a break.
- Make sure that she's breathing. Full, deep breaths will help her to expand the sensations throughout her body, increasing the chance of more all-consuming orgasm.
- Unless she likes it a bit rougher, start with slow, light touches.

SEXUAL Q&A: DOES SIZE MATTER?

When it comes to sexual satisfaction, especially during intercourse, does size matter to a woman?

When it comes to penis size, men are often quite hard on themselves. Surveys show that three out of four men believe that their penises are smaller than average. Yet the "average" penis size is:

- 3 to 4 inches in length for a flaccid (nonerect) penis
- 5 to 7 inches in length for an erect penis
- 1 inch in penile diameter when flaccid; 1½ when erect
- 5.1 inches in circumference

The vast majority of men are average or within two inches of the length figures. A review of sixty years of research in the *British Journal of Urology* assessed that length matters more to men than women, with 90 percent of women preferring a wide penis to a long one. This is likely in part because thickness, or girth, helps to "fill" her for more stimulation. The same review reported that 85 percent of women were satisfied with their partner's penis size versus only 55 percent of men having no qualms.

And most women, quite frankly, don't care about size. Case in point: Research has found that if a woman is sexually unsatisfied, then she will perceive her lover as small. On the other hand, if she's sexually satisfied, then she sees him as large. While the occasional woman likes a well-endowed man, in many cases, bigger does not make for better. It really comes down to each individual's preferences and what they're doing with what they've got!

DISCOVER HER BURIED TREASURE: "X" MARKS THE G SPOT TO PLEASURE

When a female becomes sexually aroused, her vaginal walls fill with blood and the vagina becomes swollen. During this time, the urethral sponge, the erectile tissue that surrounds the urethra, fills with blood and bulges, what is known as the Gräfenberg spot, or "G spot." This small mass can be felt on the front (stomach side) wall of the vagina, actually through the wall, about two inches in from the vaginal opening. The actual location of the spot may be different from woman to woman, since some G spots are more to the left or right of that approximate center point. The size of the tissue, and the paraurethral glands it contains, varies from female to female, getting as big as a half-dollar with effective stimulation. Powered by the pelvic nerve, unlike the clitoris, this erogenous zone slowly awakens for powerful reactions that can include orgasm.

While the G spot can be easily found and stimulated in some women, others have to hunt for it. Some never find it, meaning this area of their body does not have any erogenous qualities. For a lover exploring the G spot area's erotic potential, such a quest is well worth it since massaging the G spot increases blood flow to the genitals as a woman becomes more aroused. This invites new sensations that enable her to stay sexually aroused for longer periods of time.

DISCOVER HIS BURIED TREASURE: "X" MARKS HIS PLEASURE

As a man becomes sexually excited, his prostate starts to swell with the fluid that makes up semen, sending amazing sensations throughout his loins, the pleasure of which grows as he nears orgasm. Nicknamed the "P-spot," the prostate surrounds the urethra, just below the bladder. About the size of a chestnut, this firm gland of muscular, glandular, and connective tissue can be found right above the perineum, behind the pubic bone. When stimulated, it can result in an intense orgasm, with or without ejaculation, even when a man does not have an erection or experience any other kind of sensation. Stimulating this area can also help a man to maintain erection, prolonging lovemaking.

In the Bedroom Exercise: Prostate Stimulation

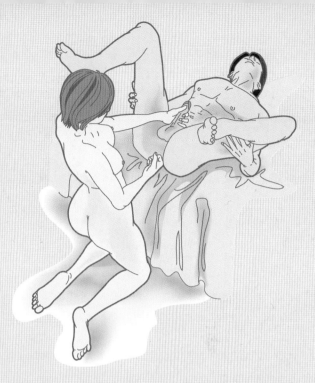

GET INTO A COMFORTABLE POSITION. Ones that are best for stimulating the prostate involve lying on your stomach (which allows for the most direct prostate stimulation); lying on your back, knees bent, feet flat on the floor or knees pulled into the chest, pillow under the buttocks; getting on your hands and knees; and lying on your side, knees pulled toward the chest.

1. Sitting between your lover's legs, slowly insert a well-lubricated sex toy or finger into his anus. As you do so, communicate with your lover, making sure that he's comfortable, especially before you insert anything a little farther.

2. As you work your way about two to three inches up, you'll be able to feel the prostate through the front (stomach side) rectal wall. It will feel like a nut or dome. Lay your finger or the toy firmly against the prostate, asking your partner to breathe deeply and to relax.

3. Once he's is more comfortable, gently press against the prostate. Ask him what feels good and what doesn't.

4. Gently massage the prostate by gently stroking it in a downward direction. Or rock your finger across it. If desired, you can lightly thrust against his prostate, slowly moving your finger or the toy in and out of the anus.

For an even more intense experience, play with his penis at the same time, especially since this can relax him. In receiving this stimulation, your lover should let you know what he needs more or less of. Know that you'll see more and better results with experience, especially as you become more comfortable with the whole practice.

A man should also explore his prostate potential on his own while masturbating. This will allow him to become more comfortable with the anal area, getting over any

concerns he has over cultural taboos involving anal play. Such concerns are quite prevalent and may impact pleasure, given that only 22 percent of men and 18 percent of women find appeal in having their anus stimulated by their partner's fingers, according to the "Sex in America" survey. A male and his lover can also get used to the idea of prostate stimulation, or bypass any issues they have with probing the anus, by indirectly stimulating the prostate via the perineum, which lies between his testicles and anus. Stimulating this muscular band of flesh, in turn, stimulates the prostate and penis.

To stimulate the prostate via the perineum, feel for a slight indentation, and begin softly pushing, tapping, or stroking against it firmly, rhythmically using your finger, knuckle, palm, or a vibrator. Change the direction and amount of pressure, moving in circles, up and down, side to side, or diagonally, all the while asking about what is and isn't quite working for him. In making this an even more riveting experience, stimulate the penis, scrotum, or anus at the same time.

While the prostate is most effectively played with via the rectum, men of all sexual orientations enjoy prostate pleasure. Every man's prostate has the potential to be a hot spot as long as he's open-minded and willing to trust his partner being in control. Before embarking on prostate play, it is best to make sure that he's fully aroused, as to avoid any discomfort or pain. A man's bladder should also be emptied, since he will feel like he needs to urinate when the prostate is first stimulated. Fingernails should be trimmed, especially if you're not using gloves. Make sure you have plenty of lubricant and that you're taking your time, since this is a delicate area you're playing with. If you're worried about cleanliness, take a shower before and after prostate play. You can also use an anal douche kit ahead of time. Condom-covered acrylic sex toys with a wide safety base can also help lovers who are initially uncomfortable with the fact that prostate play involves playing with the oft-deemed "exit-only" area of the body. Regardless of any issues you have with the anus, you may want to invest in a nice non-porous toy, such as an anal dildo or vibrator, which is curved to tease the prostate, making your job a whole lot easier.

"*I lie awake, hot, The growing fires of passion bursting, blazing in my heart.*"

—ONO NO KOMACHI, JAPANESE POET

Sexual Homework

In this chapter, we put a heavy emphasis on building arousal through manual stimulation. Lovingly attending to all of the body's erogenous zones, especially those on the genitals, is a major part of foreplay for many couples since it is so effective. Thus, for your sexual homework, we're going to look at even more ways to arouse your partner.

Give Him a Hand

1. Clamp your thumb and forefinger around the shaft of his penis, about an inch above where it joins the scrotum.

2. Pull the skin down so that your other fingers and palm rest against the scrotum (if you need to pull down any extra skin, you can reach higher up on the shaft of the penis). If he has a foreskin, pull it taut while stroking his shaft with the other hand to warm him up.

3. Now, clasp your well-lubed fingers together and use both thumbs to form circles for a figure eight on the frenulum. This tiny band of loose skin is a small bump on the underside of the penis, where the shaft meets the glans (in circumcised men, it's the sensitive scar tissue seen as a slight bump). For many men, this tissue is the most sensitive part of his penis, so liberally apply light circle massages against the frenulum, varying the speed and pressure on this point and the shaft of the penis. (Note: Your partner could ejaculate quickly if this hot spot receives too much attention.)

Raising Her Arousal Awareness

In an effort to gauge her sexual excitement, and her potential need for more arousal, lovers should pursue the following:

1. As you slowly caress her vulva, have your lover tune into the sensations and her excitement.

2. Every four to five minutes, ask her where, on a scale of one to ten, she is in her arousal. In responding, she should focus on more than the physical, gauging her overall arousal.

3. After checking in with her four or so times, think about where your arousal level was up or down and what may have contributed to that.

4. Make suggestions as to how to maintain her level of arousal while transitioning to other sexual activities, such as intercourse.

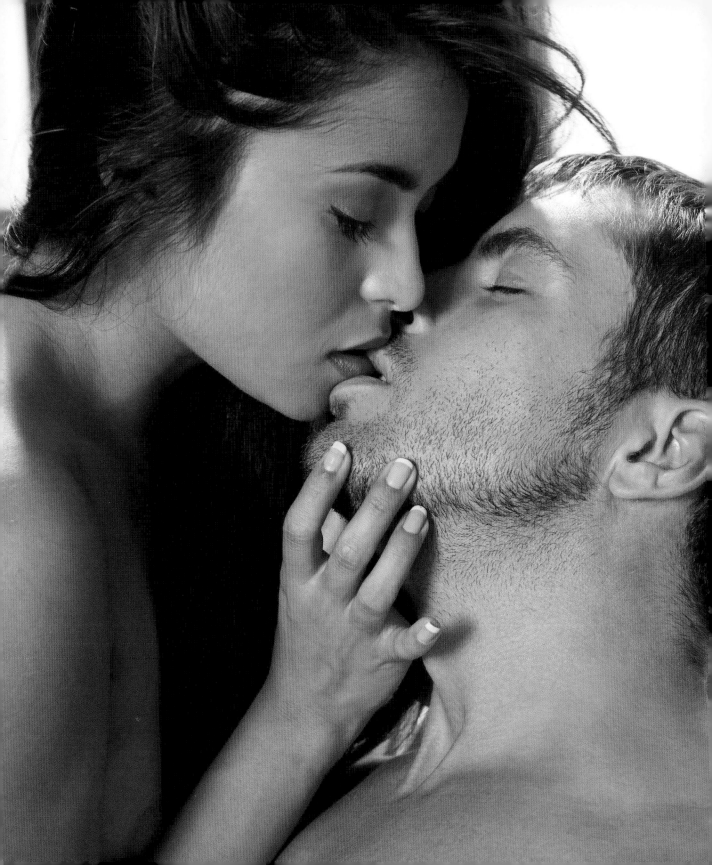

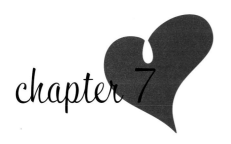

chapter 7

Oral Delights: Kissing, Cunnilingus, and Fellatio

WHEN IT COMES TO FOREPLAY, what better complements touch than the tongue? In exploring new ways to increase arousal, it cannot hurt to be reminded of the old ways. In this chapter of oral delights, we start with rediscovering the art of kissing. Over time, lovers often tend to neglect kissing, relegating such sex play to the delights of new love—and, in seeing it as so—doing themselves a huge disservice. Kissing is a true joy, which is why, according to William Cane, who surveyed thousands of people for his book *The Art of Kissing*, 87 percent of men and 98 percent of women report giggling from the pleasure derived from kissing alone.

Kissing is foreplay at its best. You can kiss your way up and down your lover—tapping sensitive nerve endings and turning on sensory centers as you go. You'll intoxicate each other during this dizzying prelude, increasing arousal with this sexy expression of affection, friendliness, and love. To add to the intensity, blindfold your lover with a scarf or a silk tie, inviting the other senses to come to life even more.

"*Love is but the discovery of ourselves in others, and the delight in the recognition.*"

—ALEXANDER SMITH

THE SCIENCE OF *Sex*

Research in Evolutionary Psychology reports that women place more importance on kissing as a way of initiating, maintaining, and monitoring their relationships than males. Men, however, appear to lock lips in hopes of increasing their chances of having sex.

Sexercise 7.1 Build Intimacy with Evening of Kissing

Kissing is a spiritual connection for some, more intimate than sex. To create this intimacy, try an evening devoted to kissing only. Focusing on the sensations of kissing alone can actually increase arousal—and guarantee that the next time you do make love, you're both wild for one another.

THE ART OF FRENCH-KISSING

Maraichignage, better known as French-kissing, can be anything from a gentle, playful mingling of the tongues to an all-out "tongue wrestle." Gently probe each other's mouths, moan with pleasure, or practically resuscitate each other. Any type of French-kissing is all in good fun, whether you are sucking on each other's tongues, pressing them together, or circling them. One tongue may become the thruster, penetrating deeply into the recipient's mouth, with lovers often taking turns on who will be more passive.

In the Bedroom:
Lip Exploration

WHILE THERE ARE times lovers devour one another with aggressive can't-get-enough-of-you, must-have-you-now kisses, usually slow, sensitive kissing works better. Start with playful, teasing touch, exploring each other's lips, and develop a rhythm. If your lover is a bit too tongue-focused too soon, kiss your partner on the neck, nibble his earlobe, or caress the back of her ear with your finger (according to Cane, 88 percent of women enjoy being kissed on the ear). Other strategies for slowing things down while building your kissing finesse include:

- Exploring your love's mouth using your tongue and lips
- Splattering your lover's face with a plethora of kisses
- Kissing one eye and the other eye and repeating (75 percent of women and 67 percent of men like this, as found by Cane)

- Use "vacuum" kisses, sucking the air out of each other's mouths while keeping the lips tightly sealed together
- Gently nibbling on your lover's lower lip
- Kissing in front of a mirror, encouraging your lover to take a look

Engage all of your senses, stay close, caress your lover's face, play with your partner's hair, and keep your hands moving. Rub the back of your partner's neck. Grab your love's hips. Pin your lover down, hands over head, as you lock gazes and exchange sweet nothings with every gasp for air. For those times you need a bit of a breather, stay connected by kissing other parts of the body. You may, for example, want to press your nose into places your love dabs perfume or cologne, giving these spots ravenous kisses.

KISSING AROUND THE WORLD

Kissing dos and don'ts vary around the world. The Japanese, for example, are known for not kissing as much as other cultures. Eskimos are noted for a "kiss" that involves rubbing their noses together. They find inhaling the breath of their lover quite erotic. Other cultures see kissing as stimulating more than only the loins.

According to ancient Chinese medicine, the mouth and tongue are related to the heart. To stimulate your heart with Chinese-style kisses, try the following:

- Use more saliva for wetter kisses, which will enable you to absorb more of your lover's energy.
- Keep your lips, jaw, and mouth loose. This allows tension to leave the body, making your breathing easier and your face more sensitive.
- Vary the degree of lip pressure, going from light-as-a-feather to firm.
- Lick your lover's gums, teeth, and palate.
- Let a kiss linger for more than ten seconds. The Chinese believe that doing so exemplifies the importance of a lover over life's other mundane concerns, serving as a reminder of why you're together.

TANTRIC KISSING

The practice of Tantric sex holds that kissing is a means of sexual enlightenment. The ancient and infamous Kama Sutra text, which encompasses a number of Tantric sex practices, instructs lovers to vary kissing so that it's slow and soft, then "hard and fast." Lovers are encouraged to vary techniques, never repeating a given type of kiss.

KISS ME ALL OVER

No matter what your kissing style, be sure to pay attention to more than just the lips. Your lover's ears, which are packed with nerve endings, beg to be toyed with. So stroke, kiss, lick, nibble, and even carefully bite and pull at them. Trace your lover's ear with a wet tongue, then blow on your wet mark. Take an earlobe between your lips for a suggestive massage. Graze the tiny hair follicles on the ear with your teeth. Softly blow into your lover's ear and on the area around it. Cup your lover's head, and massage the back of the ears with your thumbs, sending sexual energy throughout the body, as you kiss passionately. Whisper terms of endearment, use a little bit of erotic talk, utter any sound that enters your throat while you cover your love's brow with kisses.

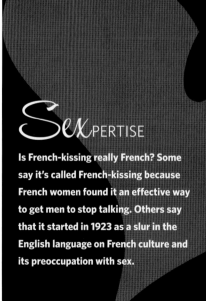

S𝒆𝓍PERTISE

Is French-kissing really French? Some say it's called French-kissing because French women found it an effective way to get men to stop talking. Others say that it started in 1923 as a slur in the English language on French culture and its preoccupation with sex.

THE ART OF ORAL SEX

Oral sex is an intense form of sex play that can be a means of seduction, a way to extend sex, or the main event itself. An extremely popular means of sexual expression, lovers can hardly get enough of the warmth, wetness, pressure, and intense sensations oral pleasuring allows for. The "Sex in America" survey found that 77 percent of men and 68 percent of women reported appeal in giving oral sex to a partner, while 79 percent of men and 73 percent of women reported appeal in receiving oral sex from a partner. Packed with orgasmic potency, this form of sex expression is effective when it comes to satisfying sex, whether it's all of the sex one needs for gratification or the stepping stone for even more.

In the Bedroom:
Tantric Kisses

LEARNING THE ART of Tantric kissing can enrich your sexual experiences. Expand your kissing repertoire by exploring the:

Rubbing Kiss: Rub your lover's lips using your tongue.

Nominal Kiss: Your lover's mouth is relaxed and closed while you actively kiss using an open mouth.

Vibrant Kiss: Your lover has a relaxed, closed mouth while you gently insert your top lip into your partner's mouth.

Crosswise: Tilt your heads slightly so that the lips are caught up in each other by making them round. (This may be something you do naturally already. According to German psychologist Onur Gunturkun, 65 percent of kissers turn their head to the right so as not to bump noses.)

Sucking: Suck the tongue and then your lover's top, then bottom, lip.

The Fifth Hold: As you press your lips together (without letting the teeth touch), gently press the cheeks with the fingertips.

Love the Way You Look: Many people are concerned about the shape or size of their genitals, fearing that they're unsightly or undesirable. Don't let your body image issues ruin what can be breathtaking sex! Your partner is engaging in oral sex because he or she wants to be with you. Your lover is between your legs for the sole purpose of pleasing you.

Keep It Wet: Whether with flavored lubricant or saliva, know that wetter makes for better when it comes to oral sex.

Take Your Time: Oral sex is like fine dining. You don't want to wolf down your meal. Not only is it ultimately unappetizing, but it deprives both you and your lover of the chance to savor the experience, all of its sensations, and potential orgasm. So as the giver, stay relaxed and breathe, taking note of the sensations against your lips and tongue. Lose yourself in your lover's moans and movements, even pleasing yourself at the same time.

Shave: Unless your lover is into brush burns, get rid of any stubble. Strive to be either clean-shaven, or keep it long, since in-between can be uncomfortable.

Warm Up: Even if oral sex is meant to be part of foreplay, get your lover warmed up first with some teasing action. Try a little oral sex while your partner is still clothed. Wear edible undies for him or her. Once naked, give your lover a tongue bath, then blow. Sprinkle honey dust across your lover, and run your tongue along the area where the thighs and torso meet.

SEXUAL Q&A: GAG REFLEX DURING FELLATIO

I start to gag when I take my lover's penis deeply into my mouth during oral sex. Is there any way to avoid this?

Deep-throating, where the entire penis goes into the mouth, can cause your gag reflex to kick in and is quite common. To control this reaction, focus on your breathing, getting into a position that puts you in control; for instance, have him lie on his back as you crouch over his penis. Another strategy is to lie on your back and to tilt your head off of the bed, to open your throat and reduce your impulse to gag. You can also take breaths on the out-strokes, since going deep causes his penis to seal off your windpipe. Finally, you can control how deeply the penis penetrates your mouth by keeping a fist on his shaft as a buffer to gagging.

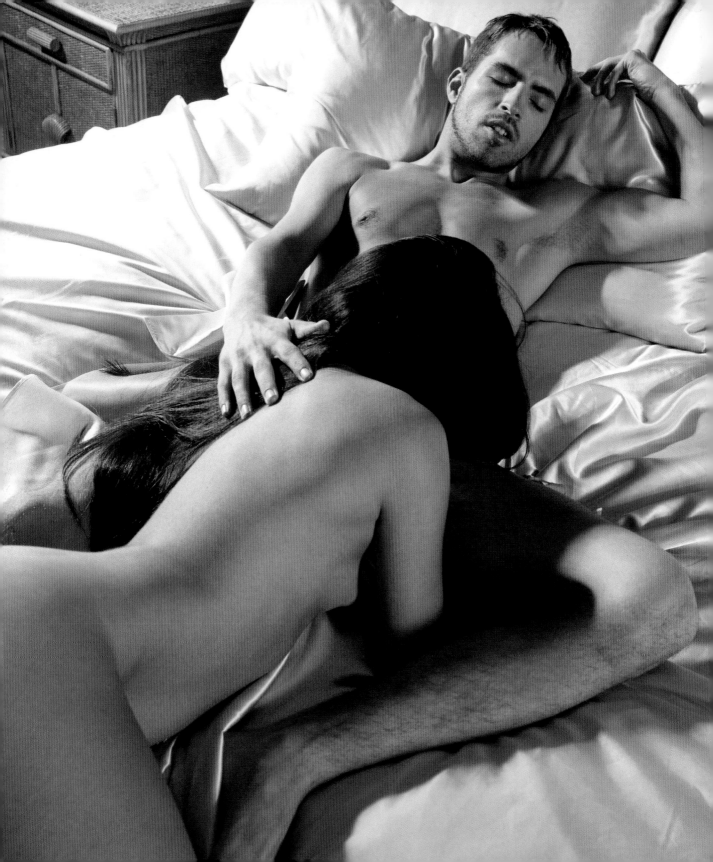

In the Bedroom:
The Hottest Licks that Will Drive Him Wild

FELLATIO, ORAL SEX ON A MAN, is such a treat for him since the skin on the penis is some of the thinnest on his body, containing more nerve endings than other regions. It is for this reason that it's vital to remember not to use teeth (unless he likes it)! Be sure to cover your teeth with your lips as you take his penis into your mouth.

1. Tighten your lips around the shaft of his penis as you press your way down to the root.

2. As you allow the penis to thrust in and out of your mouth, think of your mouth as a tight vagina.

3. With your lips wrapped around the shaft of his penis, push your tongue upward, as you would if you were trying to touch the roof of your mouth.

4. Massage the shaft of the penis with your tongue, flattening it as though you're enjoying a tasty ice cream cone.

5. Then bring your tongue to a point as you run it up and down the shaft of his penis.

6. Occasionally, focus on the head of the penis, flicking your tongue over it, or rubbing the head of his penis against the inside of your cheek or upper palate.

7. From time to time, lick the underside of the shaft of the penis with sweeping up-down motions.

8. As you bring him into your mouth again, slowly swirl your tongue around the penis' most sensitive areas as you thrust it in and out of your mouth.

9. Have your hand follow your mouth, acting as a corkscrew, going the opposite direction of your swirling tongue.

10. Flick your tongue across his hottest spots, namely the corona and frenulum, before you take him into your mouth deeper, as you build up the pace of your thrusting, pressing your tongue against his penis for greater sensation.

When you're doing any of these movements, you may enhance the experience by:

- Stroking his belly or thighs
- Playing with his nipples or testicles
- Running your fingernails up and down the area where his thigh meets his groin
- Licking and sucking on his scrotum
- Sliding a finger into your mouth to tickle his penis as you're stimulating him with your lips and tongue
- Drinking a bit of warm mint tea. Your hot mouth will heat his penis, while the menthol in the mint will cool it down as you pull your mouth away
- Resting a vibrator against your cheek as you pleasure him
- Using a finger vibrator against his perineum or scrotum

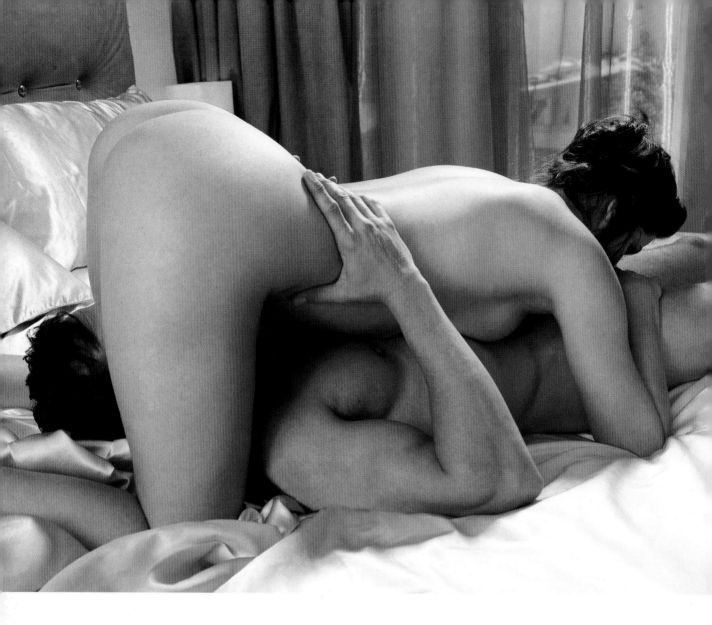

Let Go of Expectations: Just be in the moment. Don't get caught up in getting somewhere, as this may only lead to disappointment. All of us respond differently when it comes to oral sex, and we react differently from time to time, depending on a number of issues. Your lover may or may not have an orgasm. A person may or may not ejaculate. Any of that is fine and is no indicator of just how adept you are with this amorous effort.

Discuss the Ejaculation Matter: Many women, in particular, are hesitant about having oral sex, much less bringing their lover to orgasm, for fear that he will ejaculate in her mouth. This could be because she doesn't like the taste, has sexual health concerns, isn't crazy about the experience, or sees it as a form of degradation. Couples need to discuss if it's okay for him to ejaculate in his partner's mouth. If it's not okay, they need to strategize about the point at which the penis should be withdrawn from the mouth.

Address Smell and Taste Concerns: Lovers often worry about what they smell and taste like during oral sex. It's important to realize that many things can affect a person's scent and flavor. When it comes to the vulva, the smell and taste of it are dependent upon a woman's diet, the pH level of vaginal secretions, and the stage of her menstrual cycle. Strong foods, like asparagus and garlic, may increase a woman's scent. Citrus foods, like lemons, oranges, and grapefruits may sweeten it.

A man's taste and smell are very much related to his diet. To improve the taste of his semen, try acidic foods, such as fruits, for a sweeter taste. Citrus (especially lemon), cranberry, and pineapple, as well as juices made from such, are often recommended. Cardamom, cinnamon, and peppermint are also said to make him tastier. Certain vegetables can work to his benefit as far as taste, including celery and parsley, while other ones don't, such as broccoli, cauliflower, asparagus, and beets. Foods that can further affect his semen taste for the worse are red meat and fish, since these are alkaline-based. Garlic, onion, chemically processed liquor, drugs, and nicotine tend to negatively affect his semen taste. The high bacterial content of dairy products may also have a negative effect. Last, men should be mindful of consuming strong tasting foods and spices, such as curry, which end up getting secreted by the body, changing the flavor and overall odor.

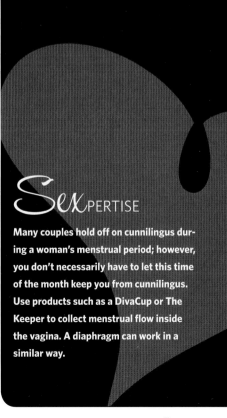

$\mathcal{S}ex$PERTISE

Many couples hold off on cunnilingus during a woman's menstrual period; however, you don't necessarily have to let this time of the month keep you from cunnilingus. Use products such as a DivaCup or The Keeper to collect menstrual flow inside the vagina. A diaphragm can work in a similar way.

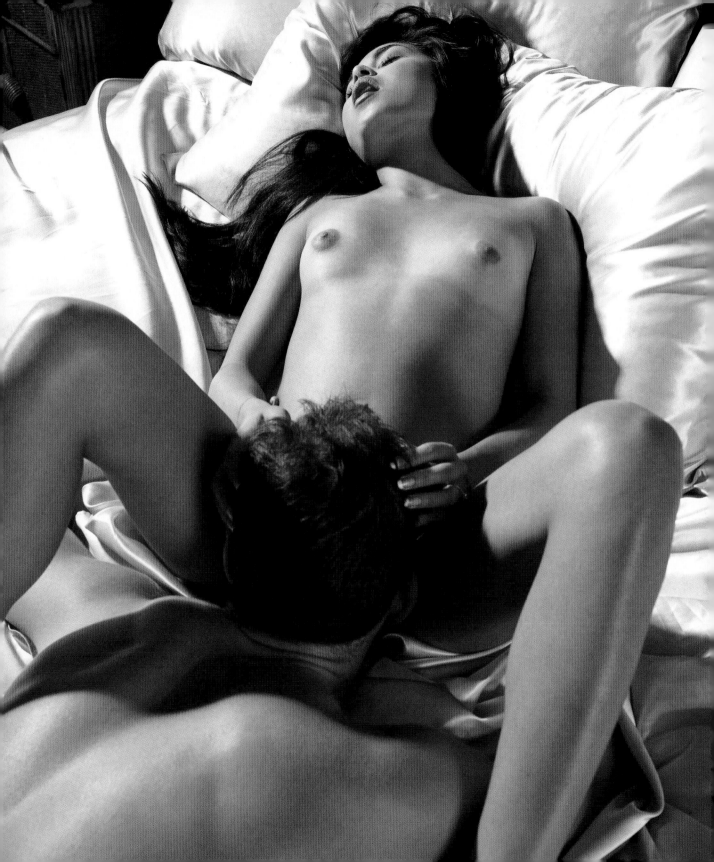

In the Bedroom:
The Hottest Licks that Will Drive Her Wild

CUNNILINGUS, ORAL SEX on a woman, is by far some of the best sex for many. This is primarily because the clitoris gets so much attention. In making sure that she gets the most out of the experience, have her sit, propped on pillows, knees bent. This positions her pelvis so that the nerves aren't compressed and so that her sensations will be much more intense.

In making contact with the vulva, approach the area like you would French kiss her other set of lips. Slowly work your way to easy, rhythmic tongue strokes.

1. Starting at her perineum, lick the full length of her inner labia, doing a circle at her clitoral head before going down the other side. No matter how excited she gets, keep a steady, slow pace.

2. Tease her, holding off on going for the clitoris. Occasionally, thrust your tongue into her vagina as a tease.

3. In focusing on the clitoris, you have several stimulation options to choose from. You can circle it with your tongue like a clock, or point it and flick it from side to side, diagonally, or up and down using fast strokes, or use a darting motion, or suck on it as you tease the clit with the tip of your tongue.

No matter which method you choose, keep your tongue soft at first, gradually intensifying your pressure as you increase your steady, rhythmic speed. (Note: If she has a bucking reaction to the intense stimulation, place your hands on her hip bones, and press.) No matter what you choose to do, you could intensify the experience by:

- Taking a sip of mint tea, for a hot-cold effect. You can then blow on the warm, wet skin to make the menthol's tingling more intense.
- Sucking on a lozenge for a vapor effect.
- Pouring and then lapping up extremely dry champagne with low residual sugar across the vulva.
- Playing with her G spot, vaginal opening, or anus for more stimulation.
- Using sex toys, such as a finger vibrator, mini vibrating tongue (which is shaped and textured like real skin), or a glass spinner (medical-grade tempered glass that is lined with pleasure bumps to stimulate the clitoris as the user rotates it).
- Stimulating other hot spots, such as her nipples. Coming up for air every now and then will help her to feel even more connected to you. It also allows you to see her radiating face.

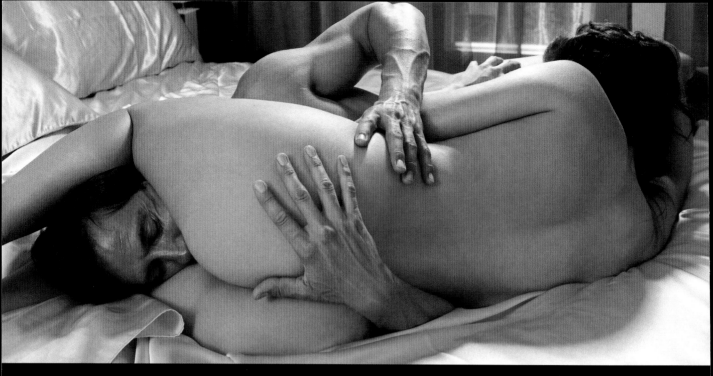

Sexual Homework

In pursuing oral pleasures, don't be afraid to change your techniques from time to time, giving things a twist or embarking upon new activities entirely. When it comes to foreplay, keeping things fresh and varied is the key to keeping long-term sex passionate. So throw some new ideas out there, or give a new maneuver a spin. You never know what can turn any particular sexual rendezvous into the best of all time.

Get Artistic—Get some chocolate paints, such as the Lover's Paintbox Body Paint, and become each other's murals, basking in the slick, smooth sensations as your run your hands over every part of each other's bodies. Write each other love messages, and cover each other with compliments. Try using the paintbrush for a more teasing effect, followed by little laps at your tasty treat for sweeter seduction.

Kitty Licks—Perform cunnilingus with a feline tongue stroke. Much like a cat cleaning its paws, you can lap at the vulva with short, repetitive licks. Save the clitoris for last, and be sure to add more pressure to this area, depending on what your partner can handle.

Passion Pearls—Take a strand of pearls, coil them around his penis so that the beads fit snuggly against it. Now place your palms on either side of his penis, and intertwine your fingers before sliding your hands up and down the shaft as you twirl the tip of his penis with your tongue.

Oral Delectable—Add a sexy twist to your oral activities: Learn the erotic art of oral lovemaking with Sinclair's Kiss & Tell Kit, Oral Sex Delights Kit, or Oral Sex board game. Any of these are sure to make you want to pucker up more often!

SOIXANTE-NEUF: DOUBLING YOUR ORALLY ORGASMIC PLEASURES

Soixante-neuf, popularly known as "69," is sex play where both lovers can perform oral sex on each other simultaneously. During such total body involvement, lovers can experience climax at the same time. In order for both lovers to experience oral-genital contact, both of you should lie side to side, heads in opposite directions. Alternatively, one of you can lie down with the other lying on top in the opposite direction.

The "half 69" is yet another option that is good if there are significant height differences between you and your partner; one lover lies on his or her back while the other is over her on all fours, facing the opposite direction. (Note: It may be better for her to be on top since many women feel choked in being on the bottom during 69.)

"For it was not into my ear you whispered, but into my heart. It was not my lips you kissed, but my soul."

—JUDY GARLAND

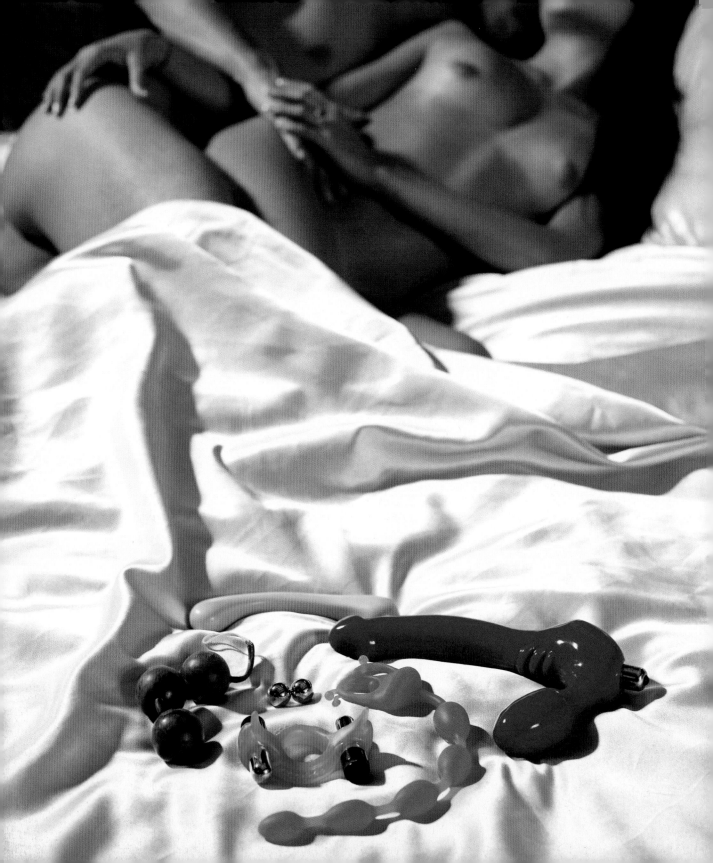

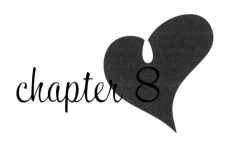

chapter 8

Sex Toys to Enhance
Arousal and Pleasure

SEX PLAY TAKES ON a whole new meaning when you invite this third party into your bedroom. It's the best kind of threesome around—you, your lover, and your favorite sexual enhancement product. But for many lovers, overwhelmed by the selection of sex toys out there, where to start is the big question. So you may be among the millions of couples who are in the dark when it comes to the thousands of products, often called "sex aids" or "marital aids," that can light up your sex life. Some are staple items that every sex-toy chest must have. Others have hit the market more recently, playing off of today's latest technology and turning you on in ways previously unimaginable.

You may also be uncomfortable with the idea of using sex toys, let alone shopping for one. This is in part because, historically speaking, sex toys have typically been regarded as "kinky," "perverted," or "pathetic." Not to mention the pervasive belief that sex toys are used only by certain types of people, namely the lonely, losers, or the seedy sort.

*"Love and compassion are necessities, not luxuries.
Without them, humanity cannot survive."*

—THE DALAI LAMA

Today, sexual enhancement products are available almost everywhere. In major corporate outlets and small retail stores alike, you'll find sex toys that offer a positive, healthful way to revamp your sex life. Sex toys are for everybody, whether you're in a relationship or not, with a partner or not. They have the potential for more alluring sex in so many ways. Namely, they can improve the quality of the sex you're having by improving the way you connect to your partner, the sensations you experience, or the orgasm(s) you relish.

Many enhancement products are even endorsed by health practitioners. This is in large part because these playtime treasures can help to get you out of a sexual rut, rekindling your relationship. They can introduce enthralling sensations, whether enjoyed solo or with your partner, and keep things varied and novel. Meant to complement your sex life, sex toys can add to the intensity of your lovemaking and increase your sexual mastery.

INTRODUCING SEX TOYS

Before shopping for a sex toy, make sure that your partner is on board with your efforts first. While some lovers like the occasional bedroom surprise or receiving a sex toy as a gift, sex toy shopping is best done as a team effort. Buying a sex toy can be a very personal experience, based on your desires, preferred sensations, curiosities, and aims. Shopping together allows you to get to know each other in new ways as you reveal your likes and dislikes, sexual yens, and vulnerabilities. In charting unknown territory both in and out of the bedroom, you'll bond as you choose your pleasures.

In broaching the subject of sex toy shopping with your lover, sensitivity is vital, since some partners may take offense to the very suggestion of sex toys, worrying that the sex isn't good enough. Worse yet, if they buy into the previously discussed old-fashioned notions about sex toys, they may fret over what kind of "degenerate" you've become. So in proposing sex toy shopping, let your lover know where you're coming from. Stay positive. Explain why you're interested in enhancing your sex life with toys and why you feel it's important that this is a team effort. Framing your sex toy shopping as an erotic escapade will make your suggestion less threatening. It will also motivate your lover to provide assistance.

Shopping for sex toys can also be terribly exciting. You never know what you're going to find or what's in store for the two of you. Sex toy shopping can be a form of foreplay, getting you piqued for sex as never before.

*Sex*PERTISE

Research has found that users of sex aids have sex more frequently and experience more satisfying sex with their partners. A 2004 Berman Center study found that almost half of females ages eighteen to fifty-five had used a vibrator. These women were more interested in sex, reached climax more easily, and were likelier to have a better quality of life. The study further found that 30 percent of couples use vibrators. Vibrators are quite popular in that they can:

- Improve sexual functioning
- Enhance your emotional and sexual intimacy
- Boost pleasuring
- Enhance eroticism
- Allow for mutual sexual and emotional satisfaction

SELECTING YOUR SEX TOY

A sex toy can be almost any object used to enhance sex. They can range anywhere from the homemade to expensive designer products. There is no set standard as far as what is and isn't a sex toy, as humans have shown a willingness to get intimate with almost anything. For example, a recent survey of sex toy experimentation conducted by the *Portland Mercury*, found that respondents had masturbated with beer cozies, G.I. Joe figurines, leather gloves, uncooked beef franks, vibrating pens, plungers, Hello Kitty(s), vibrating toothbrushes, Sharpies, warm cantaloupes, and condom-covered cucumbers.

While the sky is the limit when it comes to sex toys, do practice safe sex-toy use. Items that aren't made for pleasuring can cause injury, infection, or end up stuck in places they weren't meant to go. With the thousands of sex toys at your disposal, be sure to stick to quality products from well-respected outlets that have your interests at heart.

Thankfully, there are plenty of such respectable stores out there, such as the Sinclair Institute, Babeland, and Good Vibrations. A number of reputable sex educators and therapists also sell trusted sexual enhancement products through their own personal websites. They're all out to make your shopping experience as easy as possible. Many of these online stores will often highlight products that have been popular with lovers and/or categorize them; for instance, "sex toys for him," "vibrators," "adult novelties," "dildos," "bestsellers," "new items," "waterproof," or by brand or dollar amount. Such organization makes it easier for you and your lover to process your selections.

In buying your first sex toys, you may want to start with less expensive products—at least until you have a better idea of the types of enhancement products you enjoy. You may also want to start out simple, since most products do not come with any instructions, let alone a user's manual. In shopping, keep in mind:

- What you want the toy to do
- Where you want to use it
- Whether it can be used in a number of different ways (e.g., for his and her pleasure)
- What about it arouses you

YOUR SEX TOY INGREDIENTS

When shopping for sex toys, quality is a must, as you'll likely be putting these products on or in your or your lover's body. Your bodies deserve nothing but the best. Here are some significant ingredients found in sex toy—and what you need to know about them:

Silicone: Despite being more expensive than other toys, silicone sex toys are very popular since they're hygienic, plastic, hypoallergenic, durable, and available in many attractive colors. Whether hard or soft, all of these high-quality products can bend easily and retain heat nicely, making them very body friendly. They also conduct vibrations amazingly well. For lovers interested in a toy that feels and looks more realistic, similar to CyberSkin, go for the VixSkin silicone toys.

SEXUAL Q&A: PHTHALATES

I've heard that I should avoid sex toy products made of phthalates. What is that exactly, and what's the concern?

Pronounced "THAL-ates," phthalates are plasticizing chemicals used by the chemical industry for making dyes and for softening plastics. These esters are used to make many of the products we deal with daily, like shower curtains, medical equipment, cosmetics, clothing, building materials, and tubing. When it comes to sex toys, they're added to polyvinyl chloride (PVC), since they can cheaply and easily make the products more flexible and durable. Unfortunately, they're what cause toys to change color, develop a nasty smell and taste, and get sticky. While scientists are still trying to determine if phthalates are harmful to humans, studies have shown that large doses of the chemical are harmful to rats, resulting in fetal death, malformations, and reproductive toxicity. A report by the Danish Environmental Protection Agency, however, advises that using a sex toy with phthalates for one hour or less per day poses no health risks, unless you are pregnant or nursing.

Still, some lovers would rather be safe than sorry. If you want to avoid phthalates, steer clear of toys that smell like plastic or that list PVC, diethylhexylphthalate (DEHP) or diisononylphalate (DINP) as one of its ingredients. These tend to be jelly-rubber toys and are best covered with a condom before touching the body. Instead, shop for sex toys that are made of hard plastic, Lucite, acrylic, glass, metal, or elastomer. Most of these materials are firm and smooth, offering good pressure. They're also long-lasting and sometimes cheaper than silicone sex toys. Lucite and acrylic are known for being shatter-free and hard to break (though they can crack). Glass toys are super in that they retain heat or cold really well and require only a dab of lube for an incredibly slippery effect. For a softer toy, elastomer is nice in that it is hypoallergenic and soft. (Its drawbacks are, however, that it is slightly porous and cannot be disinfected.) Lastly, ceramic sex toys are nonporous, dishwasher safe, and durable.

CyberSkin: While CyberSkin products are attractive for feeling fleshy and looking realistic, this is a material that is best to avoid since it poses a number of problems. In being porous, CyberSkin sex toys cannot be disinfected or used with a silicone lube. They may contain rubber softeners, like phthalates, which may be associated with negative health consequences. If you choose CyberSkin products, however, know that condoms can make for safer play and easier cleanup. Powdering the toy with cornstarch after use will prevent it from getting sticky.

Jelly Rubber: Jelly rubber toys are soft, porous (even when silicone is one of the ingredients) materials that may contain phthalates or latex (which some people are allergic to). They are good at conducting vibrations.

Vinyl: Less porous, more solid, and longer-lasting than jelly rubber, vinyl is an attractive alternative for some lovers.

S*ex*ercise 8.1 Get Comfortable with Your Toy

You've picked out your sex toy. As with any other product you use on your body, you want to fully grasp how the merchandise works. Plus, you want to seduce yourselves with it. Nearly everything in life is much more incredible when you allow yourself to luxuriate in it—from a bottle of wine to a steamy hot tub. So in getting the most out of your new toy and the novelty of the first time experience, take your time with it, including the following:

1. Make sure your sex toy has no sharp edges or seams. (If it does, return the product.)

2. Figure out how it works before you get started; you won't get very far if the device requires batteries and you don't have any.

3. Wash the toy before using it. (If it's not waterproof, avoid getting water near the battery case.)

4. Test it. Let yourselves become aroused by your sex toy. If it vibrates, first test it on the palm of your hand, playing with the pulsation settings and applying different types of pressure. You may note that holding the toy too tightly or pressing it too much into your hand will only send more vibrations into your hand, which is not something you want to have happen when you're playing with an erogenous zone. Now imagine what these different pressures might feel like on your hottest spots. What would your beloved like the most and where?

S*ex*PERTISE

Since they're nonporous, silicone sex toys are great in that they can be easily cleaned. The most effective way to disinfect these toys is by boiling them for five to ten minutes (Note: Only toys with removable vibes can be boiled). You can also stick them in your dishwasher, or scrub them with warm water and soap. As long as they're treated with care, silicone toys have a longer lifespan than toys made of other materials.

To keep all of your other sex toys clean and safe, you can use:

• Soap and warm water
• A cleaner, such as Buzz Fresh wipes
• A latex condom over the toy

 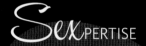

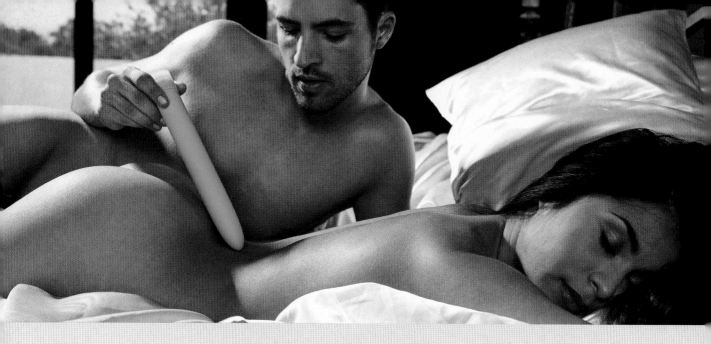

In the Bedroom: Take Your Time

DON'T RUSH TO THE most reactive erogenous zones right away. Instead, run the toy along the side of your partner's body, starting at the arch of the foot and working your way up the calf, then the hip, then the waist . . . then circle down the other side, perhaps taunting the nipples or other sensitive areas along the way. If the device vibrates, don't turn it on just yet. See how your lover feels as you press the toy firmly against the skin, making time the ultimate tease as you trace the body.

Slowly, work your way to your lover's erogenous zones as arousal deepens, gliding over parts of the genitals you plan to toy with in a bit. At times, let your touch linger. Other times, massage the area just enough to torment him or her before moving on to the next hot spot. As you get closer to honing in on an area, such as the clitoris or perineum, use some lube. This is especially important if your lover is well-shaven; otherwise, your partner will likely chafe.

If your gadget vibrates, turn it on, first running it over parts of your lover's body that might be clothed. Start at a low setting. This is in part because a lower speed may be

all that you need in some spots and in part because you're still flirting with the erogenous zones. As your lover gets more aroused, adjust the speed, working your way up if desired or necessary. Stronger vibrations work better for some lovers.

As you grow more familiar with your sex toy and each other's responses, experiment with different pressures and speeds. Also consider how they relate to different positions. You may find that you become much more easily aroused getting played with on all fours than you do on your back. Likewise, you may want to add other enhancements for more and greater sensations.

More than anything, make sure that you're communicating with each other. Tell your partner what felt good where, if you would like more or less intensity, or if the stimulation needs to be more direct versus indirect. Ask if your love would like more lube.

DILDOS VS. VIBRATORS

There is no clear distinction between a dildo and a vibrator. Most people distinguish the two by the fact that the vibrator vibrates, yet many dildos are now being advertised with vibrating features. Given that dildos and vibrators today offer so much more than the originals, allow yourselves to think outside of the box when it comes to exploring these toy options. Get creative with a dildo, as some models can be attached to furniture, such as a chair or bed, beach balls, and other objects for your pleasuring. Consider dildos, such as Lelo's Ella, with one end for stimulating the G spot while another end is for erotic stimulation. Or check out a clitoral massager that requires nothing more than a tight pair of panties. Women can slip one of these devices between their clitoris and panties, relishing secret pleasures as they go about their daily tasks.

DOUBLE-YOUR-PLEASURE TOYS

Since we've covered some of the popular sex toys for solo pleasure in Chapter 5, in this chapter, we're going to feature products that largely benefit couples' pleasuring. Furthermore, we're going to showcase toys that often get overshadowed by the vibrator, as well as some of the latest technology.

Oscillators

Oscillators are toys that oscillate—or swing—an area of the body, such as a female's clitoris and labia, back and forth. Offering different levels of intensity, popular brands include the Eroscillator 2 Plus and the Better Sex Synergy Pleasure System. Generating up to twelve thousand oscillations per minute, these toys can be used by both men and women to rev up pleasure and achieve more intense orgasms. Oscillators are known to intensify clitoral, G spot, testicular, and perineal pleasures, as well as provide comfortable nipple and penis massage.

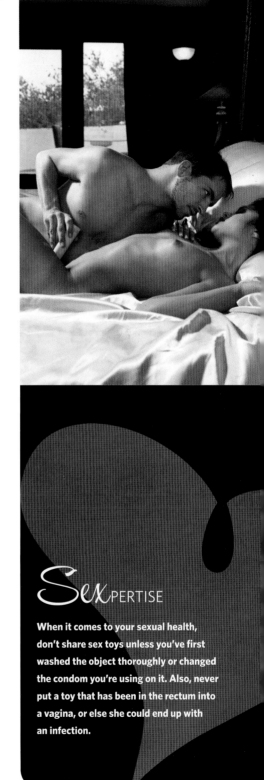

$\mathcal{S}\mathit{ex}$PERTISE

When it comes to your sexual health, don't share sex toys unless you've first washed the object thoroughly or changed the condom you're using on it. Also, never put a toy that has been in the rectum into a vagina, or else she could end up with an infection.

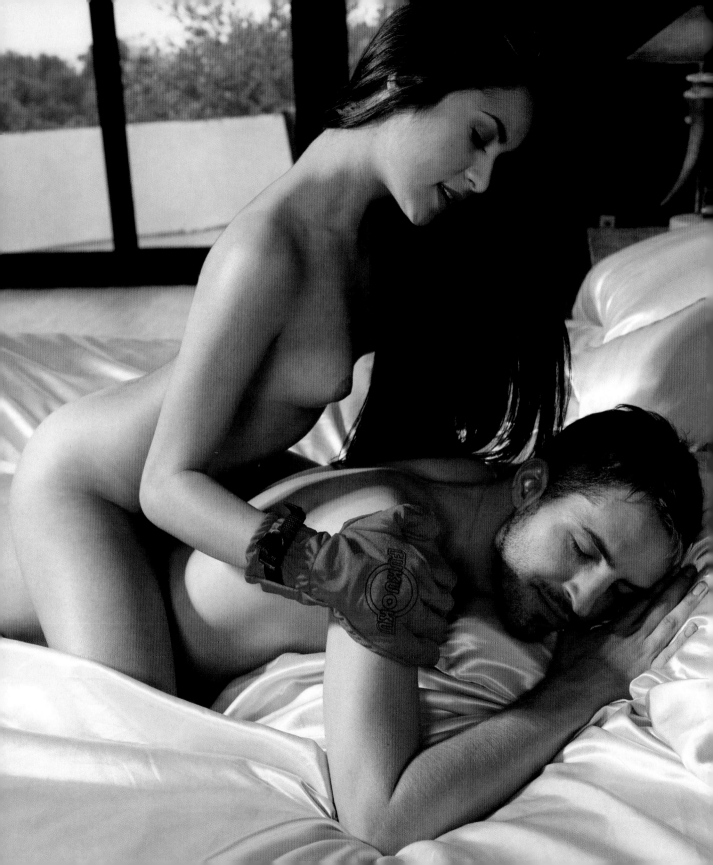

Massage Gloves

Magic hands take on a whole new meaning with massage gloves, such as the Fukuoku Five Finger Massage Glove. Each fingertip is charged with its own minivibrator, with the glove producing up to nine thousand vibrations per minute anywhere you want. When the vibe is set at the very tip of your finger, your whole digit vibrates! This is especially great for when your fingers are strained and tired from lots of loving or when you want to give a marvelous massage. Available in waterproof Lycra, this gadget can also make for some wonderful underwater or shower play. Try giving each other a hand, mutually masturbating each other as you each wear one of the set's gloves.

Pleasure Balls

The modern day version of Ben Wa balls, pleasure balls are used for vaginal or anal play and aim to tease. Using lube, slowly insert each ball into the vagina or anus, and begin squeezing your pelvic floor muscles around the balls for continuous stimulation. Available in latex, handblown glass, plastic, and gold-plated, some are linked by a silk string or chain that can be pulled on as a lover approaches climax, magnifying the orgasmic sensations as each ball makes its way out of the anus or vagina.

Love Rings

Known also as penis rings, cock rings, and erection rings, love rings work by constricting blood flow out of the penis. Keeping the blood in the shaft of the penis results in a thicker, harder, longer-lasting erection. Men love the way these rings look and feel. The toy version of a medical device called the constriction ring, this gadget can enhance a man's erections, especially if he's having trouble attaining or maintaining an erection. In doing so, the heightened penis sensitivity changes the way he experiences orgasms and ejaculation. These rings can be easily removed during or after intercourse.

When it comes to doubling the pleasure, vibrating love rings are ideal in simultaneously stimulating the clitoris and scrotum, often resulting in powerful orgasms for both lovers. Sensations are sent throughout the penis as she experiences direct clitoral stimulation. Such versions of the love ring leave your hands free to caress, grope, massage, or spank your partner. They also give you something to hold, pull, tug, or grab onto during sex (just don't squeeze or pinch too much on any one point!).

Love rings come in all types of material, primarily surgical-grade latex, leather, and latex-free rubber. In experimenting with love rings, simple, flexible, adjustable sorts are recommended for beginners in that they are easy to pull on and take off. They also tend to be more stretchable for a looser feel that may be more comfortable at first. In using the love ring, whether you plan to wear it yourself or put one on your lover, all you need to do is stretch the ring with your fingers, much like you would a rubber band, and pull it over the head of the penis and down the shaft (Note: Make sure your fingers are dry—you don't want your grip to slip, which could cause a snap to the penis!). Once the love ring has been fitted around the root of the penis and balls, carefully let the ring contract back to its original size.

Love Rings PLUS

As you become more familiar with love rings, you may want to try one with snaps, buttons, straps, and buckles to better adjust the fit. The benefit of these rings is that they never slip. Yet it can be all too easy for pubic hair to get caught. Using a dab of lube on the ring or penis before wearing the ring can diminish any hair issues or pinching of the skin. Velcro or beads that can slide are an easier alternative and are less likely to cause pain, but they can slip. Adjustable rings, which you can open up all the way, can be slipped over the penis and behind the scrotum, before tightening for a comfortable fit. Solid rings are recommended only for those who know what kind of feel they like when it comes to love rings. These must be put on before a man gets an erection and cannot be removed until he loses his erection.

An important thing to remember in using a love ring is that you should not leave the ring in place for more than thirty minutes. If you feel pain or discomfort at any point, remove the device immediately. Also, don't try to use any homemade love rings, such as those made out of rubber bands, as they can be hard to take off and may cut your skin.

In playing with vibrating penis rings, be sure to experiment with different positions and angles, since you will have varied results. Rotating the love ring so that the vibe is in a different place can also provide different types of stimulation on the perineum, scrotum, clitoris . . . whatever you choose to delight.

Sexpertise

You may wonder how to store your sex toys discreetly—especially if you have children. If this is your dilemma, consider keeping your goods in a jewelry box, a toy box with a lock and key, or an intimate-accessory bag that can be easily stored on a shelf in your closet. No matter where you decide to store your toys, be sure to:

• Take your batteries out of the product to preserve battery power and the toy itself. Batteries can corrode inside of the toy.

• Store toys in separate compartments so they don't ruin each other; for example, jelly rubber can dissolve silicone.

Double-Penetration Dildos

For lovers who are into simultaneous stimulation, double-ended dildos, such as the Feeldoe, are one way partners can experience simultaneous vaginal-anal, vaginal-vaginal, or anal-anal penetration. When approached safely, especially with condoms and lubricant, this slow, controlled type of sex play can leave both lovers satisfied in a variety of positions as their orifices are penetrated by each bulbous "pony" end of the dildo.

DOUBLING YOUR PLEASURE WITH DOUBLE PENETRATION

Double penetration (DP) has become a mainstay of adult videos because it is a type of sexual experience that is difficult to achieve yet intensely erotic and exotic for some. The term "double penetration" usually refers to a woman being simultaneously penetrated vaginally and anally. When adult videos promise double penetration (also known as an "American sandwich"), that is usually what they mean. Yet it can also refer to partners being anally penetrated at the same time. A woman can also be penetrated vaginally while her lover is penetrated anally. Two other types of double penetration are "vaginal double-penetration" and "double anal penetration." Those terms refer to two phalluses entering the same orifice at the same time (one from the rear and the other from the front). Double anal penetration is particularly difficult because the anus does not stretch as readily as the vagina to accommodate insertion.

In the case of a female experiencing double penetration, her sex organs are filled deeply and completely. The walls of the vagina and the anus receive a type and intensity of friction that women cannot attain from any other sex act. The emotional experience of DP can be equally intense.

DP Inflatable Balls

Another double penetration option for sex toy enthusiasts is an inflatable ball, usually nine to eighteen inches in diameter, that's made of sturdy rubber and designed to support the weight of one or two people—and with an attachment for a dildo on it. When used with your lover, this toy allows for many unique positions, such as double penetration for a woman, who can lay face down on the ball for vaginal penetration while her partner penetrates her anally.

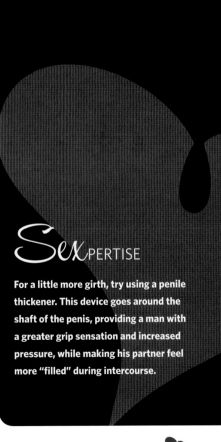

S*ex*PERTISE

For a little more girth, try using a penile thickener. This device goes around the shaft of the penis, providing a man with a greater grip sensation and increased pressure, while making his partner feel more "filled" during intercourse.

Board Games

Game nights can add a playful element to sex, especially since it can be equally nice to lose or to win. Plus, playing with a board game or a deck of sex cards can make for more diverse date nights, keeping things amusing and unexpected. In being "dared" to try this move or reveal this secret or have this kind of sex, you can let go in ways you've never imagined possible. Among the many games available are those under the names of "Fantasy and Romance," "Sexy Casino," "Sexy Slang," "Oral Sex," "Truth or Dare," "Kama Sutra," and "Spin the Bottle."

Sex Books

Whether to become more sexually enlightened, learn a few new tricks, or to get aroused, sex books and audio books can offer you hours of inspiration and excuses for exploration. Enjoy some quality bedtime reading learning about sacred sex, sex and culture, sex and relationships, or different types of sex, such as quickies, for greater sexual response. Become aroused with book erotica, from art to photography to comics. Seduce one other by reading aloud passages from erotic novels and short stories, including those about spanking, three-ways, and woman-on-top.

Adult DVDs

From softcore to hardcore, there are a number of adult sex movies for your viewing pleasure. Some are educational—such as videos on the G spot, sexual positions, the taboo, advanced sexual techniques, and Tantra—while others are strictly for entertainment. Some have no plot while others, which tend to be female-directed (for women by women), have much more of a story line. No matter what your forte—classic, fetish, same-sex, anime/hentai (Japanese erotic animation)—you're guaranteed to find it in the adult entertainment industry. Whether looking for ideas or libidinal exhilarations, adult DVDs or digital downloads offer you an opportunity to play the voyeur—and enhance your own sex life in the process.

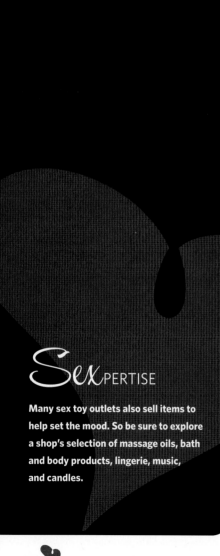

S*ex*PERTISE

Many sex toy outlets also sell items to help set the mood. So be sure to explore a shop's selection of massage oils, bath and body products, lingerie, music, and candles.

WIRELESS SEX TOYS

Many toys are Internet-enabled and can be used over the phone or the Web for cybersex. Only in their infant stages, some of the following are among your most basic ones.

Remote-Controlled Toys

Wireless vibrators, including love rings, can entertain lovers who are up to thirty yards away from each other. These gadgets, such as the Wireless Remote Egg Vibrator, can be inserted or worn anywhere you fancy—whether out on the town or in the privacy of your own home. Your partner can then have fun adjusting the different vibrating and pulsing functions for your pleasure.

Audio-Controlled Devices

These vibrators, such as the Talk2Me, work by plugging the toy's transmitter into an audio source, such as a telephone, microphone, television, or computer. The vibrator then reacts to vocalizations made into its transmitter's built-in microphone, turning these sounds into vibrations. The smaller part of the vibrator reacts to bass sounds, while the bigger part resonates with treble notes.

Cell-Phone Vibes

These toys are vibrators that work wirelessly with your cell phone. Such a vibe is activated by calls made to and from your cell phone, with the call triggering a patterned, vibrating sequence that lasts for the entire phone conversation. Great for long-distance relationships, gadgets such as the Boditalk are compatible with all cell phones or can be used as a regular vibrator without your cell. Other cell-phone vibes rely on text messaging. The Toy Bluetooth vibrator, for example, is a wireless vibrating bullet that is worn internally and linked to your mobile phone. It is subsequently controlled by text messages sent to your phone, resulting in vibrations.

Teledildonics

Using technologically-advanced vibrators, teledildonics are gadgets that enable your partner to control your pleasure over the Internet from any PC anywhere in the world. Devices such as the Sinulator allow your lover to adjust the speed and stimulation for your pleasure via a transmitter and receiver. Set up a webcam to let your lover watch you climax as well.

THE RIGHT SEX EQUIPMENT

Sexual performance takes on an exotic flair when you've got the right gear. Whether helping to suspend, prop up, bend, or move and stroke you or your lover in brand new ways, sex equipment, including furniture, can make for novel sexual positions while hitting all of your hottest spots.

Door Sex-Swing

The door sex-swing can be suspended wherever there's a door. Just hang this gadget's acrylic tubes over the top of the door, and close the door. Then, slide the loops onto the receiver's legs and adjust them on the thighs, balancing yourself with the arm handles.

Super Sex Sling

For him or her: Lovers can experience longer-lasting foreplay or sex with the super sex sling. A thick pad goes behind the neck. A fully adjustable suspension strap can then be positioned and secured with the use of Velcro cuffs. The product makers claim that the super sex sling helps to prevent leg, hip, and back strain, as well as fatigue.

Positioning Sex Strap

For improved penetration and stimulation during rear-entry intercourse, this padded strap goes around the receiving partner's lower waist. The receiving partner's bottom can then be comfortably lifted, with the top partner using adjustable handles to leverage him- or herself. The end result: deeper penetration (including for G spot access) and better thrusting.

Love Rocker

The Love Rocker is portable sex furniture that is part bed, part chair. The swinging partner, who is lying or seated on the unit, can be gently and effortlessly swung back and forth toward the "thrusting" partner for better penetration. This means less work for both lovers, resulting in more relaxing, less tiring, and longer-lasting sex. The unit can be assembled or disassembled in minutes and discreetly stored in your closet.

Love Pegasus

Love Pegasus is the brand name of five different types of padded platforms that can make for better sex: Tilt-Incline Duo, Incline, Platform, Rock-A-Box, and Tilt. Such sex furniture, made of soft cushions, enables partners to comfortably have sex in different positions. Many lovers find that the platforms increase their chance of experiencing orgasm, since they lift the pelvis for better G spot stimulation.

Loving-Angles

In going from lounge furniture to adult playground, Loving-Angles offer different types of angles and support. This sex furniture can be rearranged and involves five non-slip pads that come in various shapes and angles. Supportive, comfortable, and versatile, they can be used in different combinations or individually for more pleasurable sensations once you have converted the furniture for sex play.

Tantra Chair

This chair, which can be used as both "regular furniture" and sex equipment, has two arcs with a dip at the center. With its gentle arc cradling the body, the chair provides both partners with comfort and support. Your entire body is supported as you attempt new positions such as those of the Kama Sutra, with lovers feeling weightless. Lovers can experience amazing pleasure as the female controls the depth and angles of her pelvis during sex, bettering her chance of experiencing orgasm.

Monkey Rocker

This rocking seat is equipped with an attachable hand assembly in the front, a cushioned seat, and an attachable dildo in the middle. It works with your movement, so you control the pace and type of stroke you want in different positions.

"We may have our private opinions, but why should they be a bar to the meeting of the hearts?"

—MAHATMA GANDHI

Sexual Homework

Remember, it pays to play—and this chapter summarized just a handful of the countless products available for your sexual experimentation. Sex-toy makers are eternal inventors, always coming out with something innovative and wilder than ever imagined. So in striving for continued better sex, full of new life, be sure to always check up on the latest! Consider, too, how you can turn a number of items around your house into sexual enhancements.

Make it an Arabian night: Explore all of the different ways you can use a silky scarf, such as . . .

- Wrap the scarf around your face so that it covers the lower half. Seeing only your eyes suddenly makes you mysterious. Your lover will surely be up for an exotic adventure.
- Blindfold your lover and then feed him or her chocolate-covered strawberries, grapes—anything sweet and sensual. And don't be shy in giving your love a taste of you every now and then, whether it's your lips, nipples (perhaps dipped in powdered sugar), or other parts of your body.
- Experiment with tactile titillation, and run different textured scarves over each other's bodies. Doing so provides different sensations.

- Use a scarf as part of a strip show. You could be completely nude and wrap it like a garter around your thigh. Or you can use it for a seductive song-and-dance number, using the scarf as though you were holding a cane.
- Wrap it around your lover's neck like a collar, and tell your partner that you're the one in charge and that your love is to follow your every command.
- Tie your partner to the bedposts using scarves, straddle your partner, facing away, and bend over to deliver fantastic oral sex. In this near-69 position, with the perfect view (of your buttocks), your lover will be longing to return the favor.

Sexy Dice: Let die, such as glow-in-the-dark foreplay dice, guide your foreplay, directing you and your lover to specific sex acts or erotic foreplay activities. Allow yourselves to sexually unwind with the hot suggestions and commands that are "thrown." Or tease each other with sex kits for him and her—sure to double your pleasure!

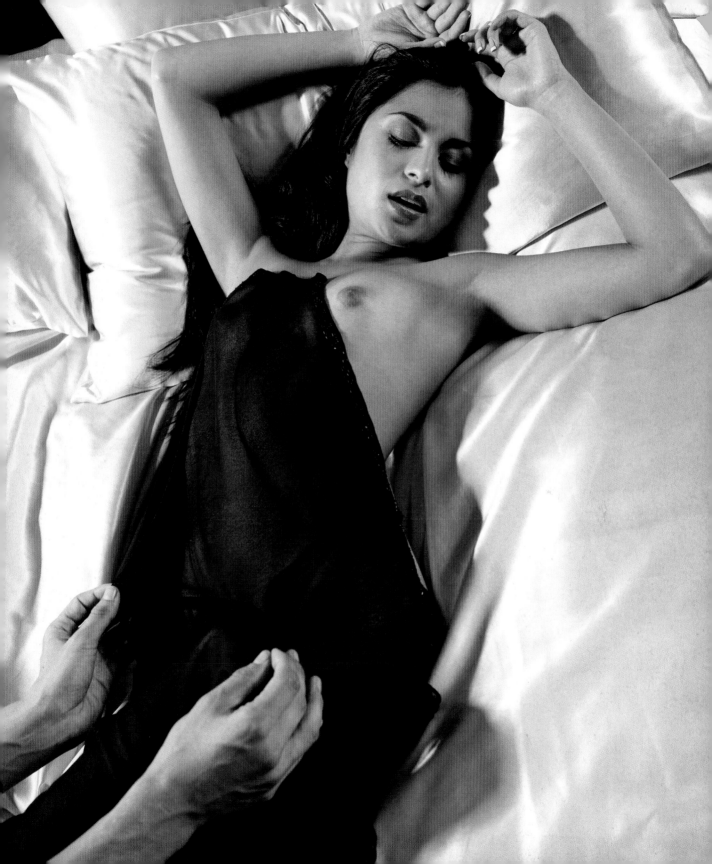

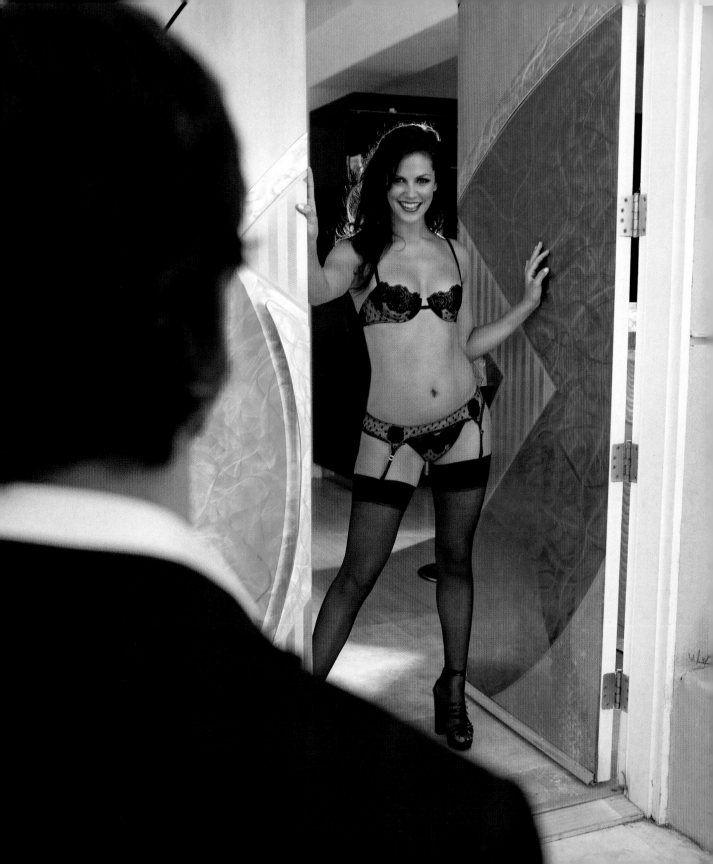

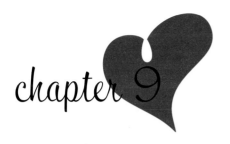

chapter 9

Exploring Your Erotic Curiosities: Fantasy, Sexual Scenarios, and Role-Playing

IT'S A PROFOUND SEX TRUTH that cannot be said enough: The key to more satisfying sex lies between your ears, not your legs. Your brain is your biggest sex organ— and that's why a large part of your greater intimacy efforts need to involve teasing your mind.

Even couples who have great sex need to work to sustain satisfying sex. Such lovemaking cannot be taken for granted. Luckily, striving to eroticize your sex life is hardly "work." These erotic exertions are nothing but fun—as long as that's the way you frame them.

"The only transformer and alchemist that turns everything into gold is love."

—ANAÏS NIN

YOUR EROTIC IMAGINATION

When it comes to your sexual imagination, the sky is the limit. With everything under the stars a potential turn-on, let your erotic ideas run wild, feeding your libido, boosting your arousal, and giving you and your lover renewed vigor for bedroom explorations. Realizing your erotic curiosities simply requires a little ingenuity, trust, and communication.

When it comes to sharing our erotic mental imagery with our lovers, many of us become timid and shy. We don't know what to share or how to go about it. Afraid of offending our partners or being perceived as a bit bizarre, we bite our tongues. Such silence hurts us, sexually speaking. We can end up feeling sexually stifled, becoming frustrated and resentful that our sexual needs aren't being met. That may make for relationship troubles in and out of the bedroom, so don't be shy.

SHARING YOUR SEXUAL THOUGHTS

Most sex experts will tell you that the biggest obstacle to couples sharing their erotic fantasies is getting past the embarrassment of doing so. Just the thought of sexual storytelling—especially when it involves sexual role-playing—is enough to make some lovers blush. You're exposing some of your deepest, most personal thoughts, perhaps with a rawness your lover may have never seen before.

Unveiling the depths of our sexual imagination involves some risk, even if we do not wish to actually act out certain scenarios. That in itself is part of what makes such erotic exchanges so sensuous. This risk factor can invoke your most passionate sexual moments as you reveal yourselves to one another. To get past any embarrassment you may feel, you need to remind each other—and yourself—that you have the right to sexual happiness and expression.

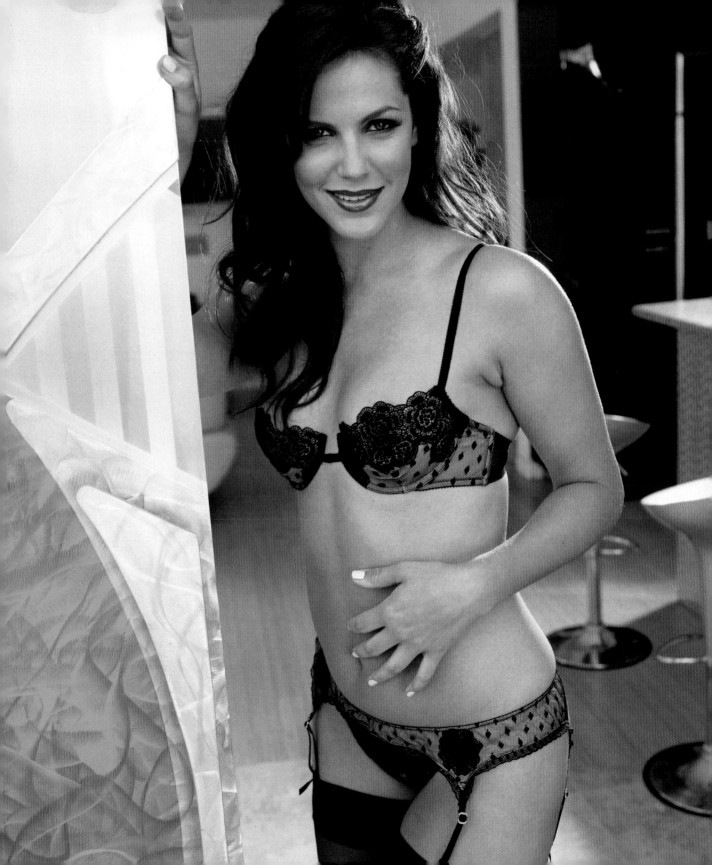

$\mathscr{S}$exercise 9.1: Make Your Sex List

Start by making a wish list of your sexual wants. Do this when you're in an erotic mindset, away from the rest of your daily life.

The ideal time to do this is when you're masturbating. As you stimulate yourself, explore the thoughts that enter your mind, taking care not to police them. Don't sell yourself short by editing your own erotic tales. It's often the forbidden that garners the greatest sexual reactions and stirrings.

Once you have an idea of what you want, whether that be a specific sex act, scene, or a novelette for role-playing, think about what you want to say in a way your partner will be the most receptive to your sharing. Rehearse it out loud so that you can feel more comfortable with it, so that it doesn't feel so foreign. Ask yourself why this scenario arouses you—past experience, the thrill of the taboo, etc.—and answer yourself, as you may very well be asked the same thing by your partner later when you share your sex list. Knowing the answer will help both you and your partner understand your vision of sensational sex.

In getting started, you can use the following as a guide, making sure to add your own erotic flavor by filling in the adjectives, verbs, and other delectable details:

 "I can't wait till our next private moment, since I've been having these visions of my (adjectives) mouth making its way down your (body part) . . . your fingers racing over my (adjective) (body part), hungry for my (adjective) (part of genitalia) . . . sending tremors through your body as my lips (verb) your (adjective) (part of genitalia), my tongue doing its magic . . . . I can't wait for you to work your swollen, aching (part of genitalia) between my (body part), my (part of genitalia) dripping, begging for a taste of (partner's name) . . . . Hearing you (verb) as you remove my (article of clothing) with your teeth, your head (adverb ending in "ly") madly between my legs turns me on like nothing else . . . especially as I please your every whim by (verb ending in "ing") . . . ."

SEXY STORYTELLING

There is more than one way to share your sex list with your partner. You can tell it as a story, which may be best if you're feeling shy. Instead of admitting that you want to try "X," you might frame it as something you just happened to read about or overhear. Or you can be quite frank in your intentions, playfully challenging your lover to a sex storytelling contest: Which of you will develop the most erotic story? In all cases, you become a storyteller, planting the seeds of seduction while not taking as much responsibility for your lurid, shocking, or devilish desires. There's nothing wrong with taking this approach if it allows you to unmask your deepest desires.

Still, while storytelling provides a lot of safety in one sense, it can be quite nerve-wracking in another, especially if telling tales has never been your forte. You may worry that your story lines are too unoriginal or unimaginative. Or you may draw a blank altogether.

SEX-WRITER'S BLOCK

Know that it's okay to "borrow" fantasies. And outright quoting a line or two of your favorite red-hot passages for your own private purposes isn't going to hurt anybody. Here are some ready sources:

- Erotica books by authors such as Nancy Friday, Erica Jong, and Caleb Knight
- Sex-tryst confessions in sultry nude magazines
- Free online erotica websites
- Writing collections such as Penthouse Forum
- Sex and relationship Web blogs
- Movies with erotic story lines

Take the liberty to punch up your work—or whatever written lines you've borrowed. Get a thesaurus of sexual terminology or an erotic words glossary. Keep a sex-dream journal of your nightly visions. Remember, sexual scenarios are all around you. See what amorous animations register with you. Better yet, think about what would arouse your lover's libido.

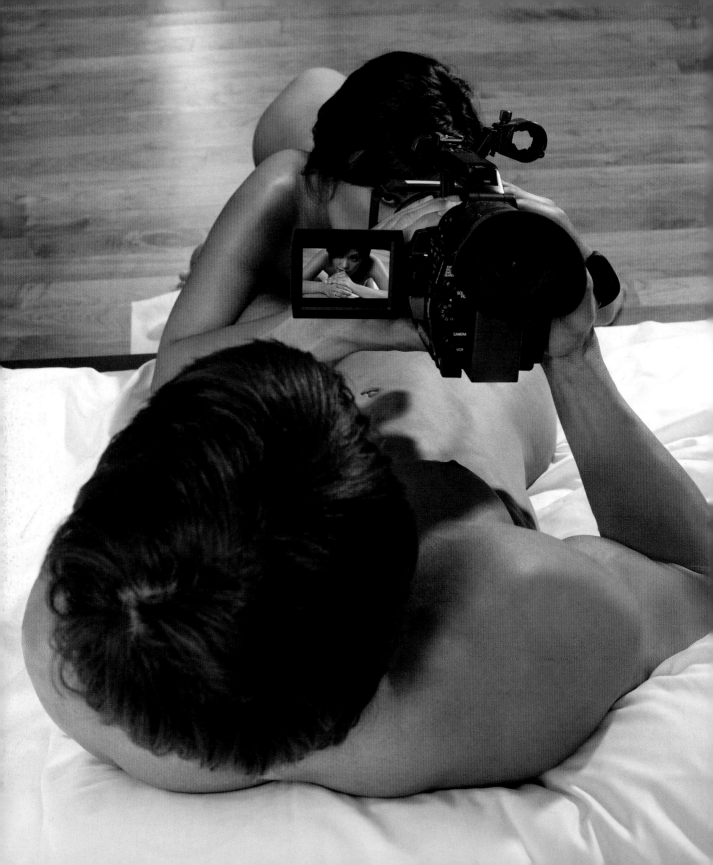

WRITE WHAT YOU KNOW

The first bit of advice aspiring authors always get is to "write what you know." So you may want to do this, at least the first couple of times you tell a story. Vividly describe chronicles of amazing moments you and your lover have experienced together in the past; for instance, talk about that steamy shower you took on your honeymoon. In painting an erotic picture, take care to set the scene, outline what had you aching for one another, and be sure to emphasize the sex itself. Use powerful, graphic descriptions in making your passion points. Then go ahead and build on that story, adding what you wish had happened next.

TAKE A SEXY DOCUMENTARY APPROACH

Pretend you are writing your own erotic movie or "real sex"-type TV show. Go ahead and get X-rated! Describe a sex act you've always wanted to try, or let your lover know what you've always wanted someone to do to you. Make yourself the object of the story, detailing all of the ways you want to be touched. Or stroke your lover's ego, and get into all of the ways you want to play with your lover, using explicit details. Strive to be provocative, such as in the following . . .

"During a recent holiday, my partner and I found ourselves without privacy, but still wanting to get all over each other in the wee morning hours before daybreak. I was pleasantly surprised when my love pulled the bedcovers over our heads, kissing me a couple of times before, much to my surprise, submerging himself into the deep depths of the down comforter, content to make me his breakfast. As he took his time exploring and probing every part of me, I was soon losing myself in waves of pleasure, panting, moaning, and trying to stifle the occasional playful shriek. Overwhelmed with adoration, I peered down into the dark gray undercover light, past my stomach, glistening with sweat, expecting to find my lover struggling, gasping for air.

But my beloved was happily lost in what had become a prime rain forest region. He ignored any of my attempts to rescue him with a pull of his soaking wet locks. He was insatiable, his frenzied head movements spraying beads of sweat. I had no choice but to surrender and went completely limp with bliss until he surfaced . . . . He stared deeply into my eyes, as a drop of sweat rolled down his nose and splashed onto my already wet face. Attempting to wipe it away only created more of a sight, with soaked strands of my hair matting my cheeks. We were a mess—a slithery, sticky sex wreck, but somehow, still, incredibly sexy to the other from this daring attempt at lovemaking . . . ."

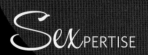

As you and your partner share erotic stories, including personal sexual fantasies, listen for any themes that may crop up over time. Does she have a thing for people in uniform? Does he seem into the idea of having sex with celebrities? Suggest a scenario to play out that's built around your lover's apparent fantasy pattern.

$\mathcal{E}$xercise 9.2 Work on a Story to Improve Role-Playing

Pique each other's thirst for role-playing by working on an erotic story together, creating a shared fantasy scenario. Make yourselves the main characters, considering how both of your needs and desires could be met. Remember to be sensitive to each other, as not to hurt the other's feelings. And, unless it's what both of you fancy, try to avoid fantasies where someone or something else steals the leading role. Once you've written your "script," talk about the story. What possibilities does it hold for enlivening your sex play? When would it best be narrated: during foreplay or in email form right before your lover is about to leave work?

"After months apart, she ached from the excruciating anticipation of finally feeling him again. And he didn't waste any time. His hands couldn't stay off of her, ripping her clothes from her as they fell hard against the bed. His fingers worked their way down her delicious curves, stopping briefly to give a tingly pinch to her ever-so-perky nipples. As he reached for her yearning, she writhed. She wiggled. She looked deep into his eyes and begged him to enter her. Still, he teased, gently stroking his penis across her throbbing clitoris. "Put it in me!" she screamed. So he put it in an inch. They moaned. He pulled out as she cried out for more. Again he went in, slowly passing her lips, one inch, then out—till they both could take it no more. As he finally plunged into her depths, they both let loose a primal scream, longing to merge more and more . . . ."

$\mathcal{I}$n the $\mathcal{B}$edroom:
The Bedroom as Center Stage

BY ROLE-PLAYING, your bedroom suddenly becomes your stage, and you and your lover suddenly become sex stars. There are many sexy benefits to role-playing, including:

- Boosting your sexual self-confidence
- Overcoming your sexual anxieties
- Feeling more attractive and sexier
- Creating greater intimacy with your lover

Role-playing can do all that—and more. But for best results, you need to set some basic common courtesy guidelines first.

INDULGE YOUR SEXUAL FANTASIES . . . TO DEEPEN YOUR EMOTIONAL CONNECTION

Storytelling is one thing; revealing your personal fantasies is another. For some of us, disclosing the details of our fantasies is enough for more enticing sex—as the disclosure itself eroticizes our sex lives. Some of us, on the other hand, bare our innermost sex secrets in hopes of actually realizing the fantasy in one form or another. Either way, mutual fantasy sharing is a great way to arouse each other. And if you are willing to take the next step, and act out your fantasies, you can take your sex play to a whole new dimension.

RULES FOR ROLE-PLAYING

Rule #1: No pressure—You don't have to do anything you don't want to do. Sharing doesn't mean acting. Each partner has the right to refuse a request and with no apologies.

Rule #2: Be nice—Be able to refuse a request to act out a fantasy without putting the other down. This can be done as simply as saying, "Thank you for sharing. It really means a lot that you were willing to suggest that. But I don't think that this is something I'm up for." You can then go on to suggest another related activity that can be seen as a bit of a compromise. Doing so shows that, while you have boundaries, you're still open to eroticizing sex with diversity.

Rule #3: Never say never—While certain sexual scenarios may seem out of the question, don't commit yourself to never considering a sexual adventure. Human beings are known to evolve as sexual beings, and your sexual tastes and preferences could very well change with time. Just let your partner know that this request isn't your cup of tea, but that you will certainly suggest it when and if you should ever change your mind.

Rule #4: Respond—Saying nothing can shut down future sharing. If you don't know how to respond, then say that. If you need some time to respond, let your partner know that you'd like to think about the request for a little while. You don't want to leave your partner wondering.

Rule #5: Withhold judgment—Don't criticize, laugh at, or ridicule the fantasy. Even if you have an issue with your lover's thoughts, try to show empathy.

Rule #6: Don't allow yourself to feel threatened—Fantasies should not be seen as an indicator of relationship dissatisfaction or a glaring sign that your lover is planning to do something with or without you. Couples who fantasize often find that being able to engage such thoughts, including thoughts about other people, ultimately strengthens their sense of commitment to the relationship and their ability to be monogamous.

Rule #7: Keep it couple-focused—Fantasies can be very selfish, and rightfully so. But sharing sexual fantasies via role-playing is just that, a shared experience. Your relationship should be center stage, with the requesting lover stressing that the most exciting part of acting out the fantasy is that "I'm doing this with you."

SEXUAL Q&A: SEX IN CYBERWORLD

My partner is suggesting going online for a totally different type of sexual role-playing via cybersex. Apparently, there are cyberworlds where we can reinvent ourselves and take on characters. I'm trying to be open-minded but can't quite wrap my head around it. What do these sites offer exactly? And can they really enhance our sex life?

The Internet is the wild, wild West of sex. Cybersex is taking lovers on a fantasy ride as never before. Sites such as Second Life boast millions of users. When you enter such a website, you create what's called an "avatar." This allows you to become any kind of animal, fictional creature or character, or any sexual orientation or gender. You can style your online persona any way you want—from face and body shape to clothing and accessories. You are limited only by your imagination. You can then, as your avatar, do anything you do in real life, only more so, such as own an island, fly, or have sex on a cloud. You can even act out behaviors regarded as taboo in the real world.

When you're on one of these sites, it's important to realize that you are not alone; you are interacting with thousands of people. Indeed, (massively) multiplayer online role-playing games (MMORPGs) often boast tens of thousands of users online at the same time. All this "interaction" can be tricky for couples worried about maintaining monogamy. You'll need to agree on some ground rules when you are interacting with other players, as some could be quite harmless while others can be very sexual.

Entering these sites for your own playtime as a couple can be lots of fun. You can send instant flirtatious messages to each other, eventually having virtual sex in up to 100 positions. You can also live out fantasies you might not ever consider doing in your real life, such as virtual escorts, lap dances, and sex clubs. Allowing yourselves to experiment with realistic, but strictly fantasized, sexual behaviors and scenarios could invigorate your sex lives.

TO SHARE OR NOT TO SHARE— THAT IS THE QUESTION

While sharing your sexual fantasies can be incredibly erotic, it's important to assess if you should share and, if so, when anything should be revealed. Not every lover or relationship can handle a partner divulging sexual fantasies. Lovers who are easily jealous or who see sexual fantasies as a type of infidelity are not good candidates for sharing, especially if your fantasies involve other people. Your relationship, too, needs to provide a safe space for sharing. If either lover doesn't feel respected or fears judgment, then it's simply not wise to open up. There needs to be a certain level of trust in a relationship for this kind of intimate exchange. You should be sensitive, too, as to the timing of your confession. Professing a fantasy during sex, for example, can cause your lover to erupt in anger instead of into orgasm.

Finally, realize that you don't have to share every fantasy or all of the details, even if your lover is pressing you for more. Some sexual thoughts are best left private, if even for your own personal eroticism. Some may also not resonate well with your lover, especially if they reflect your often unconscious psychological needs. Even though research by psychotherapist Brett Kahr on British and American erotic fantasies, involving data from thirteen thousand adults, has found that the most popular fantasies are those involving bondage, sado-masochism, voyeurism, and exhibitionism, many lovers regard such fantasies as shameful, remorseful, or possibly "perverse."

PLAYING PRETEND: ACTING OUT SEXUAL SCENARIOS

Make date night a play night. Start with scenarios and characters that resonate with you in some way. Think about your favorite movie or comic book characters for inspiration. Recall favorite childhood stories, such as "Little Red Riding Hood." Consider historical or famous people, such as Greta Garbo, who could be amusing to impersonate.

Whatever you do, don't pick a role that is too like somebody you or your partner knows. Also, try to imagine scenarios far enough removed from your normal sex routine that you will not resort to your regular sex. You're taking sex to a whole new level here, which means escaping to a dream world where the unimaginable can happen.

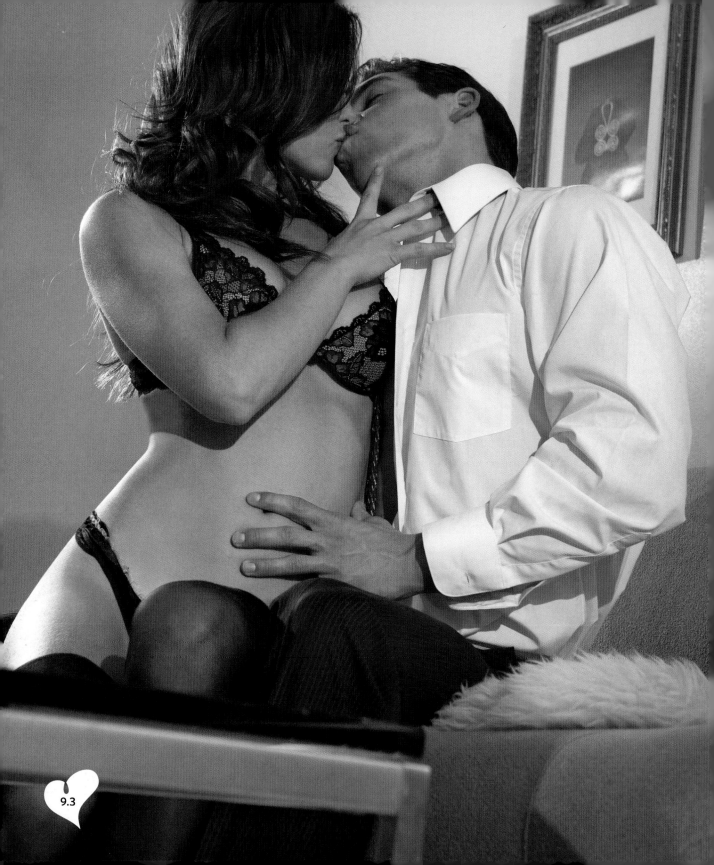

9.3

$\mathcal{S}e\mathcal{X}$ercise 9.3 Inspire Your Partner with Role-Playing Ideas

Half the fun is coming up with scenarios on your own. But to get started on your role-playing, here's a list meant to inspire you and your partner. Begin by marking the scenarios that you'd both consider trying. Then take the role-play teaser and run with it, using the better-sex tips in the next section!

Nurse and Injured Patient: It's World War II, and you've been stationed in the Pacific, attending to wounded soldiers. One of them has suffered an injury to the upper thigh, and you find yourself surprisingly aroused when, in removing the adhesives, you see more than what you bargained for . . .

Postal Carrier and Housewife/Husband: The children are off at school. Your spouse, who has been neglecting you, is busy at work. You are lonely, bored, and need more than your afternoon cocktail for escape. Seems like the postal carrier on your front porch can bring you a lot more than the mail . . . (An alternative to this home-alone-and-lonely scenario is the "Homeowner and Plumber.")

Flight Attendant and Passenger: You're on a transatlantic flight and, in encountering turbulence, have accidentally spilled a drink all over a passenger. As you lean over to dab at the mess, you can feel this good-looking passenger's sweet, warm breath on your neck. Suddenly, joining the Mile High Club (as in sex in the airplane bathroom) doesn't sound like a bad idea . . .

Hollywood Producer and Starlet: You're important in Hollywood, and people are willing to do anything—that's anything—for you because you can get them anywhere. But who knows where this young hot-to-trot aspiring starlet, who is all too willing to please, will take you?

Aesthetician and Customer: You're going on vacation and want to be clean-shaven to wear your new bathing suit. When you get to the spa, the male stylist commands you to strip down and don a disposable bikini bottom (a super option if you want something to rip off of your partner later); before you know it, he's giving you more than hot wax . . .

Call Girl and Businessman: You're on a business trip, short on time, and in need of a date for an evening function. That escort service you know always serves you well, especially since you're feeling aroused at the thought of this one call girl in particular . . . (An alternative to this scenario is a rich lady and gigolo.)

One-Night Stand: You're at a cocktail party and have just been introduced to a friend of a friend who is absolutely stunning. How can you refuse the invitation to go home together for a little bit more than a goodnight kiss?

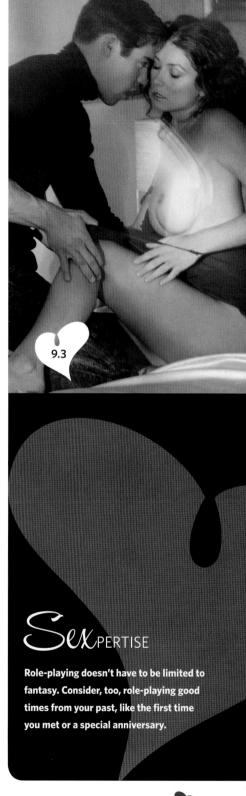

9.3

$\mathcal{S}e\mathcal{X}$PERTISE

Role-playing doesn't have to be limited to fantasy. Consider, too, role-playing good times from your past, like the first time you met or a special anniversary.

Photographer and Model: You're used to filming hundreds of models, but there's something about this one that's intriguing you as no other. You've never taken such joy in suggesting that the model take off more, give you more. You can hardly contain yourself as you make your way over to the gorgeous naked form, giving you the most seductive look, on your couch . . .

In the Bedroom:
Preparing for Your Sexual Scenario

NOW THAT YOU'VE got some ideas, you need to get busy with the planning if you want to be successful:

Plan the scenario. Outline who the two of you are (e.g., Princess Leia and Han Solo), where you are (Death Star space station), and what you're wearing (e.g., Han is in a white shirt, dark vest, and leather-and-metal belt—black pants optional). Imagine the main points of the scene (e.g., you're under attack, but with your hearts racing in the face of death, you can't keep your hands off of one another). What kinds of sex do you want to have? Will you finish the scene? Or are you okay with the possibility that you may not make it to the end of the story?

Set boundaries. Couples need to set ground rules for sharing and acting out fantasies. For example, by using a word or a sign, you can stop the scene at any time. Sexual role-playing can become intense at times, evoking feelings that may surprise you. Also, discuss anything you don't want to do or things you will do only while in character. Be able to state your needs. All of this provides a sense of safety for revealing yourselves. These boundaries essentially involve common courtesy, such as not laughing if that isn't appropriate.

Practice getting into character. This is your opportunity to act like somebody else in the name of eroticizing. You get to forget about your daily life and lose yourself in a character. You may want to try to get into the costume or try using the props privately, doing a test run of your character. Explore his or her inner workings. What's your character's history? What brings your character to this sexual escapade? What motivates your character? What drives your character wild with desire? What's a total turn-off?

Have fun and stay positive. Remember, this is all a game. You're playing, so make it feel like the sexual amusement it is! Things may go wrong. Something funny might occur. The unexpected will probably happen—and it's all okay! And it's okay to laugh. This means that you're having a good time.

Process. Talk about the experience. What did you like? What didn't work? Would you do that again? How would you do things differently? How did it feel to be that character? Could you be that person or thing again?

Ravishment Fantasy: You're so irresistible that your lover won't take "no" for an answer. The ravisher remains clothed, all the while being rough in the kissing, groping, and gentle pulling of the hair, and stripping you naked . . . (Be clear about the action stage here and just how "rough" you want things to be.)

Bank Robber and Bank Teller: You're robbing a bank and have told everybody to get down, only you want a little bit more from the one head-turning teller than just money. You may just have to take a hostage . . . (An alternative to this role-play is "Police Officer and Burglar.")

SEXUAL Q&A: ROLE-PLAYING RELUCTANCE

My partner is anti-role-playing. He thinks it's too kinky and doesn't see the need for it, plus he ays he has trouble with make-believe. I've asked him a couple of times to at least try sexual role-playing; I'm hoping for tips on how to make him more receptive as I give this request one last go.

In feeling out your partner, don't bring up the fact that you want to role-play initially. Instead, describe a sexual scenario to him, letting him know why you find it so appealing. Part of his hesitation may be that he's nervous about what he's getting himself into. So be sure to start out with a tamer scene, highlighting how sexy you think he'd look all dressed up in your character of choice. Or if he needs to keep it more real, suggest a scenario that he can more readily identify with, such as the two of you being secret lovers. Once you know whether he finds your sexual fantasy erotic, ask him if it can be realized, stressing the benefits of doing so. Role-playing can be such a good time. You'll learn a great deal about each other. You'll feel closer to one another as your relationship becomes more intimate. It will keep things novel, which is something every couple wanting passion for the long-term must pursue.

Finally, let him know that you want him to be part of making things a reality beyond simply being a player. Tell him that you want his input in building the scene. Reassure him that you're willing to negotiate and compromise in making sure that this is enticing for both of you. Lastly, if none of this works, remember that there's always Halloween or a good costume theme party. Take advantage of these events. Getting dressed up in a seductive costume, such as a nurse's outfit, or as an angel to his Greek god, may just have him singing a different tune!

In opening the door to your erotic curiosities, you reveal a new world of passion possibilities to you and your lover. From telling erotic stories and sharing fantasies to making suggestions for sex play and acting out sexual scenarios, changing your rendezvous repertoire will expand your sexual horizons. It will bring you closer together, taking your lovemaking to new heights.

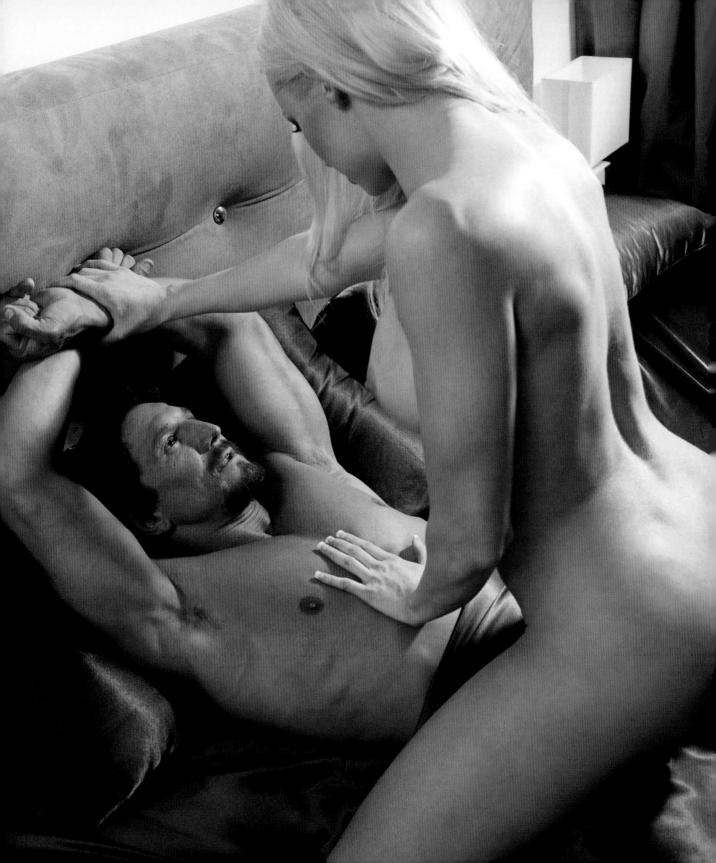

> "My chief occupation, despite appearances, has always been love."
>
> —ALBERT CAMUS

Sexual Homework

The human imagination is endless. This is such a blessing because, while we covered a number of ideas for spicing up your love life with fantasy, you have an endless number of scenarios for your titillation. So allow yourselves to get creative on occasion, with the following sexual homework also great starting points for making some of your sexual fantasies come true:

Role-Play in Public—Decide on a fantasy scenario that you can act out in the real world. Plan, for example, to be in a quaint café at the same time—and in complete character as strangers who have never met. Have fun flirting with each other, using fake names and French accents, as you attempt to seduce the other into coming home with you over a glass of wine and a baguette. Allow yourselves to be naughty in ways you would never dream in reality.

Switch Roles—Have fun playing the other. Keeping a sense of humor, take on your lover's personality, mannerisms, sex appeal, dress, verbal expressions—basically anything that makes your lover the person you love and adore. Try having sex through the eyes of the other, using this as an opportunity to express what you know or think your lover likes. See this as an opportunity to celebrate each other while still being experimental and having sex that's outside of your normal lovemaking.

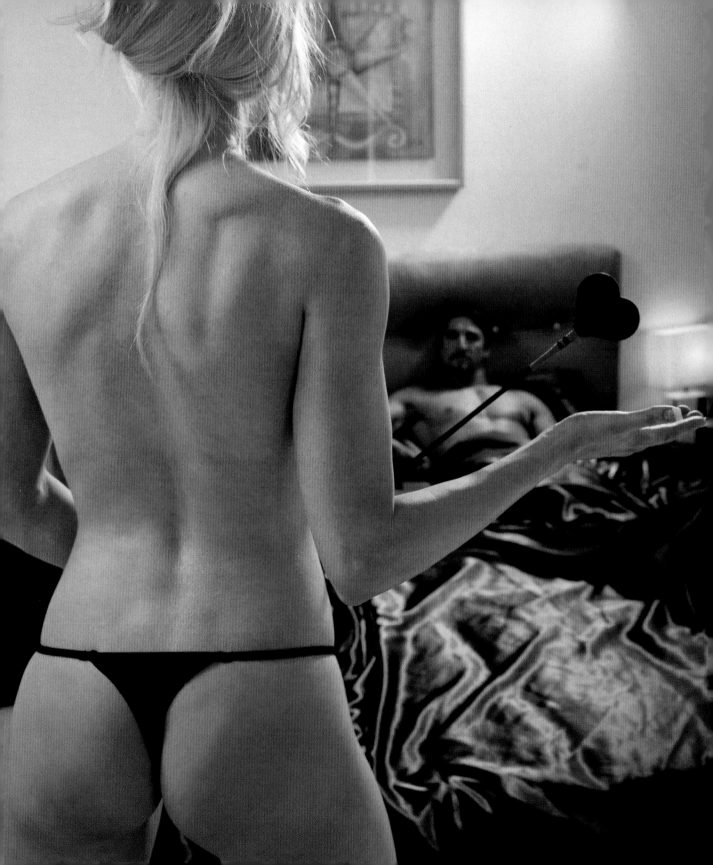

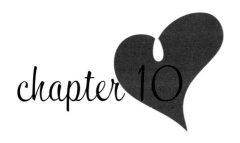

chapter 10

From Leather to Love Spanks: Incorporating Adventure to Enliven Your Sex Life

MOST OF US CONSIDER our sex lives private affairs—yet, even so, many of us feel obliged to indulge only in "standard" or "normal" sex. Otherwise known as "vanilla sex," "normal" sex describes a heterosexual couple engaging in the missionary (man on top) position without the benefit of enhancement products.

There's nothing wrong with vanilla sex, but beyond "normal" lies a world of possibilities that can revitalize your sex life. Open that door to new sensations and pleasure, and you and your lover can enjoy increased self-confidence, trust, and eroticism—and feel closer than ever. Some couples are afraid to even sample this kind of sex play, yet going beyond vanilla sex is often what it may take to have more exhilarating sex. A little adventure in and out of the bedroom can invigorate your sex life, making you feel more sexually alive than ever. So give yourself permission to at least see what all of the fuss is about.

"If we do not try, we will not know."

A LITTLE BIT OF KINK

The word "kink" has different meanings when it comes to sex, depending on who you talk to. It can refer to a single unusual sexual behavior or way of life, or to a group of "atypical" sexual practices. But in striving for satisfying sex, it helps to think of kink as "gourmet sex"; try it and you can become sex gourmands.

When it comes to kink, couples need to be in it together. It takes care and planning to navigate erotic indulgences that include the likes of fetishes and bondage. So it's important to approach the broadening of your sexual repertoire as a team.

It's also important to understand that not all of these behaviors enhance sex, especially in their most extreme forms. They are not required for great sex. Some lovers are, understandably, uncomfortable with the mere thought of sex play that can involve, for example, leather or brandishing whips. Others, however, find such sex play quite savory, with the element of eccentric eroticism half the turn-on.

In this chapter, we'll demystify sexual behaviors that are often misunderstood. There are plenty of ways to test the waters without completely emerging yourselves. You'll learn what you need to know to explore the more wholesome side of kink. You'll pick and choose your favorite flavors of nonvanilla sex to see what works for you.

SEXUAL CHARMS

Sexual behaviors and objects can be quite charming—some more than others, and for some people more than others. Some individuals become quite sexually fixated on the behavior or object—and that's when it becomes a fetish.

The word "fetish" actually has quite an innocent, fascinating background. Originally from the Portuguese word fetich, fetish was the word used by Old World Portuguese explorers to describe any religious artifact that tribal cultures thought had magical powers. It wasn't until the nineteenth century, however, that "fetish" was used to describe something that aroused an individual. (The exclusive attraction to a body part, such as the feet, is known as "partialism.")

Sexual fetishism means that you are aroused by an object that typically isn't considered a turn-on, such as gloves, lace, or fur. The high-heeled shoe, for example, is more than just a shoe. It is the means to emotional and erotic gratification. While fetishes are normally cast as sexual longings and experiences, fetishists experience emotional, even spiritual, responses to the object of desire.

THE
SCIENCE OF *Sex*

A paraphilia, literally meaning a "love" (philia) beyond the "usual" (para), refers to atypical or problematic sexual behaviors that are obsessive and compulsive. Such behaviors often interfere with love relationships and intimacy. A paraphilia is regarded as a preoccupation with a sexual behavior or object to the point that the individual is dependent upon it for sexual satisfaction. There are about thirty different paraphilias, with the prevalence of this behavior much greater among men than women.

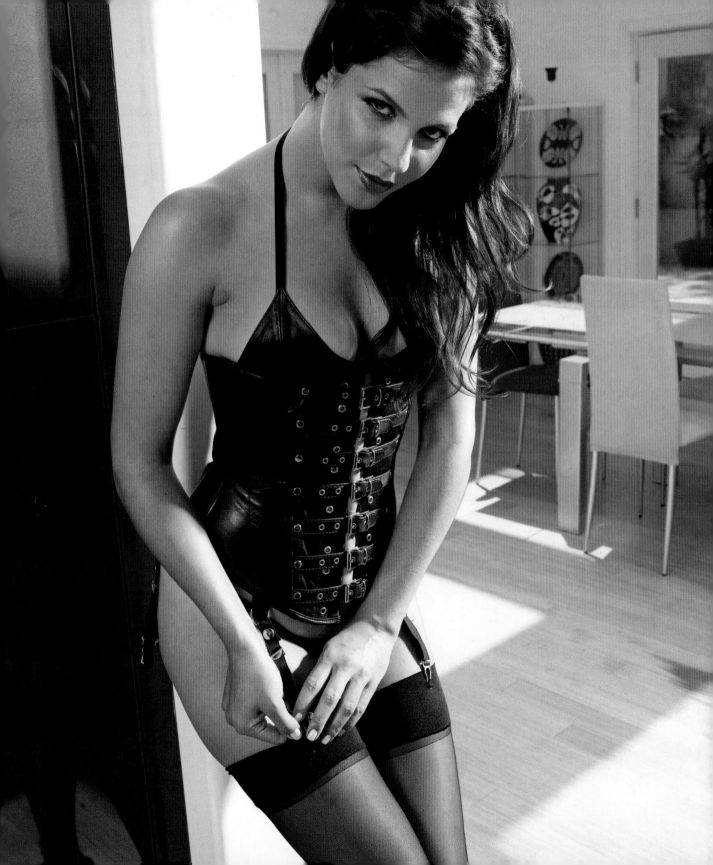

Most people have much milder relationships with favored sex objects or behaviors. For example, many people are aroused by something that isn't explicitly sexual, like the smell of leather. Such "fetishes" are so unnoticeable, however, that most people don't realize that they have them. This may be, in part, because their fetishes are also harmless—which is where your potential for wholesome kink comes in.

SEXUAL Q&A: HOW FETISHES DEVELOP

My lover recently revealed that he has a fetish. I was wondering how he came to have such and if he can/should be treated for it?

A fetish develops when a person learns to attach erotic significance to an object that is not in itself sexual in nature, often because of an inability to cope with a sexual relationship. It may stem from a fear of rejection; the body part is seen as a safe focus for erotic behavior because it is nonthreatening. Typically, however, fetishes are mostly harmless. They're only problematic if they become an obsession, affecting other areas of life, most notably intimacy and healthy relationships. Sometimes even orgasm becomes impossible without the fetish. That said, most people with fetishes aren't so extreme. They can have satisfying sexual encounters without having the fetish object present. Often the greatest harm a fetish can cause is not with the fetishist but with the reactions the fetish evokes in other people, who reject this human behavior as bizarre or unhealthy.

Nobody knows how or why fetishes form. Psychoanalytic theory has proposed that a fetish is the result of sexual shame. At an early age, a person feels so embarrassed seeing a sexual organ that his eyes focus on something else, such as a stocking, for instance, which later becomes his fetish. Another belief is that an event very early in life shapes one's sexual identity; for instance, while crawling, a baby may sniff someone's feet, becoming permanently fixated on feet later in life. The fetish gets locked in the brain, and the individual seeks it out when older in remembering initial arousal. Still, other academics have proposed that fetishes are a part of human nature. Much like people who are fanatics in collecting baseball cards or stamps, a fetishist has a stronger internal impulse to be aroused by an object or body part. The object begins as something that simply comforts or fascinates them, but then becomes more erotic as they reach adolescence and adulthood, and masturbate thinking about the object.

Unfortunately, if a person or his or her partner is bothered by a fetish, it isn't something that can be "fixed" overnight. It is most easily treated with the help of a certified sex therapist. In fact, in extreme cases, there is no evidence that a fetish can be cured. Forcing someone to give up the fetish could actually lead to, in the very least, depression. So in seeking help, a person needs to decide if he wants to get rid of his fetish entirely or if he wants to simply train himself to become sexually excited by other things and to keep the fetish under control. He should consider this because, to a certain extent, there is something to envy about a fetish. A person is practically guaranteed arousal by the object; the thought of it is almost too easy when it comes to stimulation! Furthermore, his fetish can be used to his lover's advantage when intimate.

Exploring different sex charms can make for more sexual adventure, entertainment, and sensations. While you may not fully realize or even understand the power of irresistible attraction that defines a fetish, exploring fetish-like fascinations could be, in the very least, a bonding experience as you and your lover investigate what charms have any magical effects, if any, on you.

TYPES OF SEX CHARMS

Professionals who specialize in understanding fetish behaviors will admit that, just when they thought they'd heard it all, they learn about a new behavior or object that has become a person's private amulet. Given that there are nearly innumerable sex charms out there, attempts have been made to categorize them, with the following being just a handful of these classifications. Such sex charms can offer you hours upon hours of sex play, should you choose to explore them:

Materials: Articles of clothing and materials made of rubber, silk, fur, or leather are common fetishistic objects. Think about how good it feels to slip into a fabric like silk or to make love on satin sheets. Humans like things that feel good on our skin, that make it feel vibrant. So consider how different substances may feel against your body. How can you experiment with it during lovemaking?

Accessories: While some may not like hearing this, using a sex toy could make you a fetishist. This is because accessories, from sex aids to masquerade eye masks, have been considered sex charms when used on a regular basis. Remember, almost anything can be turned into a sex toy or accessory, even fishnets, a French maid costume, or biker gear. Don't be afraid to consider how the many things you come in contact with regularly may somehow safely ramp up your sex life.

$\mathcal{S}\textit{exercise}$ 10.1 Ramp Up Your Sex With Everyday Items

Try having sex on bubble wrap, allowing yourselves to get wilder as the sealed plastic air pockets burst around you. Let go enough to laugh as your new "set of sheets" explode around you. Talk about what you liked and disliked about that experience and what you'd like to try next time.

Mess: People love getting "down and dirty," with some lovers taking that quite literally when it comes to involving food and/or fluids, such as mud, whipped cream, pudding, or shaving cream. So take a bath in milk. Or equip yourselves with ample amounts of lotion, and pour it all over each other during sex. Or let yourselves become kids again as you smear frosting all over each other's bodies.

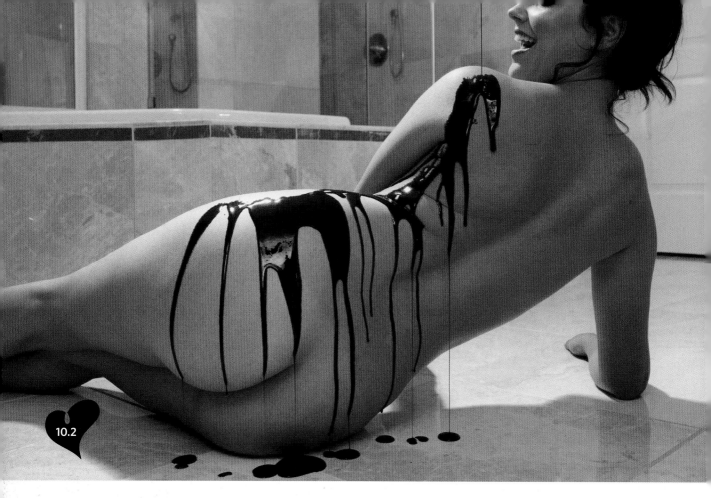

10.2

Se𝓍ercise 10.2 Use Food to Add Some Flavor to Your Sex

Lay down some tarp, and have a food fight. Messy fun, such as a good pie fight, can help you to release tensions, with the best part being that you can lick your favorite foods off of each other as part of cleanup.

Body Hair: Some people love playing with body hair or are obsessed with removing it with or without a partner's assistance. Incorporating pubic-hair maintenance into your love life as a form of foreplay or as the main event can invigorate intimacy. Another great thing about turning your bedroom or bathroom into a barber shop is that every grooming can be a unique experience.

$\mathcal{S}$eXercise 10.3 Amp up Arousal with a Sensual Shave

Shave one another. The two of you have many depilation options, primarily trimming, shaving, plucking, hair removal creams, and waxing. Once you have decided on your method of choice, you can take this kind of action practically anywhere in your home, with the bathroom counter a favorite for many. Such salon-style sex is especially arousing when the one being groomed is hoisted up beside the bathroom sink, knees splayed, while the groomer leisurely goes to work, delicately and thoroughly washing every square inch of the genitalia (including anal area), meticulously trimming each hair, sensually lathering the groin with shaving cream, and then skillfully making his love baby-smooth once more . . . .

$\mathcal{S}$eXercise 10.4 Swing and Sway into New Positions

You may want to try a sex bungee swing, a safe way to add a little bit of fun risk to your sex life. This harness system, which is suspended by bungee cords, can be attached to any ceiling that is a minimum of eight feet high. Lovers can then be flipped and twisted into a number of "weightless" sexual positions. Whether you're being twisted, rotated, or spun, you can enjoy a nice bounce as your lover bends you over for more vigorous thrusting.

EROTIC POWER-PLAY: TAKE YOU R SEX LIFE TO THE NEXT LEVEL

Erotic power-play is a general term for a wide variety of sexual activities— and types of interpersonal relationships—in which power plays a part. Such sex may simply be an extension of the type of sex you're currently engaging in, such as having your arms pinned above your head during sexual intercourse. It can also be a more blatant form of the power dynamics that already exist in many relationships. For example, one partner may always be submissive in bed, giving into the other's demands without protest.

In erotic power-play, you lay your relationship dynamics on the table, examining vulnerability and trust issues you're already dealing with outside the bedroom. In effect, you eroticize one partner's desire to be authoritative and the other's desire to be obedient—thereby casting your sex roles in a completely new light.

$\mathcal{S}$eXPERTISE

When it comes to hair removal, you may want to forego depilatory creams. While easy and nice for their satiny smooth finish, they are sure to kill the mood with their smell and ability to induce skin irritation. Remember, no matter what you choose to do, remove hair with great care, especially in the ever-so-sensitive genital area. Also, you may want to consider buying an intimate shaving kit, which is sold in many retail stores.

WHO'S ON TOP

In erotic power-play, you can explore the role of power in your relationship. One of you will be the "top," or dominant one, while the other will be the "bottom," or submissive one. The top is the more active partner, exercising control over the bottom partner, who has agreed to consent to pleasure. This does not mean, however, that the top exploits the passive bottom. In fact, in many ways, the bottom is in charge, since he or she ultimately decides how far things can go and when such play should come to a close. Far from barbaric, oppressive, or degrading, this consensual arrangement involves one partner leading the other. The acronym BDSM stands for the elements of this type of sex play:

B: bondage
D: domination and discipline
S: sadism, submission, surrender, or slave
M: masochism, master and mistress

Erotic power-play may also be framed as D/S, or dominance and submission. This power-play thrives off the tension between power and surrender, being overpowering and giving into authority. This is the focus more than the actual sex itself, with some scenarios never involving sexual intercourse. It seeks to emotionally and sexually gratify lovers' needs to feel desired and vital in body, heart, and soul.

Erotic sex play can be thrilling, heightening lovemaking because partners are given a greater freedom to feel. Enthusiasts claim that it guarantees passionate sex years into a relationship, with the sexual release offered helping the body. This is in part because the variety of erotic power-play activities helps couples, especially those in long-term monogamous relationships, not to become bored with monotony and routine. It appears that some behaviors currently labeled as S&M (sadomasochism) were commonly found in ancient marriage manuals, such as Vātsyāyana's original *Kama Sutra*, written in 450 AD.

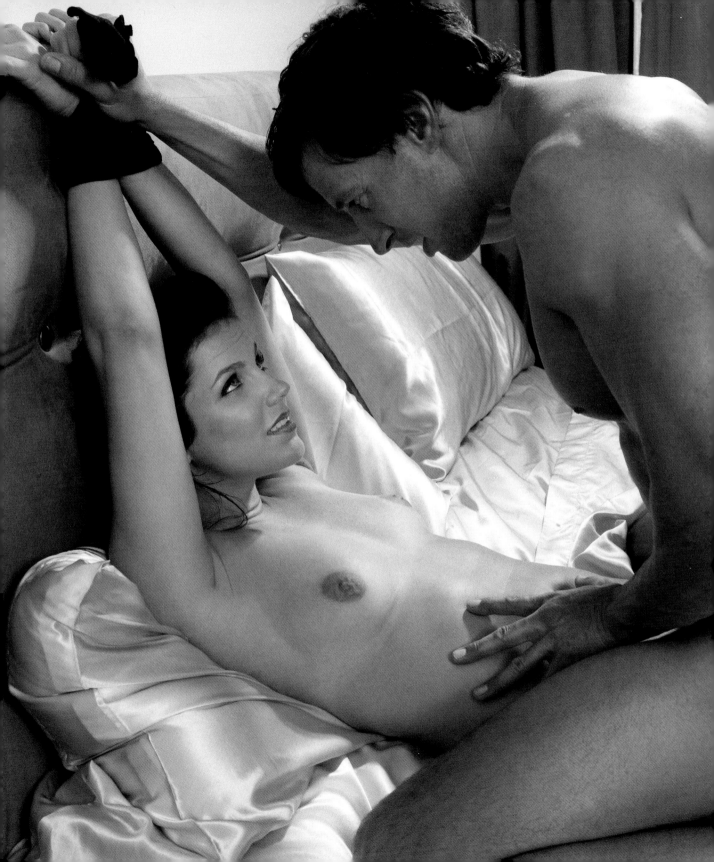

OUT-OF-BODY SEX

With mutual pleasure and growth primary goals, erotic power-play can foster greater communication and creativity—even a spiritual, enlightening altered state of consciousness and sex. Some claim to leave the body while feeling an intense psychic connection. Many feel that such sex play results in profound intimacy, with the total trust involved being sexy. Finally, couples who engage in different forms of erotic power-play describe feeling empowered in the situation, becoming more powerful and eroticized by the power they provide one another. With erotic power-play a new way of seeing the self as an object of desire, many lovers feel more wanted and nurtured, all the while pleasing the one they care about. It's no wonder that museums and galleries have showcased various visuals, equipment, and enhancers that portray these intimate exchanges.

FEELING OUT YOUR
EROTIC POWER-PLAY POTENTIAL

You may want to experiment with your roles in the bedroom. You may have fantasies involving power dynamics that you want to act out. You may want to test your physical and emotional limits. Or perhaps you're intrigued by the sexual potential power-playing holds, having seen glimpses of it in music videos, movies, or erotica. You may be curious about the sex play and how it can enhance your sex life, or long to learn more about your personal potential. A woman, for example, may want to free her inner temptress in testing how dominant she can be in bed. Or her lover may want to try submitting to her. This is actually quite common, with submissives often instigating power-play. This includes specifying what they want, need, and expect from the exchange.

Experimenting with power-play can reveal facets of the self that were never known. It also allows us to let go of ourselves in the name of gratifying sex while becoming emotionally naked. Better sex requires exposing yourself to some degree, with power-play scenarios facilitating that as you learn to let go in brand new ways. As you open up to one another, you become more intimate, and it's this union of mind, body, soul that may result in the best sex.

My spouse wants to try erotic power-play, but I'm a little apprehensive, despite being aroused by it. I feel like, if anybody found out, we'd be seen as sex freaks. My spouse says that plenty of people engage in this type of play and that most of them are in the closet about it. What do you think—are we alone in wanting to experiment?

Erotic power-play evokes strong positive and negative reactions from people. Those who regard such sex play favorably may be more open-minded or have dabbled in it and know its benefits. Those who are adverse to it may be fearful of the unknown, meaning they don't know anything about such eroticizing, or believe that the harsh portrayals they've seen depicting such sex games in movies represent all this area has to offer.

While people of all socioeconomic classes and groups are believed to engage in erotic power games, what sometimes surprises people is those who are more educated and successful appear to be into it more than other groups. Even more eyebrow-raising is hearing that those in high-powered positions in the real world are often ones who adore being submissive in bed. "Bottoms" might be doctors, therapists, attorneys, police officers, and corporate executives, since these individuals want to relinquish the power they have during their typical day at work. Informal magazine surveys further continually find that both men and women are turned on to the idea of at least experimenting with erotic power-play. But we really don't know much about the "who" of erotic power-play beyond all of that. Little formal research has been conducted in this area, though one sex survey conducted by the University of New South Wales, involving twenty thousand participants, did look at Aussies' fetish habits.

The survey found that those who are into bondage and discipline (B&D) are not considered damaged or dangerous. In fact, they may be happier than those who adhere to "normal" sex. B&D may actually make men happier in general, with male participants scoring lower in evaluations for psychological distress. This may be in part due to a person feeling more in harmony with the self and more accepted in being allowed to engage is this fantasized play. The investigation further found that 2 percent of adult Australians engaged in S&M in the last year and dominance-and-submission-type sexual role-play. (More are believed to have engaged in such, but are likely unwilling to label their sex play "BDSM" given the stigmas around the term. A *Playboy* readers sex survey found that 5 to 10 percent of Americans engage in S&M behaviors for pleasure at least on occasion, while The Janus Report on Sexual Behavior found that 14 percent of men and 11 percent of women had had some S&M experience. Reasons for engaging in erotic power-play stemmed primarily from sexual interest, not as a reaction to sexual abuse or being sexually "deficient" in some way. Researchers also found that people who enjoyed BDSM were also more sexually adventurous in other ways, such as trying phone or anal sex, looking at Internet erotica, or using sex toys.

TRUST IS POWER

Perhaps part of what makes the benefits of power-play so powerful is that such sexual exchanges cannot take place in just any relationship. You need to have a certain level of respect and trust. You need to know that each other's boundaries are respected and that things will come to an end as soon as the request to conclude is made. On a more personal level, each lover needs to love his or her self. Not loving yourself can make you extremely vulnerable in these power-play situations, especially if you have physical or emotional limits that will become hypersensitivities. You need to own the power you have in liking and accepting yourself and knowing what you want. You need to see yourself as a desirable, sexual being, full of sexual self-confidence.

Before embarking on an erotic power-play adventure, it's important to realize that you as a couple have your own style and preferences, from scenarios to instruments of pleasure to clothing. You may experiment with bondage, spanking, or cross-dressing. While those who are heavily involved with the BDSM scene get into its ritualistic nature, forms of address, and modes of behavior, you do not need to take your sex play to this extreme. You also don't have to worry about such sex play being addictive or destructive, as some wrongfully argue. You can pursue consensual erotic power-play on a number of levels. Consider:

Bondage

In restraining for pleasure, bondage involves tying a partner's arms or legs together with a restraint such as handcuffs. It can also involve tying arms and/or legs to an object. Bondage can be so elaborate and require so much skill in some cases that tying up a partner is an art form known as "ligotage."

Discipline

In controlling a submissive's behavior, discipline may be in order at times. So rules and forms of punishment to control the behavior must be agreed upon. Punishment can be physical, such as spanking, or psychological, such as humiliation; it can also include a loss of freedom via restraint, such as tying your lover to a bedpost.

If you and your lover think that you want to just stick to bondage play, realize that the main forms of B&D involve physical or symbolic restraint or constriction of any body part and "punishment." This is often accompanied by fantasy role-playing. S&M, or sadomasochism, involves more intense sensations.

THE
SCIENCE OF *Sex*

For certain lovers, the pain-for-pleasure component makes for more rewarding sex in some ways. This is something some individuals have trouble understanding, but think about the last time you had rough, unbridled, passionate sex. It may have resulted in bites or bruises you noticed the next day. When you experience pain, your body reacts with a surge of its natural opiates, namely dopamine, a hormone and neurotransmitter, and endorphins, neurotransmitters similar to morphine. Both of these lessen the pain's intensity, while producing a rush—a high—as we slip into a comforting, trance-like meditative "subspace" that removes the conscious self away from the pain. Pain actually evokes the activation of the reward areas of the brain, as is the case when the brain responds to good food or certain drugs.

Sadomasochism

During sadomasochism (S&M), the sexual sadist feels sexual gratification in inflicting pain or humiliation on another, while the sexual masochist is sexually satisfied from experiencing the pain and suffering. Yet such sexual power exchanges are not about physical pain, or at least not the level of pain that most people associate with S&M; in truth, the majority of S&M play involves only as much pain as an individual can handle. Consider, for example, that the pain from biting, scratching, or pinching your lover during passionate sex is very different from being punched in the face. Couples also vary according to how intense they want sensations to be. While many erotic power-play activities may seem abusive or coercive, BDSM is not a form of sexual violence. Reinforcing this is the fact that such erotic power-play should be pursued only if it is SSC, as in "safe, sane, and consensual." Furthermore, enjoying such a power dynamic in an erotic context does not mean that sadomasochism, whether it involves causing or receiving pain, is desired in other nonsexual situations.

DECIDING YOUR ROLES

Whether you and your partner think that B&D or S&M is more your style, in both types of sex play, partners need to seriously negotiate and script their sex scene, dialogue, and props ahead of time. Perhaps the easiest place to start is in defining and setting limits to your roles. When your sex life dares to toy with erotic power-play, understand that your interactions are all role-based. This is a script for the bedroom. Being dominant or submissive is not to become your primary identity. Furthermore, your main goal in your role is seduction—not being harsh. Remember, both lovers need to negotiate each role's limits.

Top/Dominant

Don't be mistaken in thinking that, as the Top, all you need to do is act bossy and give orders. Your Bottom is entrusting you to take care of both of you during you sex scene. This means that you need to be educated about everything the scenario entails. You need to competently know what you're doing and be able to keep dominance in its place. Becoming a new, powerful self can be transforming and liberating, and all of that needs to be handled responsibly.

As a Top, you direct the behavior. You're more concerned with applying sensation and take an active role in the physical scene. You aren't going for emotional or mental control over your partner. In deciding if this role is for you, ask yourself if you enjoy nurturing and caretaking? Do you get sexually excited over the rush that comes with control and power?

*Sex*PERTISE

Algolagnia, pronounced "al-goe-LAG-nee-uh," is the sexual gratification derived from inflicting or experiencing pain.

Bottom/Submissive

The Bottom is frequently the partner who specifies the basic conditions of the session and gives instructions, directly or indirectly, in the prelude to the session; the Top often respects this guidance. The Bottom may also try to control the Top by provoking reactions or "misbehaving" to attract interest. So you need to be able to express how you feel, and use the "safe word" that has been decided upon. This is a word—any word you and your partner decide upon—that, when stated, means that all activity is to stop immediately.

In deciding if being submissive is for you, ask yourself if surrendering control gives you a rush. Do you like the idea of being told what to wear, poses you should assume, or how to serve and please your partner?

Don't feel as though you're going to be locked into the role you choose the first time you pursue such sex play. Switching roles is something many couples do at least in the beginning, with lovers experimenting with either role during a single or different sex sessions. Likewise, your preferences aren't set forever with these talks. You may find later that you prefer that your partner be more aggressive than gentle. Or you may learn that you like the intensity of certain sensations so much that you'd like something harder or faster for a little pain. While couples negotiate a great deal ahead of time, some improvisation is often required, too. Some simply prefer to have a "looser," more stringent story line in place.

$\mathcal{S}$ exercise 105 Establish Rules for Your Power-Play Activities

Discuss what appeal erotic power-play has for you. State any fears and concerns you have, especially in clarifying your limits and describing how you see your role as a dominant or submissive. Share your fantasies as far as what it would be like to be a top versus bottom and why you'd prefer one over the other. Let your lover know what falls within your comfort zone. Do you have fantasies of being tied up or being spanked? Or does being flogged pique your arousal? After discussing all of the physical and emotional benefits and risks, draft an informal contract that will act as a promise as to how you will treat and view each other during this type of sex play. Be sure to spell out all of the ways you'd like to be pleasured, as well.

FIGURING OUT YOUR ROLE-PLAYING SCENARIO

While some couples relate to each other as just a Top or Bottom, others prefer acting out a story line by taking on characters. Fantasy is a major element of erotic power-play, driving up the lust many thrive on and acting as a form of empowerment as lovers find strength in the need to give a well-delivered performance. Those often enjoyed within the context of erotic power-play include:

- Drill Sergeant and Military Officer
- Ruler (think Cleopatra) and Slave
- Pirate and Captive
- Trainer and Puppy
- Head of Household and Nursemaid/Governess

In other scenarios, a Bottom may choose to be a sex object, martyr, cherished possession, or even an inanimate object, such as a foot stool. The Top may be a criminal, tyrant, giant, or rebel. Couples may also choose to experiment with gender and sexual orientation.

SEXUAL Q&A: EROTIC POWER-PLAY

My lover and I are about to role-play a BDSM scene, and I'm going to be the top. I'm a bit nervous, though, in that I want to make myself believable as the dominant one. Any suggestions?

You can make your role-playing believable and enjoyable by considering the following:

A. What submissive behaviors turn you on? Contemplate what your lover can do as your personal servant that would turn you on, such as giving you a foot rub, doing housework, or brushing your hair. Pinpoint what thrills you, and let your lover know that you expect those desires to be fulfilled.

B. Stay true to yourself. This is a safe space for you to let out feelings of aggression, your need for control, or your sexual desires. While a little bit of theatrics couldn't hurt, the more you look like you, the more you'll sell your role as dominant.

C. Set boundaries. Think about how far you want things to go, and then, with your partner, agree upon limits as to what both of you can handle, and abide by them. (You can always see if you can handle more at a later date.) Make sure that both of you are comfortable with these rules and that neither is being pressured into anything.

D. Keep the action all about you. If you tend to be a pleaser or the main giver in bed, it's easy to put your partner's needs above your own; however, this doesn't complement your role as the dominant. Be self-indulgent, making sure that your pleasures and needs are being met.

E. Be easy on yourself. There are times when you may fumble, and that's okay. Learning involves making mistakes on occasion.

KNOW YOUR SEX PSYCHODRAMA

With your story line decided upon, you need to now negotiate how you're going to relate to one another during the scene. Details of the psychodrama must be sorted out, including:

- What will you call each other? For example, in a slave relationship, the submissive may refer to the dominant as "Master."
- Will you take on character voices, such as changing your pitch, acquiring an accent, or using a foreign language?
- What kind of costumes would add to the role-play (e.g., waist-cinchers, corsets, posture collars, and hobble skirts)?
- What enhancements would reinforce the power dynamic? For example, "ownership" could be indicated by a Bottom wearing a velvet ribbon or a studded black leather collar.
- How elaborate will you go with forms of bondage?
- Will there be any physical pain involved? If so, how much?
- What kind of time frame are you aiming for?
- What will enhance versus ruin the scene for you?

More than anything, determine your safe word(s), such as "forest" or "firefly"—things you don't normally think of in the bedroom. This is the most important aspect of your sex play by far. Again, when this word is uttered, all activity is to immediately stop. In the case where one lover is gagged, a special form of eye contact or a hand signal should be given in the place of a word.

As you can see, communication is critical. And this doesn't just apply to what must be discussed before you get kinky; it also must continue throughout the scenario. The Top needs to check in with the Bottom regularly, which can be done while in character. Being dominant requires observing the reactions of the submissive. The Bottom, in turn, needs to communicate his or her needs, especially as things get more intense—which they may. A huge part of the draw to erotic power games is the amount of intensity involved on both the physical and psychological level. What many don't realize, until they're in their role, is that this includes an intensification of the self.

In becoming a Top, you're in charge of the scene's suspense, mystery, and anticipation. These revolve mostly around whether to indulge your submissive with exhilarating sexual sensations or whether to punish him or her for "bad" behavior. A great deal of the way you communicate is through commands that involve psychological restraint, such as "Get down" or "Don't make a sound." Among your goals are to tease and torment, magnifying sensations even more when they're finally delivered. Or this could involve the torture of sensory deprivation, where you do not stimulate at all or only provide extremely light, gentle stimulation. If pain is allowed, reserve it as a form of "punishment." Likewise, the Top should reward good service, giving compliments, showing appreciation, and always honoring your commitments. This may include the "privilege" of switching roles as a reward for a job well done. Finally, realize that, in controlling the scene, it doesn't have to be all sexual. You can play up this power dynamic for what it's worth, demanding that your Bottom do sensual things for you, such as giving you a pedicure.

Dominance

Regarded as the more "mental" side of BDSM, dominance and submission involves behaviors, customs, and rituals that reinforce one partner's power over the other in either an erotic or lifestyle sense, such as a "sex slave."

EROTIC POWER-PLAY TOYS

While erotic power-play can involve items around the house—a wooden spoon, clothespin, or rope from a clothesline—to keep things safe, it is generally recommended that lovers invest in some erotic power-play gear. Yet before doing so, make sure you've set your budget. You can easily get carried away in shopping for restraints, slappers, or products aimed at heightening sensations!

Restraints

In practicing bondage, you have your options of handcuffs, ropes, scarves, neckties, medical tape, and chains. Products, such as Liberator Shapes, allow for unique positions and also have clipped cuff attachments to make this experience more comfortable for the partner being restrained; these products offer a wide array of restraint choices such as soft, velvety, fully adjustable wrist and ankle cuffs, but still make ensure that the submissive cannot get away.

Some restraints can work with your mattress, such as Sportsheets, if you want to safely pin your lover to the bed. Others, such as door jam cuffs, can move the action off of the bed, temporarily strapping a lover to the door. Some restraints are sold with kits, which include a blindfold, gag, or soft floggers. No matter what, make sure that the product guarantees quick and easy removal, and that you have items, such as the key to handcuffs, easily accessible.

In restraining your partner, it's important to make sure that he or she feels no stress on the muscles or joints and that the restraint is safely secured but isn't too tight. If either is the case, help your lover change positions or adjust the restraint. Also make sure that the blood flow and breathing are not restricted in any way, and never tie anything around the neck. This should include when the Bottom moves. Do not leave arms or legs suspended up for too long, since the lack of blood flow will cause unpleasant tingling and numbing. Never leave your partner alone, and always have a pair of surgical scissors handy in case of emergency. If you're the Bottom and are uncomfortable in any way, let your partner know!

Slappers

Many lovers enjoy a good spanking, and when it comes to toys for a nice, stinging swat, there are a number of items to choose from, including rulers, wooden hairbrushes, spoons, straps, belts, switches, kitchen spatulas, crops, bamboo rods, paddles, doeskin whips, canes . . . When purchasing any of these, consider what the object is made out of, including the material used to make the tassels, as some will deliver more sensation than others. Some are also made with separate tops to create a more dramatic spanking sound. The Bottom can wear briefs or panties, making it easier for them to withstand the impact of harder spanks.

In assuming the position, the Bottom can be facedown on the bed, hanging over the back of a chair, bending forward, on all fours, or bending over an ottoman, table, or the Top's lap. Start soft, perhaps with your hands, focusing on the "sweet" spots—the fleshiest parts of the cheeks—and exploring how much the Bottom can take. In between blows, fondle your lover's genitals. Lovers can gradually handle harder strokes when the Top alternates with softer soothing strokes, since spanking results in an endorphin release.

S*ex*PERTISE

Mummification involves restraining your lover's entire body using elastic bandages or plastic wrap.

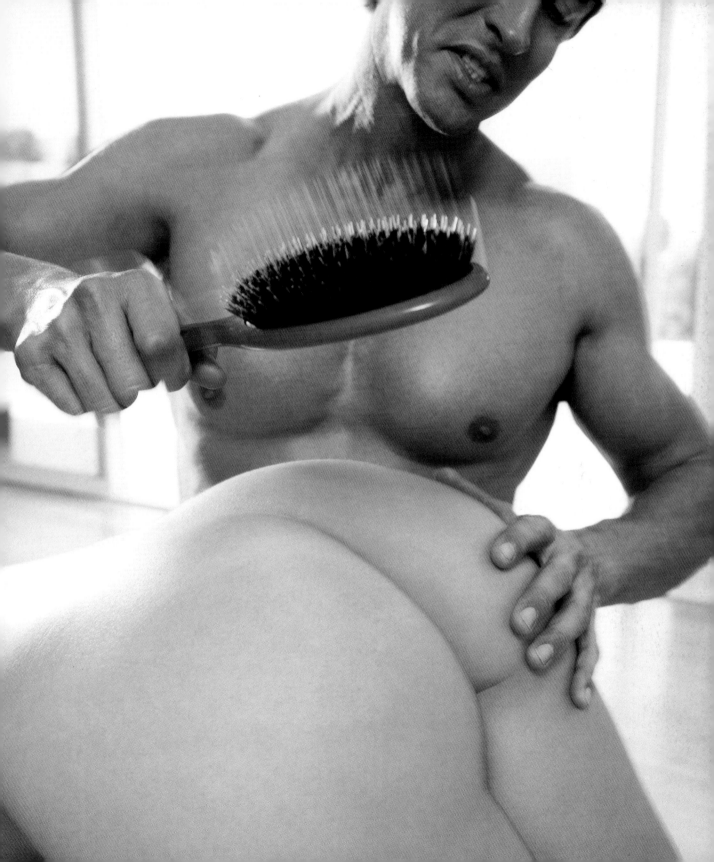

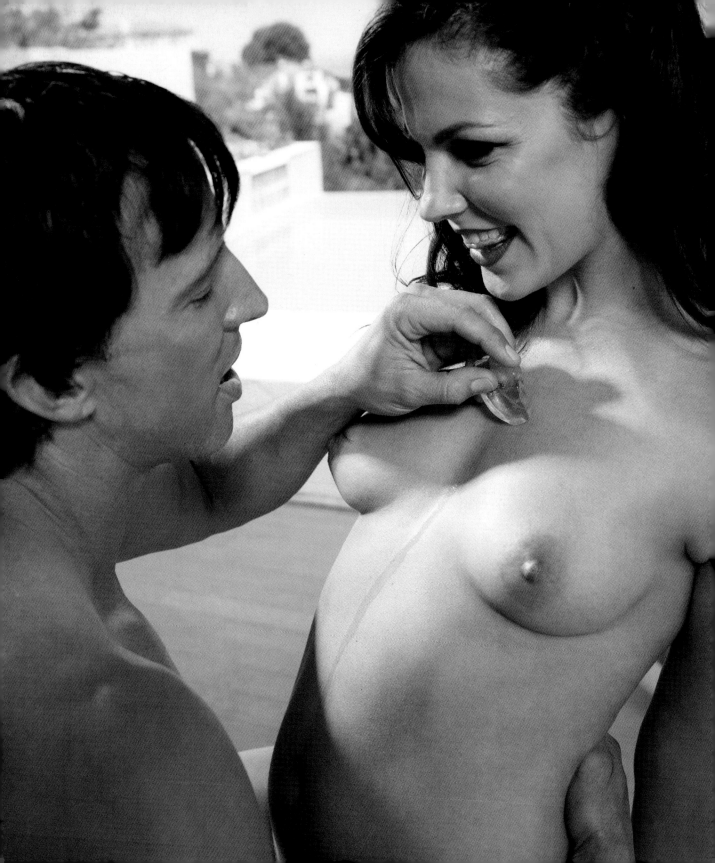

Sensation Play

You have your own preferences when it comes to types of sensations, whether that involves pinching, biting, scratching, or tickling. A great deal of erotic power-play involves magnifying what we feel in being stimulated in such ways.

Hot and Cold: In playing with temperature, a Top can pour hot wax from a paraffin candle (since this candle burns at the lowest temperature) on a lover's midsection, or run an ice-cold spoon or ice cubes over the Bottom's nipples before sucking on them. (Note: Holding the candle closer to the skin will make it hotter and riskier.)

Suck and Pump: In providing more "suck" sensation, a Top can use vacuum cups on the Bottom's buttocks, nipples, or penis for a temporary hickey. Each plastic or glass cup is attached to a hand pump and pumped before being placed on the body. Be sure to follow up each hickey with some delicate oral action of your own.

Point and Shoot: In bringing nerve endings in the skin to life, the Top can use a Wartenberg wheel. This stainless steel or plastic medical device has a wheel with rotating pointy, sharp pins that stimulate the flesh without puncturing it.

In following any of these suggestions, or in employing some of your own tactics, keep your partner turned on, intermittently stroking his penis or her clitoris while using these accoutrements of pleasure. Doing so heightens the eroticism and the overall sensations for the entire body.

At the end of your erotic power-play session, be sure to cuddle and express affection to each other. Loving each other with kisses and hugs brings back the balance in your relationship. Such "aftercare" is necessary in restoring your regular relationship and in processing the scene. Don't be surprised if there are tears of grief or joy from having acted out the scene. Such sex play can be cathartic and bring lovers closer together. Be sure to support each other with loving touch and reassurances as you come down from this sensual experience.

EXHIBITION AND VOYEURISM

The terms "exhibitionism" and "voyeurism" refer to a wide range of behaviors that range from completely harmless in a consensual adult relationship to crimes punishable by law. In hearing either word, however, most people tend to think of the actions that will lead to arrest, not realizing that most people engage in exhibitionism and/or voyeurism on a regular basis.

THE SCIENCE OF *Sex*

One U.S. study, "Sex in America", found that 93 percent of men and 74 percent of women like to watch their lovers undress. (Note: When watching another is done without that person's willing consent, the voyeurism then becomes a punishable offense.)

Voyeurism

Voyeurism is deriving sexual pleasure from seeing another person nude (e.g., a stripper) or engaging in sex (e.g., an adult star). Voyeuristic pursuits may include going to a strip bar or peep show or looking at "live cams" on the Internet. In a relationship, voyeurs like to look while a partner engages in sexual behaviors or undresses.

Exhibitionism

Exhibitionism, too, ranges in behaviors, most of which are harmless. A number of people like to reveal their bodies by wearing sexy clothes or by skinny-dipping. Such behavior becomes illegal, however, when it involves exposing one's sex organs to somebody who hasn't given consent, such as when a person flashes someone.

While many people don't like to think of themselves as exhibitionists or voyeurs, that's not to say that such behaviors aren't going on or that they don't belong in your erotic efforts. You have your own values around nudity, whether that's how much you'll strip down or how much you'll enjoy someone else taking it all off. In figuring out how such can boost your sex life, talk to your lover about what's appropriate and not—then pursue what works for the two of you!

$\mathcal{S}\mathcal{U}$ercise 10.6: Explore Erotic Power-Play Outside the Bedroom

For this exercise, you're actually going to take things outside of the bedroom. While you can't flash your partner in a public place, you can go commando when you leave the house. Throughout the evening, give each other private peaks, revealing that you're not sporting underwear. Look for opportunities where you may be able to slip a hand up her skirt or down his pants, all in the name of fun and foreplay.

Whether erotic power-play, voyeurism, or exhibitionism, "kink" behaviors can add a whole new dimension to your sex life. Couples can explore such sex play, taking it to a level they are comfortable with while testing their sexual boundaries, for greater eroticism. Many lovers find themselves surprisingly delighted by the mental and physical pleasures these sex acts offer. The sexual rewards reaped are in large part due to couples keeping an open mind in their interpretation of the stimulation. After all, the ability to experience sexual pleasure comes down to the meaning you assign to any form of sexual intimacy, from the "tame" to the "explicit."

$\mathcal{S}\mathcal{U}$PERTISE

Incorporate fetish dice into your play. One die tells you to spank, tickle, or paddle while the other one tells you which body part(s) to fawn over!

> "O Love, O pure deep love, be here, be now. Be all; worlds dissolve into your stainless endless radiance."
>
> —RUMI

Sexual Homework

This chapter summarizes a number of sexual behaviors that some books have been devoted to entirely. The behaviors can be overwhelming in many respects; taking action can be intimidating at first. In making sure that you get your feet wet, the following sexual homework has been assigned to you.

Bondage Put to Action—Using soft restraints, such as Velcro cuffs or stockings, gently tie up your lover. Feel free to use your partner's body to pleasure yourself. Have fun teasing each other to the brink of orgasm, taking turns "torturing" one another to near climax, only to back away just shy of orgasm. Thrive on the erotic pleasures that can be had in consensually—temporarily having control over one another—playing up the theatre B&D is known for. Get dressed up, use props, and role-play, as the dominant partner delivers light doses of pain, such as spankings or pinching, or verbal abuse while calling the sexual shots. To recap, make sure that you've discussed each other's needs, wants, and limits. Plan your script so that you're working on a plot, where boundaries have been agreed upon. Have a safe word established. Remember, if you're the Bottom,

being passive, relishing in the sensations that can come only in not needing to take any responsibility for your pleasuring.

Spanking—Packed with nerve endings, the buttocks is a major erogenous zone that can handle a great deal of stimulation. You can make the most of this asset by giving your partner a good spanking (or by asking for one yourself). Once your partner is aroused, smack or slap the buttocks. (Other areas that can handle such touch are the thighs and back of the calves; you want to avoid hitting the spine and kidneys.) Start with a slow, steady rhythm, taking your time building up to a faster pace. You can alternate such stimulation, plus give your lover a slight break from the action, by running your tongue over the area and then blowing on it. Consider other ways to bring the zone to life; for example, follow a slap with the light touches of a feather. As the spanker, be sure to check in with your lover, asking if your spanking needs to be harder, softer, faster, slower . . . As the receiver, do not hesitate in letting your lover know if you're uncomfortable or in too much pain, as well as what feels good.

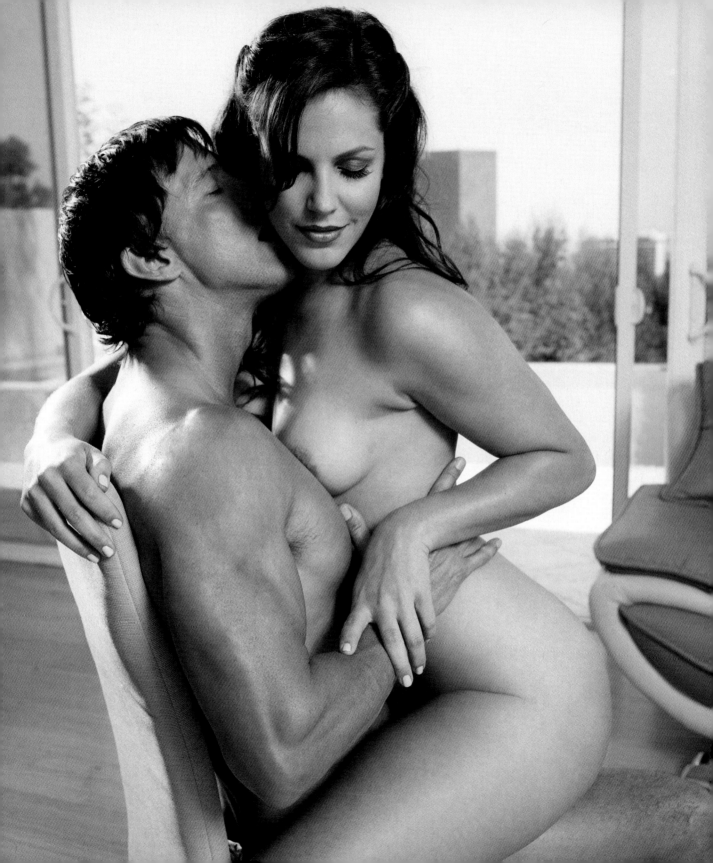

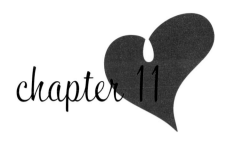

chapter 11

The Top 10 Sexual Positions: Enjoy the Most Climactic Coupling to Build True Sexual Intimacy

WHILE EVERY COUPLE has its favorite tried-and-true sexual positions, it never hurts to add a couple more to your repertoire. Trying new sexual positions not only helps in avoiding monotony, but also keeps the sparks alive in the bedroom. The excitement and adventure that comes with trying new positions is made even better as you discover new ways to touch and please each other.

There are hundreds of sexual positions available for your sexual pleasuring. Yet between being nearly impossible or not very climax-inducing, some of these positions aren't in your best interest when it comes to sexual fulfillment. The following ten positions can invite some of the most exhilarating, intimate sex you'll ever have.

"I realized what was hidden within me and conversed with You in secret. Though we were united, we still were apart. Though awe hid You from my searching eyes, ecstasy brought You close to my innermost being."

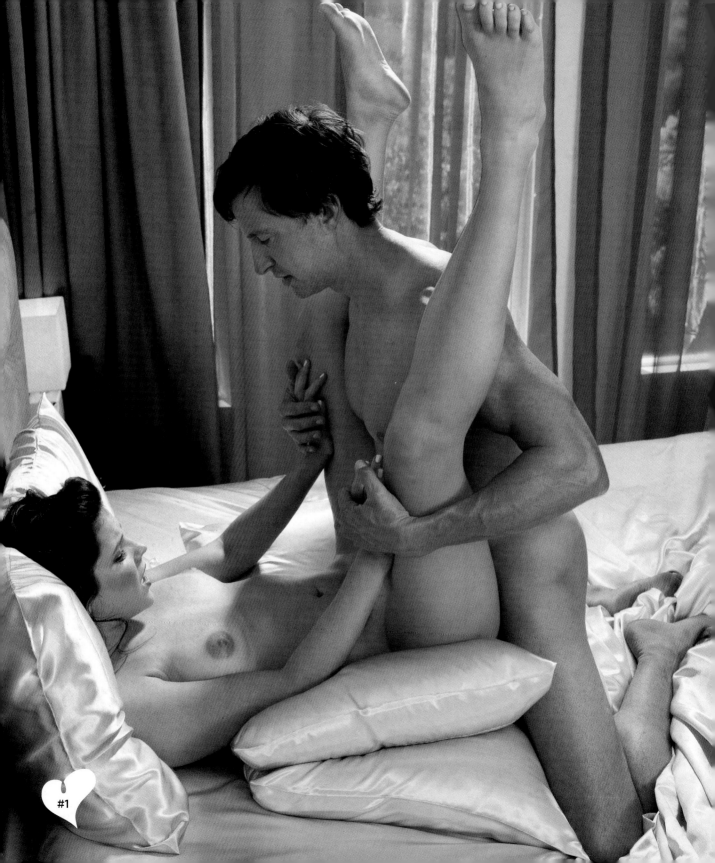

POSITION #1: Deeper Penetration Position

Normally, we don't think of the missionary position for deeper penetration. Traditional missionary tends not to allow the penis to plunge as deeply into the vagina as other positions. Yet we're going to try a variation of the missionary for deeper penetration since lovers adore this position for a number of good reasons:

- You get to gaze lovingly into each other's eyes
- You can see your lover's face during climax
- You can whisper and moan into each other's ears
- Men have great access to their partner's body and enjoy having control over the intensity and depth of the thrusting
- Women may like feeling taken care of as they are easily caressed and are not doing most of the work

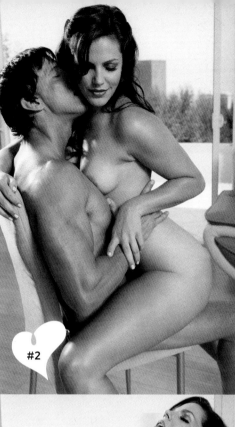

#2

In modifying missionary, slide pillows under the woman's buttocks for a better angle, as she spreads her legs. Her partner should then hold her legs in a "V" shape, supporting himself with her calves as he penetrates her. Not only will lovers find that the man is able to go deeper, but it may feel as though he's filling her up, thanks to the narrowing of her vaginal canal while in a raised-leg position.

Partners may also find that he's better able to stimulate her G spot and clitoris in this position. He can do this by rocking back and forth against her pelvis. He can also swivel his hips, finding a rhythm when he tucks his pelvis under and pushes up against her groin every couple of swivels. She can further make sure that her clitoris is stimulated by grinding her pelvis into his.

POSITION #2: Lap Dance Position

You can become sexually aroused from the occasional lap dance, especially if you're up for a long sex. In this position, neither partner has to worry about their arms or legs getting too fatigued, as the woman controls the angle and depth of entry. Have him sit on a chair or the side of the bed, and straddle him. This is super since lovers will want to let their hands roam, stimulating any erogenous areas on their upper bodies or holding each other's faces during a passionate embrace. This position is also great for new partners in that a man can learn what kind of rhythm she prefers.

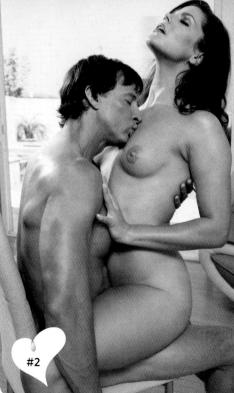

#2

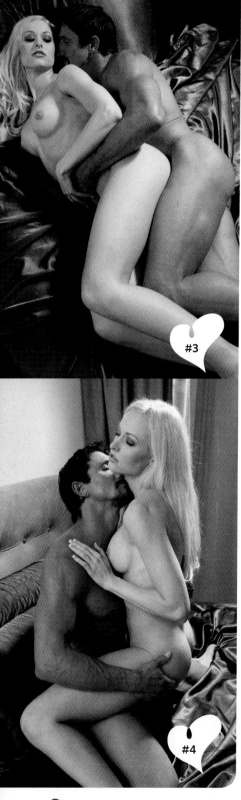

#3

#4

POSITION #3: Full-Body-Contact Position

Side-by-side positions are ideal for those times you're in the mood for easy, smooth, calm, relaxing sex. What makes them even better is that they allow for full-body contact, for greater intimacy, while providing effortless access to the clitoris. So try a spooning position for leisurely sex, piqued by the idea that you could be at this for quite a while—kissing, teasing, hugging, touching, massaging . . .

POSITION #4: Cowgirl Position

Woman-on-top is one of the hottest positions around since many lovers are aroused by the mere thought of this position since it:

- Puts her in charge of the depth, angle, and speed of thrusting, the confidence from which could send her sex appeal into overdrive
- Allows either lover to directly stimulate her clitoris with fingers or a sex toy.
- Enables him to experience more blood flow to his erectile tissue, increasing his pleasure and stimulation
- Allows her lover to take in the sight of her breasts and curves, turning him on even more as he watches her vagina slide up and down the shaft of his penis
- Makes it possible for him to play with her body and breasts, running his hands up and down her sides
- Enables her to play with herself, which adds to both lovers' arousal
- Allow him to play with himself, enhancing the sexual excitement even more

In keeping the woman-on-top position fresh, aim for variety. You can do this by pursuing a series of positions. Start with the man on his knees and sitting back on his heels. She then straddles him. She next angles her body so that he can keep the penis pressed against her G spot, as both grind for clitoral stimulation. Eventually, he can straighten his legs to then briefly transition to traditional cowgirl before she does more of a split over his penis. She can then hold her labia open for a good view of his penis as she "rides" him. She can also wrap her thumb and middle finger around the base of his penis, like a penis ring, to harden his erection even more, as both lovers tease each other, getting to the brink of orgasm before holding off for more.

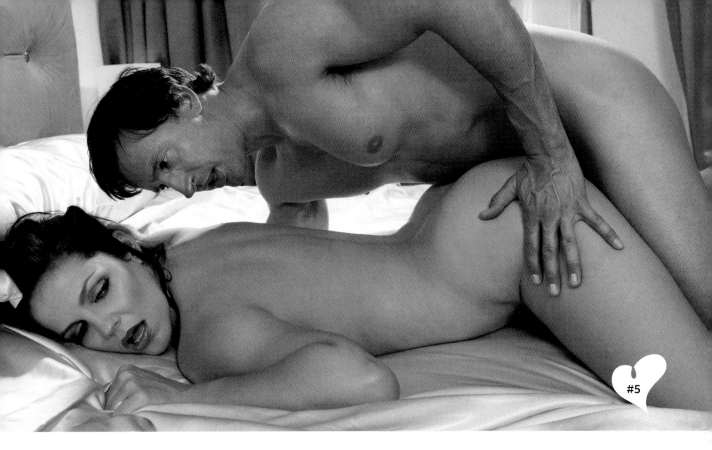

#5

POSITION #5: Au Naturel Position

The rear-entry position is a favorite way to merge for many since:

- Either partner can stimulate the clitoris
- The position offers deeper thrusting
- He can kiss and touch her body, playing with her hair, running his fingers down her spine, caressing her breasts, or playing with her nipples
- He can slap or massage her buttocks for more sensation
- He can play with her anus
- She can play with his scrotum, buttocks, and thighs
- She can play with herself

For a slight variation of the traditional rear-entry, try having her rest on her arms before bringing her legs in between his, back arched. Once he has hit her G spot area, she can bring her legs together as she squeezes her buttocks and pelvic floor muscles for a tighter grip. For a deeper thrust, she can lower her chest, spread her legs, and arch her back; for a shallower thrust, she should flatten her back. For more sensation, either lover can swivel the hips, pushing back at the other with each thrust.

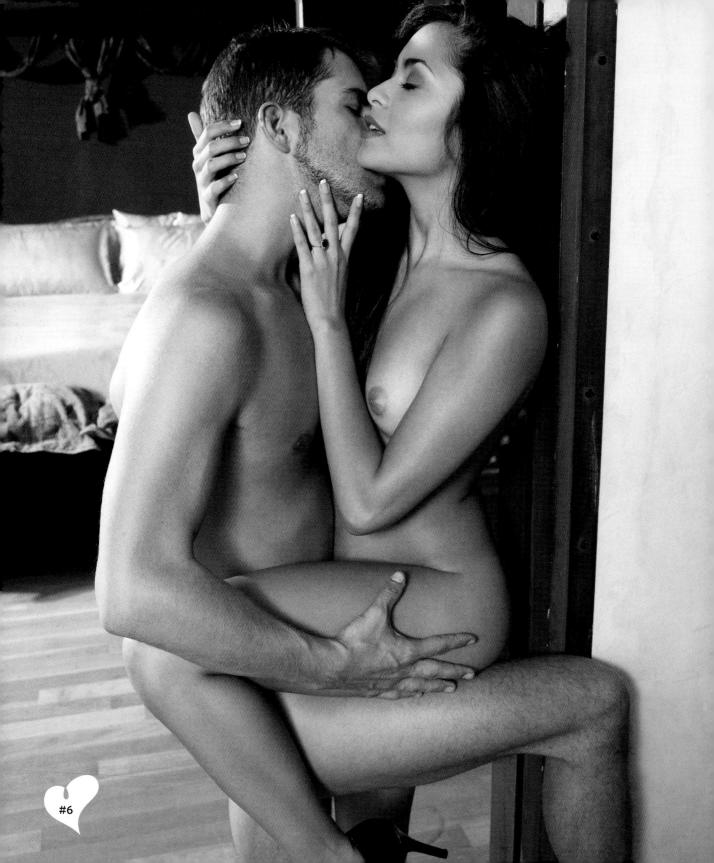

#6

POSITION #6: Off-the-Bed Sex

Every now and then, lovers want to have sex out of the bed, with standing positions allowing for lovemaking almost anywhere. Between full-body contact, great mobility, impulsiveness, and total unrestraint, lovers can have sex anywhere. One fun variation of standing sex is for a man to stand facing his lover, who is standing on the edge of a couch, a secluded bench, or another elevated object. She is to adjust the width of her stance (bending her knees if need be), so that he can glide between her legs. As your pelvises merge, gyrate, letting your hands run wild as she strokes the back of his neck, he massages the base of her spine, she teases his testicles, or he kisses her nipples.

POSITION #7: Loveseat Sex

The woman is to straddle her lover's lap, then lean back onto it as she pushes her buttocks up against his groin, knees bent up into his chest. (If you need help supporting your weight or maintaining your balance, stretch your arms out behind you.) She can then thrust back and forth along the shaft of his penis, pushing herself off the back of the couch and opening or closing her legs for variation. He's going to love watching her.

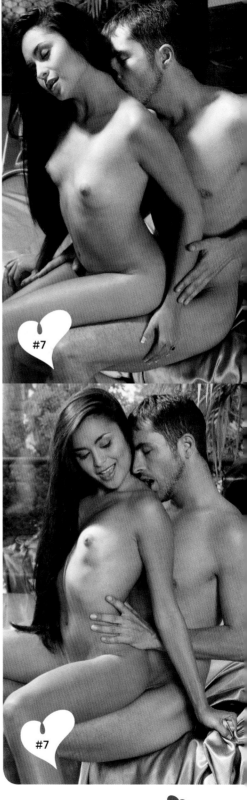

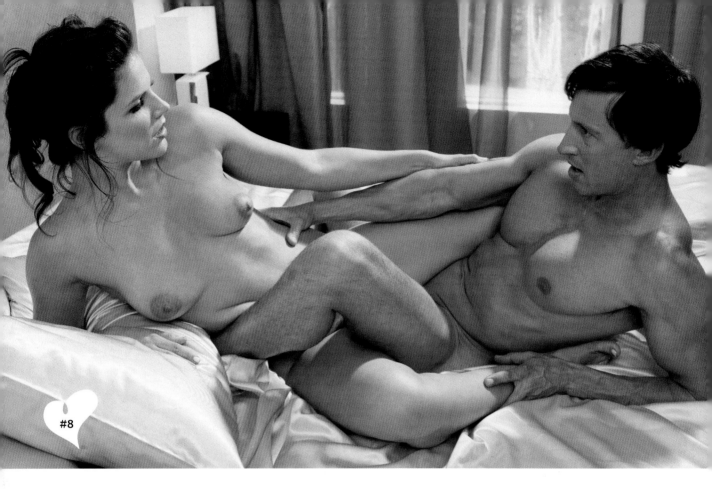

#8

POSITION #8: Challenge for Better Sex

"Getting there is half the fun" couldn't be truer when it comes to trying challenging positions. Even if lovers are unable to master a certain sexual position, they can enjoy the fact that they tried and feel closer for it. So whether or not you're feeling terribly flexible or coordinated, try this side-sex position:

Both partners are to lie on their sides, woman in front, facing the same direction but with heads at opposite ends (you'll be joined at your groins, with heads at opposite ends). After penetration, she is to wrap her legs around his torso, with her arms stretched behind her to support her body. He then circles her waist with his legs, gripping her upper thighs as he begins thrusting, eventually moving his hips in circles. In offering shallow sex, this position activates nerve endings in the head of his penis and in the lower one-third of her vagina.

POSITION #9: Exotic Sex

Yes, these require a bit of flexibility, but exotic positions evoke arousal simply by the fact that they're "outlandish." Have sex simply to be experimental, maximizing on the glamour that comes with dabbling in the mysteriously unusual. To do this position, the woman is to lie faceup, hands supporting her lower back as she lifts her legs and lower torso up to the point that they're almost perpendicular to the ground. Her partner is to then kneel in front of her, taking her ankles and bringing his knees toward her shoulders. He next takes her hands and holds her hips. She can steady her body with her hands on his thighs as she thrusts her hips and arches her back in becoming one movement with him. As you make love, the woman should notice the blood rushing into her pelvic region. Couples should feel how they fit so nice and snugly, especially as he reaches around to stimulate her clitoris.

POSITION #10: Coaxing-the-Clitoris Sex

One of the questions people ask sex experts the most is how couples can better stimulate the clitoris during sexual intercourse. Here's one position that coaxes the clitoris on two fronts. The woman lies down on a surface that puts her pelvis a foot lower than his pelvis, as he stands in front of her. She then lifts her legs, resting them on his shoulders. She then tilts her pelvis toward the ceiling so that her back is straight as their groins connect. He next puts his hands under her hips, holding her buttocks, as he thrusts and grinds up against her clitoris while she stimulates it further with her fingers or a sex toy.

THRUSTING TECHNIQUES EVERY LOVER SHOULD KNOW

When it comes to satisfying sex, thrusting is everything. This is because, whether passive, playful, powerful, passionate, or furious, every thrust causes thousands of nerve endings to be pulled and tugged in the vagina and head of the penis. No matter what position or body parts you have access to, the right kind of thrust can make all the difference between mediocre and magnificent sex. So as you have sexual intercourse, assess how the position you're in can be enhanced with any of the following:

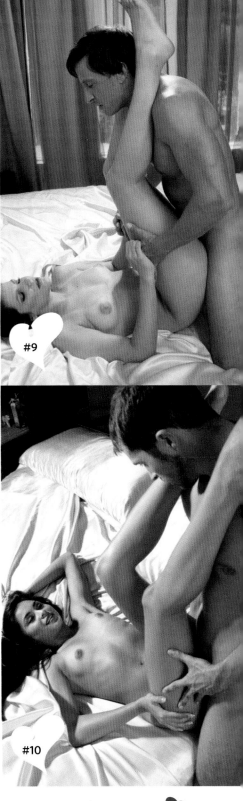

#9

#10

Keep it shallow.

Resist the urge to go deep. Sometimes it's best just to tease, so keep the thrusting limited by allowing only the head of the penis to bob in and out of the vaginal opening.

Be a tease.

Play with the vaginal opening (introitus), tracing it with the tip of the penis. Take the head of the penis, trail it along the labia, up around her clitoris, and back down a couple of times before playing with the introitus a little more.

Show off your "dancing" skills.

Don't let your hip action go to waste. Unleash it by gyrating against one another, swaying your hips, or grinding your pubic bones into one another.

SEXUAL Q&A: DEALING WITH VAGINISMUS

I am unable to penetrate my lover every time I try. Her physician cannot find anything physically wrong with her. What could be going on?

Vaginismus is a condition that makes sexual intercourse nearly impossible or extremely painful. It is characterized by a strong involuntary contraction of the vaginal muscles, mostly of the outer third of the vagina, which occurs whenever sex is attempted, making penetration sharply painful. Often an unconscious series of spasms, vaginismus is most often psychological and emotional in nature, but is sometimes due to physical reasons. It may be occurring because of previous unwanted sexual experiences, discomfort with a sexual situation, a vaginal infection, or an intact hymen in younger women. Vaginismus is almost always the result of a specific phobia concerning vaginal penetration, whether it's due to sexual abuse, having sex when a female doesn't want to, or negative thinking about sex.

In confirming that your partner is suffering from vaginismus, seek out treatment and therapy. She'll learn how to train the vaginal muscles to open and relax during sex, during both masturbation and with the use of a vaginal dilation kit. The woman (or her partner) starts by slowly, gently inserting a vitamin-E-oiled cotton swab, followed by an oiled finger, then two fingers . . . or by using different sized dilators into her vagina while relaxing the vaginal muscles. For sex therapists or counselors in the area who may be able to help, visit the website for the American Association of Sexuality Educators, Counselors, and Therapists at www.aasect.org.

Go crazy.

Lose yourselves in mad, unquenchable thrusting, giving it to each other "hard and fast"!

Guide your lover.

In making sure you get the action you need, grab your partner's hips and merge even deeper. Use your hands to steer the motions and rhythms you need to reach orgasm.

SEXUAL Q&A: DEALING WITH PAINFUL SEX

My wife and I are newlyweds and virgins, and we're having no success in trying to make love. She's in pain every time I try to penetrate her. Any ideas on what's going on?

Painful intercourse, also known as dyspareunia, is the most common sexual complaint that gynecologists hear from their female patients. This is characterized by pain or discomfort during or right after sex, which happens almost every time she has sex, and can be due to any number of physical and psychological reasons, namely:

- A lack of lubrication (vaginal dryness) due to aging, medications, late childbearing, relationship issues, or not enough sexual arousal
- A medical problem, such as pelvic inflammatory disease (PID), fibroids, hemorrhoids, a reproductive tract disorder, an inflammation of the uterine lining, a Bartholin's gland cyst, or endometriosis (especially if the pain is experienced on deep penetration)
- A reaction to creams, fabrics, perfumes, feminine hygiene products, spermicides, or latex, any of which can cause an irritation or allergy
- The need to use the bathroom. Pain could be due to a full bladder or the need for a bowel movement

In treating dyspareunia, your lover should have a gynecological exam to rule out or treat any of these etiologies. She should stop using any products that may be the problem. Make sure that you and your partner are using plenty of lube and that you spend a lot of time on foreplay. If a woman is not fully aroused before penetration, her uterus may not be raised, and his penis may be coming into contact with the cervix, which can be painful and/or uncomfortable. Also, try a position, such as woman on top, that gives the woman more control over deep penetration and any pain it might be causing. A woman should work with a physician and therapist to learn arousal techniques and explore feelings about her partner, as well.

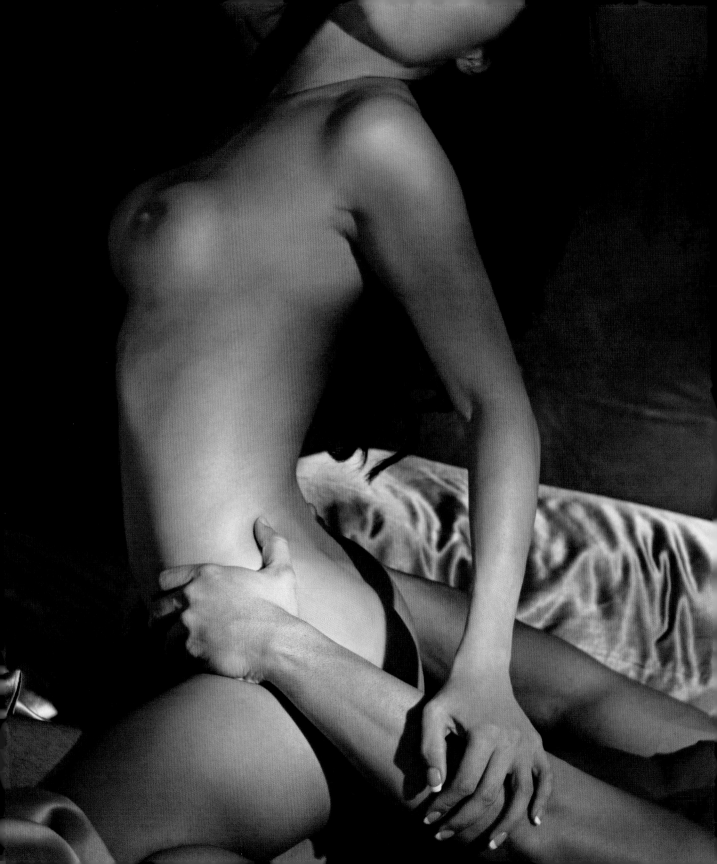

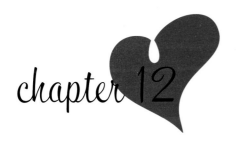

chapter 12

The Art of Anal Loving: Exploring the Pleasure Zone that Can Enhance Your Sexual Life

LOVERS HAVE BEEN INDULGING in anal pleasures throughout history. From Greek ceramics to East Indian temple sculptures to Persian paintings to African carvings, humans have long acknowledged and celebrated anal intercourse. While overwhelmingly regarded as a taboo practice today, people still engage in anal play for variety, to spice up their sex lives, or because they find it a terribly exciting, gratifying form of eroticism.

"*Every time you are able to go beyond the body's superficial desires for love, you are bringing your body home and moving toward integration and unity.*"

—HENRI NOUWEN

For those who have dared to explore such pleasuring, the anus is a trove of delights and orgasms, with lovers experiencing sexual intimacy in a completely new and exciting way. On a psychological level, such sex is thrilling in that you are challenging the taboo. You may love going into taboo territory and being "naughty" with each other. On a more physical level, you might like the tight feel of the anal region since this erogenous zone is packed with sensitive, responsive nerve endings. You might love the fullness anal sex offers, and the increased intensity that comes with thrusting of the anal canal. This reaction is in large part due to the fact that the anus and anal canal are engorged with blood during sexual arousal, becoming even more sensitive when stimulated. Anal enthusiasts adore the deep feeling of sexual pleasure that they claim can only come from stimulation of the anus.

For some people, the anus is the greatest hot spot on their bodies, eroticizing their sex lives like nothing else. For males, receptive anal sex is especially gratifying given the rectum is the easiest way for him or his lover to access his prostate for incredible stimulation and orgasms. Some females like anal thrusting since it can indirectly stimulate her G spot for greater pleasure. It is no wonder that anal pleasuring can result in amazing sex as couples realize a deeper romantic and sexual connection.

TALKING ABOUT "FORBIDDEN" PLEASURES

More people would probably experiment with anal sex if it was as simple as saying "Bottoms up!" But, despite having racy thoughts about doing this, many lovers are wracked with fears and worries when it comes to this kind of sex play. Many don't understand that this is a form of sexual behavior enjoyed by all types of people of all different sexual orientations. Some think that playing with this often-deemed "exit only" zone is unnatural, wrong, or dirty, so they end up denying themselves a form of sex that could make for some of the greatest sex of their lives.

It's really important for lovers to be proactive in sitting down to diffuse each other's concerns. Talk frankly about fears, keeping things positive by discussing fantasies and desires when it comes to anal play. While it may be a daunting conversation in some ways, it can be incredibly stimulating in others as you reveal what makes your spine tingle at the idea of anal play. Being able to share your innermost thoughts on this "licentious" lovemaking also puts you in charge of your pleasuring.

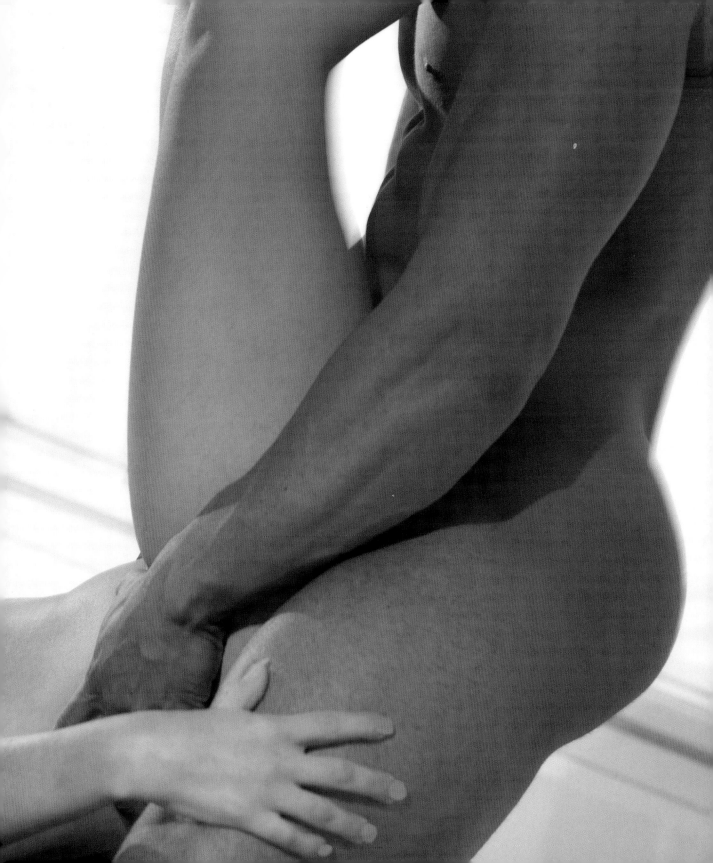

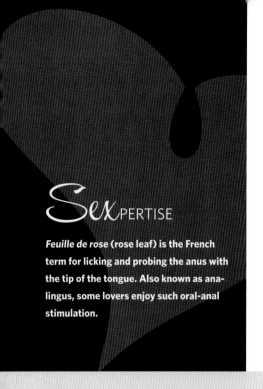

Finally, couples need to equip themselves with the facts in order to not only be well-informed on the "how to" of this sexual practice, but also to challenge myths and misconceptions about anal pleasuring. Lovers need to come up with a plan of action for dealing with their concerns. Anal sex is an adventure that requires a lot of trust, confidence, and responsibility, with both partners needing to feel comfortable and in charge. You'll need to address major issues that often discourage or turn lovers off to anal sex. You also need to confirm that both parties are interested. If one partner feels coerced or pressured into anal sex acts, the body will not cooperate, with the anus becoming tight with tension upon penetration. And that doesn't do anything when it comes to pleasuring.

In pursuing anal pleasuring, lovers need to continue to communicate throughout the entire experience, knowing that they can rely on an established safe word such as "Peaches" for "Stop!" or "Slow down."

SEXUAL Q&A: ANAL SEX FOR PROSTATE STIMULATION

My wife and I have been exploring new ways to excite each other, and she recently surprised me by asking if she could use a strap-on dildo on me. I was somewhat taken aback and uncomfortable, especially since I would not be in control. However, I have decided that maybe this is something we can both enjoy since it's one way to stimulate my prostate. Do you have any tips on dildos and harnesses?

Kudos to you and your wife for considering something new to try! Some men report feeling homophobic or "butt-phobic"—or both—to consider the sensual pleasures anal play can provide. In starting your anal adventure, you and your partner can have a great deal of fun selecting a dildo (you have your choice of glass, rubber, silicone, or latex), since they come in a wealth of sizes, textures, colors, and styles. Know that a silicone dildo may be overall the most resilient and the easiest to clean, it retains heat well, and becomes more flexible with time and use. In choosing a size, keep in mind that the dildo will be about half an inch shorter once in the harness. Dildos typically range in size from 4 to 12 inches in length and 1 to 2 inches in girth.

In selecting a harness, know that they come in leather, vinyl, denim, nylon, or webbing, and in two basic styles—with a leg strap encircling the thigh or with a center strap running between the legs. The latter is used like a jock-strap, giving users a lot of control while still giving access to the vulva or anus for stimulation. If your wife wants to double her pleasure when stimulating you, she can wear a harness with a vibrating penis ring or a pearl massager, with its "pearls" in the shaft, that can be slipped between the harness and her body.

During anal intercourse, check in with one another, and trust the power dynamic that this sex act invites. The person providing the stimulation needs to ask for instruction, while the receiver needs to give direction, such as "A little faster," "That's too much," or "More pressure." The recipient needs to let the giver know if something doesn't feel right or is painful. The giver needs to stay mindful of any power rushes that can come with being in a dominant role and having complete control of another. Sex play loses all of its fun when it turns rough, emotionally and physically harming the other.

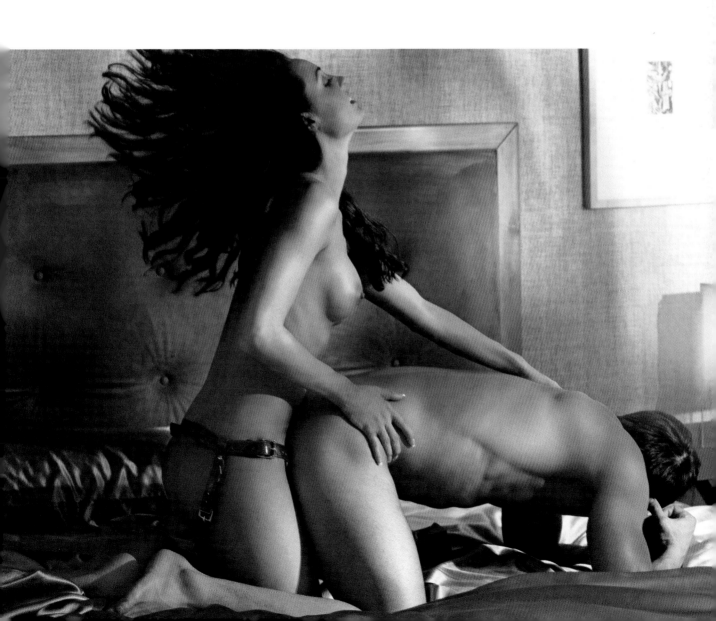

ANAL SEX SAFETY

When it comes to anal sex, there are several rules to keep in mind:

Never double-dip: The mouth and vagina are "no go" zones until the penis, fingers, or sex toys are washed with hot water and soap or a wipe. Failure to keep things clean can spread bacteria, which can lead to infection.

Use protection: Condoms keep everything cleaner, easier, and safer, plus help to protect a male against prostate infection. If transitioning from anal sex to oral or vaginal sex, changing or removing condoms enables lovers to avoid spreading infections from the anus to the mouth or vagina. So in practicing anal sex, use a latex or polyurethane condom to protect yourself from sexually transmitted infections. Tears can occur in the rectal lining from penetration, even when anal penetration is at its safest.

Stick with plain condoms: You want a condom with a plain (versus stimulating) texture to avoid any discomfort, abrasions, and irritation. To further protect the rectal tissue, stay away from condoms with nonoxynol-9, since this spermicide is an irritant.

Wash your toys: Sexual enhancement products should be cleaned after every use. Also, ones that are inserted into the anus need to be thoroughly cleaned before being used in the vagina, and the toy should be washed if you switch to use your toy on your partner.

EXPLORING YOUR ANUS

When it comes to anal adventures, you may want to explore your body on your own first. Getting to know your anal area in a private space will make it easier for you to enjoy this erogenous zone with a partner. You'll know what to expect and be better able to let your lover know what feels good and what doesn't, plus what you need to be stimulated.

$\mathcal{S}$exercise 12.1 Ways to Start Exploring Your Anus

During your next solo session, get to know your anal region. Some people like to do this in the shower with a soapy or lubricated finger. You want to take your time in this kind of exploration, allowing yourself to get turned on while relaxing your anal sphincter muscle for nicer, easier penetration. Make sure that you're in a relaxed space where you'll be free of interruptions, where you can note your likes and dislikes.

If you have trouble with the idea of using your finger, or would like a little bit of assistance, try using rectal dilators or a small anal toy. Rectal dilators are a set of instruments that get progressively larger. You use them by inserting the dilator that is the smallest in diameter first. When you are comfortable, you can move on to the next size, then the next, until, over time, you've tried the largest. Alternatively, a sex toy such as a "butt plug," with a flared base, can also help (it is important to use a toy with a flanged base so that the toy does not accidentally completely slip inside). This sex toy, which is available in different sizes and shapes, can help to relax the anal muscles. Slowly insert the lubricated butt plug into the rectum, breathing deeply as you notice the feelings of fullness. If you'd like, thrust the toy in and out of your rectum, especially as you rub your clitoris or run your hand up and down the shaft of your penis. (Note: This toy may slip or shoot out of your anus as you become aroused or climax.)

With or without a lover, you may want to experiment with different butt plugs, since they come with a variety of features, including being ribbed, smooth, or bumpy. Some are fancier than others. Some are simple dildos while some vibrate. Some even inflate. The inflatable butt plug can be expanded up to three inches in diameter and up to four inches in length.

PREPARING FOR ANAL SEX

Whether you're getting to know your anus on your own time or with a partner, you want to be prepared. Make sure that you have all of the following within easy reach ahead of time: safer sex products, lubricant, baby wipes, a towel, and sex toys. You also want to be sure to do the following:

Go to the bathroom: Having a bowel movement before teasing this area is going to make things a lot cleaner and more comfortable. (It will also decrease the chance of an accidental bowel movement following withdrawal; if a bowel movement occurs, or if feces is present when the inserting partner withdraws, don't make an issue out of it. Just clean up with disposable wipes or a dark, wet washcloth.)

Wash up: Thoroughly clean the anal area during a bath or shower, or with a warm, soapy washcloth. If you want to be even cleaner than such bathing affords, you have a couple of options. First, some lovers like to shave or wax their anal region, feeling cleaner from hair removal. Some individuals like to use an enema, which involves introducing water or a liquid solution into the anal canal in order to flush fecal matter out of the colon and rectum. It also stimulates your bowels, which is a really great idea for those times you plan on having lots of anal sex or are into using bigger sexual-enhancement products.

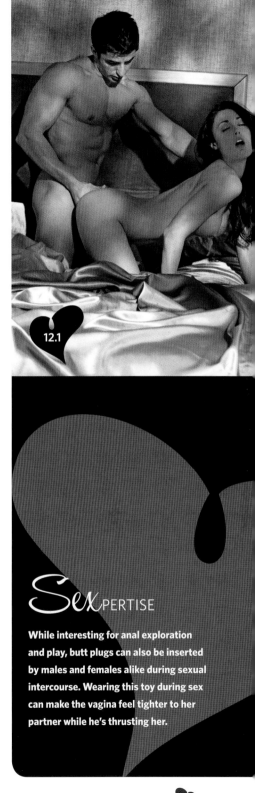

12.1

SEXPERTISE

While interesting for anal exploration and play, butt plugs can also be inserted by males and females alike during sexual intercourse. Wearing this toy during sex can make the vagina feel tighter to her partner while he's thrusting her.

Trim your nails: You want fingernails that are smooth and free of torn cuticles and rough edges, lest you tear the anal lining. Those who can't bear the thought of parting with their long nails should wear latex gloves, with a cotton ball stuffed into each fingertip, to prevent harming the rectal lining. Shorter nails are, however, recommended.

Love your lube: Anal sex is not as easy as penile-vaginal intercourse since the rectum has no natural lubrication. Without lubrication, your delicate anal tissues can be easily torn, and your experience will not be nearly as comfortable. So use lube, preferably a thicker one or silicone, which lasts longer—and lots of it.

Relax: Being stressed and full of tension is going to do you no good. You want to unwind and calm your nerves. While many people may want to do this with alcohol or drugs, these will only make things sloppy and heighten any risks. If you must have a glass of wine or another such drink, limit yourself to one serving. To relax, take your time and channel most of your efforts on tuning in to your body, focusing on your breath. This is a must if you're the receptive partner, since you'll want to come back to the breath.

Get sexually excited: You must be highly aroused and in the mood before anything comes near your anus. So aim for plenty of foreplay. Build excitement, getting yourself excited at just the thought of what you're doing. Stimulate your other erogenous zones, especially ones in the groin and buttocks area, since this will invite more blood flow to the nether region. If you're the giver, lick the outer folds of the anus, teasing it with the tip of your wet, warm tongue. Or stimulate the anal area with a Swizzle Stick or an anal vibrator, both of which are specially designed for anal play. Some have small balls at the top of the shaft to tease the anal opening, preparing it for more pleasure. Leave the tip at the anal opening, letting the vibe slide in gently when the body is ready. Go ahead and have an orgasm ahead of time since this may relax you for anal stimulation.

Assume position: Couples use many of the same positions they use for coitus for anal sex. Positions that make for easier anal sex, some of which we just reviewed, include rear-entry position or missionary, with pillows to support and tilt the pelvis. Side by side (spooning) is considered best for beginners, since it gives the receiver total control of the pace and movement. Being on top is ideal for recipients needing to feel in charge. Lovers looking to get more creative can adjust missionary so that the receiver's legs are pushed toward the head. They can also have the receiving partner squatting on a chair, holding onto the back for support. Or both can sit in a chair, facing the same direction, which gives the receiving partner control over penetration.

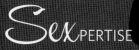

S*ex*PERTISE

While specific anal lubricants may sound ideal for anal play, be wary of the ingredient benzocaine. This local anesthetic numbs your anal area, which actually hampers your ability to engage in anal play safely. Not feeling pain can lead to damage. It can also diminish the quality of the wonderful reactions you're hoping for.

In the Bedroom:
Probing for Pleasure

ANAL SEX REQUIRES, in many ways, its own form of foreplay since it's vital that you warm up the anus first. The anal sphincter muscle is quite tight, and you'll want to be mindful that you're not squeezing it. Practice relaxing the anal area. You can do this by clenching and holding the muscles of your buttocks for a couple of seconds, then releasing for five seconds.

Gentle finger stimulation helps to relax the body, preparing the anal sphincter muscle for more penetration. (Alternatively, you can use a toy meant for anal pleasuring with a flared base or extra big handle for grip—important features in making sure that the product doesn't get sucked and stuck inside!)

1. You're going to start by applying lubricant to the anal opening and your finger(s) or toy. (Note: People with tighter anuses may want to start with the pinkie finger.)

2. Now as you begin to insert a finger into the anal opening, know that the anus has two sphincters, or rings of muscles, that will resist penetration. A person has control over relaxing the first one, which is at the entrance. The second ring, the internal sphincter, is about a quarter inch in and is under involuntary control. This sphincter is the one that makes penetration difficult and painful when a receiver is tense or fearful.

3. You may notice that your initial sphincter muscle will begin to spasm as the finger goes in. As the recipient, breathe through any desire to squeeze the anal opening shut, staying relaxed. Instead, take control and squeeze your anal sphincter muscle. This will allow you to feel the difference between a relaxed and a clenched rectum, plus will help prepare you for dildo insertion.

4. As your anal opening relaxes, have your partner push his or her finger in a little deeper, just up to the first knuckle. Take a break here as your anus gets used to the sensation. If you experience any pain, have your partner remain still; if the pain doesn't subside, have your partner remove the finger slowly and either add more lube or halt all action entirely. If you wish to try again, use a smaller finger or toy, or take a rest from this activity and play with other hot spots for a while.

5. As the "giver," check in with your partner, encouraging your lover to breathe deeply. As he or she exhales and the sphincter muscles relax, slowly, carefully slip your finger deeper inside, pressing against the front (stomach side) rectal wall.

6. When your partner is ready, begin thrusting in and out of his or her anus, asking your lover if you need to go deeper, faster, slower . . . or if more pressure is desired.

In the Bedroom:
Transitioning to Anal Sex

FINGER PENETRATION of the anal region may be all some couples want to try, or all that they're ready for in initially exploring this erogenous zone. Sooner or later, some couples like to try having anal sex, with the following instructions making for the most comfortable experience:

1. Once you've warmed up the anus with some fingering, lubricate the condom-covered penis or dildo, and slowly, gently insert.

2. As the recipient, you can try to open up your anal opening by pushing the anal muscles outward while your lover is gently inserting the penis or dildo. Be sure to breathe during insertion.

3. Both partners should stay motionless at first, especially the first couple of times they try to have anal sex. As the inserter, be sure to check in with your lover with questions such as, "Are you uncomfortable?" "Should I go slower?" or "Let me know when you can take deeper penetration." Don't be surprised if you need to adjust the angling or slow the pace, always remaining patient with yourselves.

4. Whether it's needed, stimulate other hot spots, such as his perineum or her mons pubis, perhaps with a vibrator, while penetrating. This relaxes the muscles and adds even more sensations.

5. The receiver should give the signal that he or she is ready for thrusting. As the giver, begin slowly, with a controlled pelvic rhythm, being attentive to not tear the condom or anal lining.

6. Continue thrusting, accelerating the pace only if your recipient is enjoying it and can handle it. Be careful to not become overzealous; hard action isn't for everybody. Lovers must be physically and emotionally ready for that kind of sex play.

As you're thrusting, enjoy watching yourself going in and out of your lover. Relish your lover's hips and buttocks as you feel each other's pleasure. As you get more anal-sex savvy, aim for your lover's G spot or prostate, which is located about two to three inches up the front wall (stomach side) of the rectum.

In all honesty, anal sex may not be possible the first couple of times you try it, namely because of pain. There is nothing wrong with this. If you feel pain, you should stop, since that's your body letting you know that it is in distress. You don't want to come away from this experience damaged, so tell your partner when to stop. The thruster should then withdraw slowly, since doing otherwise can damage the anal lining and tissue.

Some people get nothing from stimulating this part of the body, while others like to engage in anal play on occasion, and still others prefer to do so regularly . . . . It's up to you and your partner to decide if this type of play works for you as a couple.

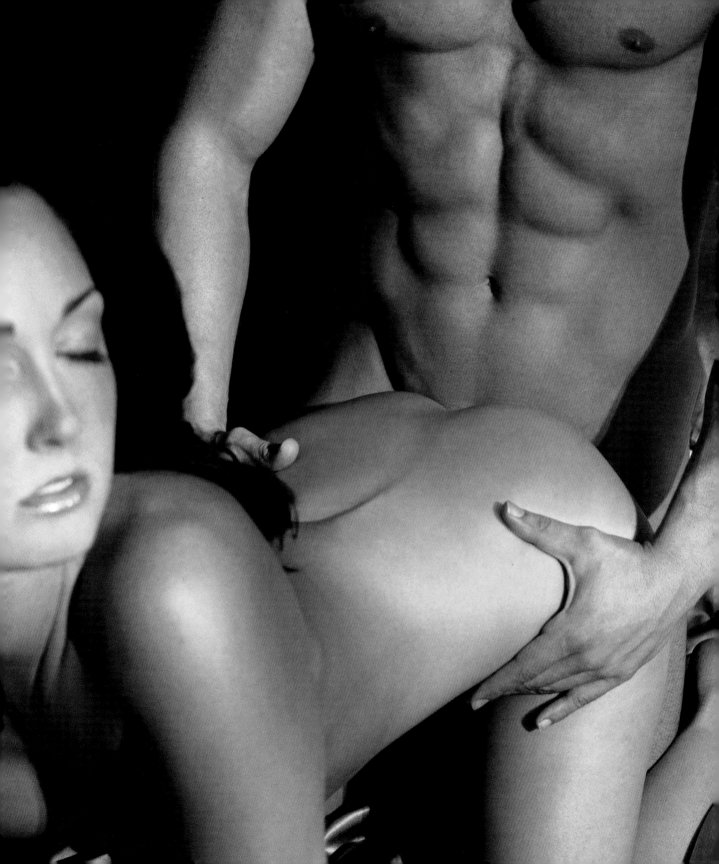

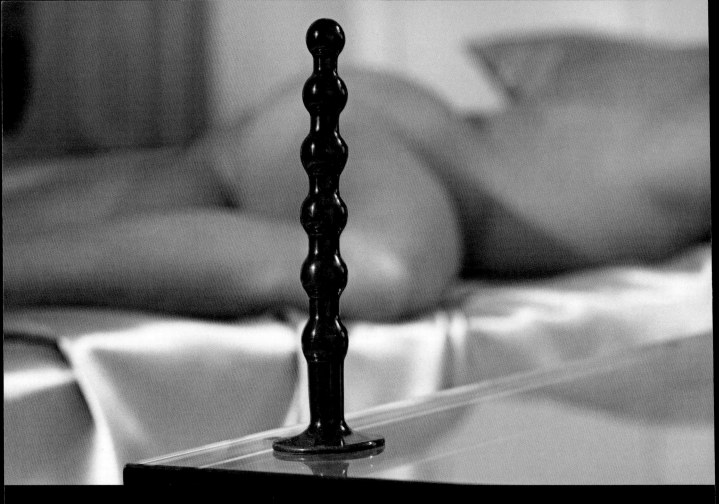

Sexual Homework

Postillonage—This French word captures the act of pressing and poking the anus with the finger. Take some massage oil and pour it on the crevice of your lover's buttocks. Do not penetrate the anal opening, but caress and stroke it. If the partner being pleasured is female, slide your penis up and down the crevice (but do not penetrate). You can practice this sliding action after penetrating the vagina or alternate it with vaginal penetration.

$\mathcal{S}\!\textit{e}\!\mathcal{X}$ercise 12.21 Tips for Incorporating Love Beads

For variety, try using love beads. Usually made of latex, wood, or hard plastic, these firm or soft climax or anal beads, as they're also known, usually involve four to ten balls on a nylon, plastic/rubber, or cotton cord, often with a ring at the end. After covering the beads with thick lube, typically silicone, slowly insert them into the anus, ball by ball, to stimulate the nerve endings. You can simultaneously have vaginal intercourse or manually stimulate your partner's genitals. Then, leave in place until your lover is near climax. As orgasm nears, intensify sensations by slowly and gently pulling out each bead. (If the string cannot be sterilized be sure to buy a separate set for vaginal use. Also, you can keep a condom over the beads, knotting it at the end to keep the balls, especially those made of soft or jelly rubber, clean.)

In many ways, sexual intercourse, or coitus, is regarded as the most intimate of sexual behaviors. It is for this reason that it has typically been considered the ultimate goal of sexual intimacy. Yet in recent years, the term "sexual intercourse" has broadened to include a wider range of behaviors, such as anal intercourse, motivations, and intentions. According to a survey of North American sex therapists, sexual intercourse typically lasts three to thirteen minutes. This is important to keep in mind since, for many people, satisfying sex does not come down to the length of sexual intercourse, or even the act itself, but the quality of the overall lovemaking experience.

"The truth about intimate relationships is that they can never be any better than our relationship with ourselves."

—JAMES HOLLIS

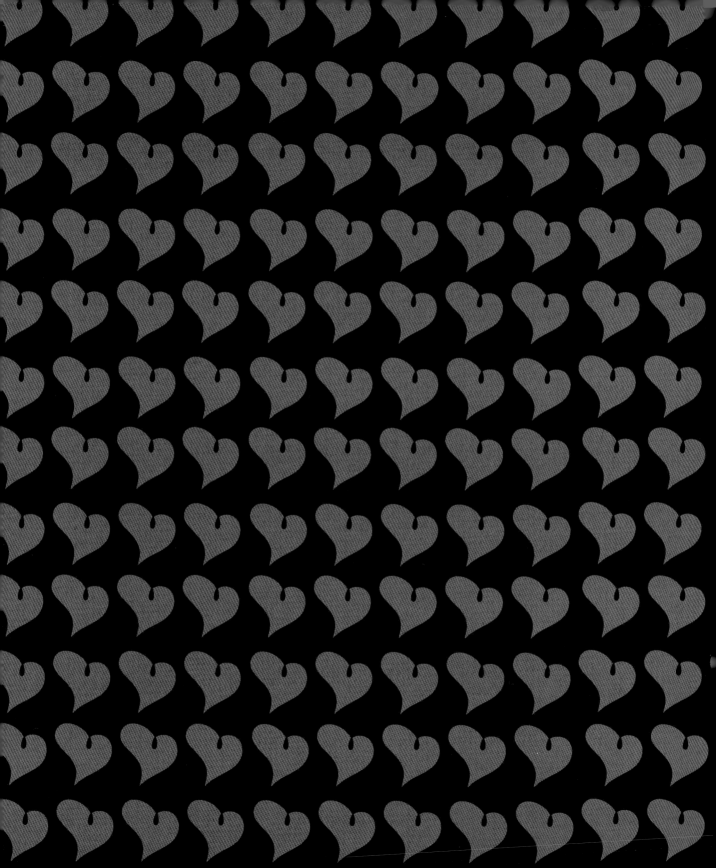

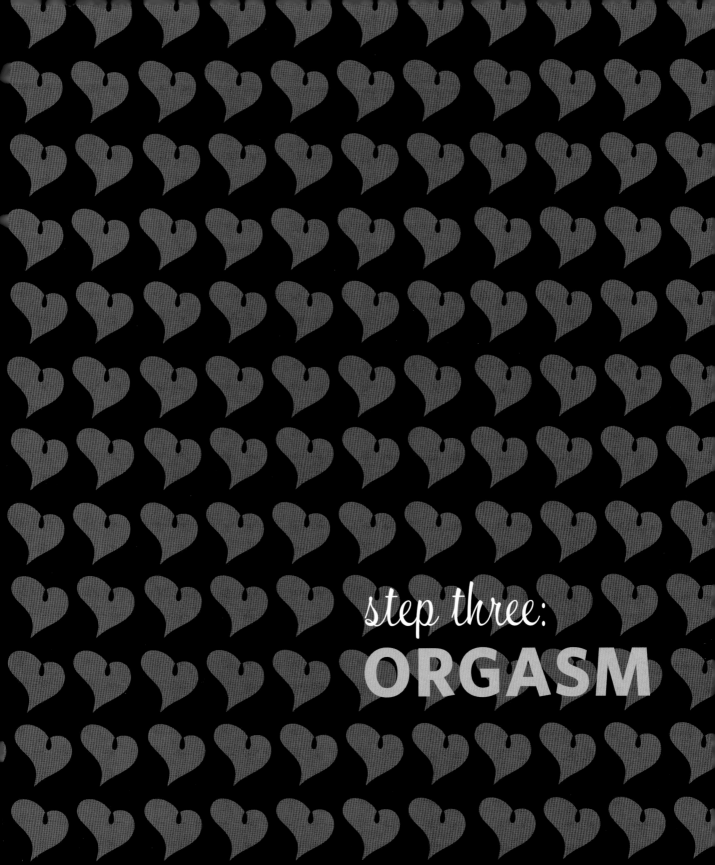

step three:
ORGASM

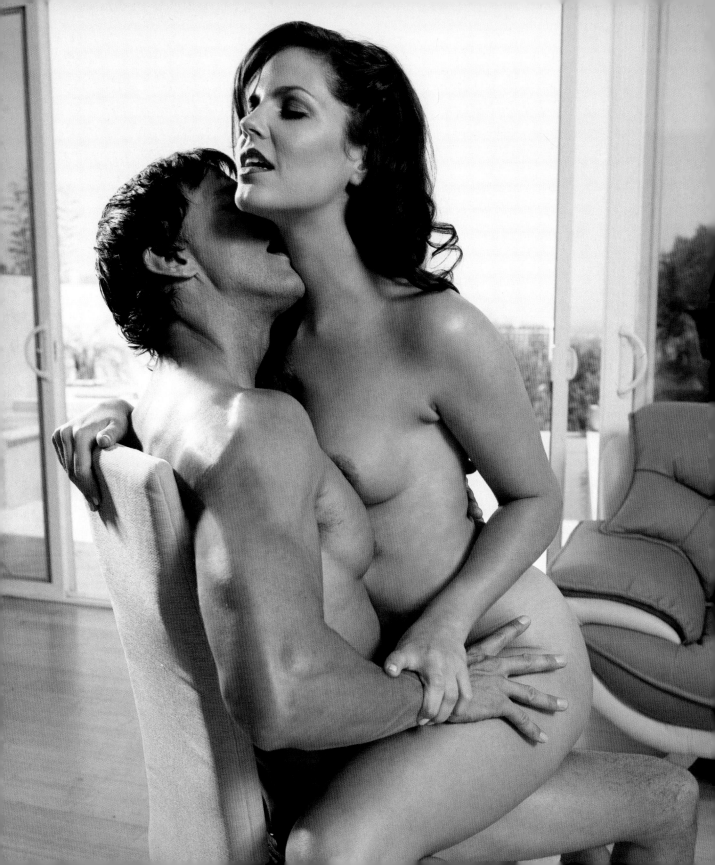

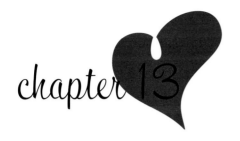

chapter 13

The "Big O": Climactic Tricks to Intensify Orgasm

LEARN THE NATURE OF ORGASM AND CLIMACTIC TRICKS TO INTENSIFY ORGASM

ECSTASY. EXPLOSION. WHISPER. Lightheadedness. Warmth. Peace. Wonder. Rush. Tingling. Trembles. Slow-burn. Laughter. Bursts of energy. Soul-touching. Genital sneezes. Energizing. Mellowing. Color. Light.

There is no one way we humans experience climax—and no one way to describe it. Our orgasmic potential is practically endless, with climax nearly impossible to define. A few academics have, however, tried to capture the essence of orgasm. Among their efforts are definitions that orgasm is . . .

" . . . the expulsive discharge of neuromuscular tensions at the peak of sexual response."

KINSEY ET AL., 1953

"A brief episode of physical release from the vasocongestion and myotonic increment developed in response to sexual stimuli."

—MASTERS & JOHNSON, 1966

"There is the heat of love, the pulsing rush of Longing, the lover's whisper, irresistible—magic to make the sanest man go mad."

"The zenith of sexuoerotic experience that men and women characterize subjectively as voluptuous rapture or ecstasy."

—MONEY, WAINWRIGHT & HINGSBURGER, 1991

In defining this incredible, largely indescribable phenomenon, academics emphasize the physiological buildup—the muscular tension and pelvic fullness—that works to a peak for orgasm. They describe the body's sudden release of all of its tension and the accumulation of blood in the genitals. This is orgasm as a sensory motor reflex, a rapid succession of involuntary, alternating contractions and partial relaxations, or spasms, of the body's pelvic muscle groups. But as anyone who's ever experienced an orgasm knows, it's so much more than that—as we'll see in this chapter.

ORGASM FOR BETTER BONDING

Beyond the bonding that comes from the act of lovemaking itself, during orgasm, the body releases a couple of hormones believed to produce reactions associated with attachment. Vasopressin and oxytocin, your "cuddle chemicals," are unleashed, allowing for a sense of fusion, closeness, and attachment. Oxytocin, in particular, plays a major role in your feelings of closeness and intimacy. This neurohormone is secreted by neurons and goes into the bloodstream, brain, and spinal cord in response to sexual stimulation, spiking three to five times higher than normal just before climax.

For her: In the female, this results in a dramatic increase in uterine peristaltic movements, as powerful as those of child labor, following nipple, breast, vagina, cervix, or uterine stimulation. This uterine reaction propels sperm into the particular fallopian tube that receives the ovum, increasing the likelihood of conception.

For you both: This hormone further sensitizes the skin, encouraging touch. It also has an amnesic effect during sex and orgasm—one that can block negative memories lovers have of each other for that period of time. (The same oxytocin is released during childbirth to help a woman forget about labor pain.) So powerful is your oxytocin response that it can be conditioned by the smell you, consciously or not, associate with a lover. Oxytocin can condition your arousal response in simply using aromas.

SEX EQUALS A GOOD NIGHT'S SLEEP

For both men and women, the profound relaxation that typically follows lovemaking, especially after orgasm and/or ejaculation, may be one of the few times people actually allow themselves to completely let go, surrender, and relax. Many people indicate that they sleep more deeply and restfully after satisfying lovemaking. In the relaxing afterglow, lovers may be able to let go of distracting thoughts. This effect of stopping all thought has helped many to overcome insomnia.

YOUR ORGASMIC SMORGASBORD

Having an orgasm can be a bit like choosing your favorite delicacy. That's because we've only recently begun to openly appreciate the human body's capacity for different types of orgasms. With every research study, we learn or confirm that different types of stimulation result in various types of climax for different people. These differences in the sensory quality of orgasm have to do with different nerves receiving sensory activity from different body parts. While you may not experience orgasms or every type of orgasm out there, knowing that you have the potential to enjoy them—and any and all of the following climactic reactions—may be all you need to make it happen!

Clitoral Orgasm

Given that the vast majority of women have an orgasm from direct clitoral stimulation, you may already be familiar with this bit of bliss, also known as the "vulvic" or "vulval" orgasm. Characterized by involuntary rhythmic contractions of the pubococcygeus muscle (PC muscle), clitorally-induced orgasms are considered more reliable, accessible, obtainable, faster, and insatiable,

THE SCIENCE OF *Sex*

Clitoral stimulation is key to orgasm for many women. According to sexologist Shere Hite:

- **44 percent of women climax from clitoral stimulation by hand regularly.**
- **42 percent of women climax regularly during oral stimulation.**
- **50 to 75 percent of women require direct clitoral stimulation to reach orgasm during intercourse.**

SEXUAL Q&A: WHY HE GETS TIRED AFTER SEX

My husband always falls asleep soon after sex. This has been the case with most of my past lovers, as well. Why does this happen?

While sex can be a very exhausting activity for you both, it can take a toll on men in particular. There are a couple of major reasons for this. First, while the parasympathetic nervous system causes both sexes to feel deeply relaxed, it has him feeling especially tired since he comes down from sex much faster than she does. Soon after climax, his physiological reaction involves losing his erection almost immediately as his heartbeat and breathing return to their normal state. Second, the oxytocin and endorphins released at orgasm are thought to cause a sedative effect. A male's oxytocin levels are generally lower than a female's, except after orgasm, when it's up more than 500 percent! This may help to explain why men are sleepy after sex, as it's this same hormone that makes babies sleepy when released during breastfeeding.

In the Bedroom:
Stimulating the Clitoris

FOR SOME WOMEN, the most effective way to experience orgasm during lovemaking is via cunnilingus. According to *The Janus Report*, 18 percent of women prefer oral sex to reach orgasm. When she is the recipient of oral sex, she is likelier to experience climax prior to penetration and/or during thrusting. So take some time pleasuring the clitoris.

1. Begin with long, slow, gentle tongue strokes up and down the vulva as you press on the mons pubis with one hand. With your other hand, massage her perineum.

2. After a minute or so, begin stroking the clitoral hood with long tongue strokes, sweeping down each outer labia for a half-circle move.

3. As she becomes more aroused, take the clitoris between your lips and suck on it.

4. Maintain pressure on this area, unless she prefers otherwise, as you make fast, horizontal sweeps across the clitoris with the hardened tip of your tongue.

5. If this becomes to much, or if you want to tease her, alternate step four with more of a massaging motion, using the top of the tongue as a massager against the clitoris.

6. Continue these moves, checking in with her as to her rhythm and pressure preferences, until she is satisfied.

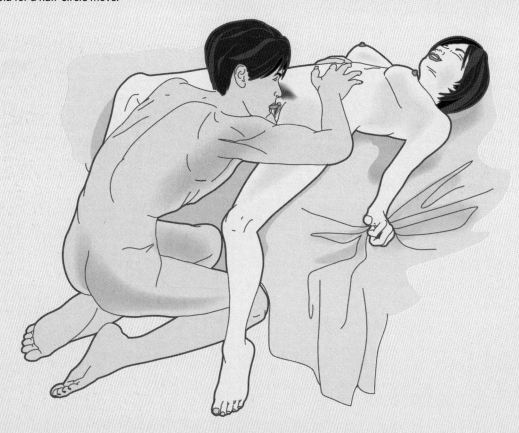

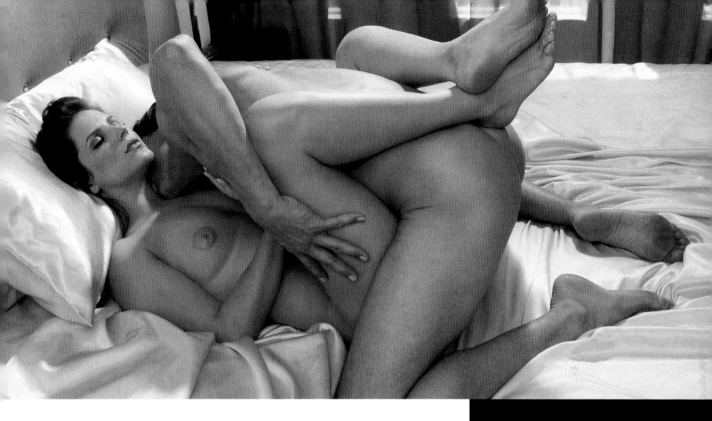

sometimes to the point of multiple orgasms. Triggered by your body's puden-dal nerve, repeated stimulation of the glans clitoris evokes a uterine reflex response, known as the clitorouterine reflex, creating sensations concentrated in the lower one-third of your vagina. This is in large part because, as you or your lover play with or around your clitoris, it swells and changes position as your pelvic region is engorged with blood. This creates a feeling of fullness and heightened sensitivity. If you've never had an orgasm before, be sure to spend time playing with your clitoris, rubbing it back and forth or in circular motions with well-lubricated fingers or a vibrator, to bring yourself to orgasm.

Vaginal Orgasm

It can—and does—happen! Direct, mechanical stimulation of the vagina with-out direct clitoral stimulation can generate orgasms in some women, according to several studies summarized in the book *The Science of Orgasm*. This is in part because your pelvic nerve provides the sensory nerve supply of the vagina, cervix, rectum, and bladder. The hypogastric nerve, in particular, conveys sen-sory activity of the uterus and cervix. This can generate orgasm when you're stimulated vaginally or rectally. The walls of the vagina also have many sensory nerves that respond to deep pressure—which can produce orgasms that last ten to fifteen seconds!

THE SCIENCE OF *Sex*

Women have shared, in interviews with Sexologist Shere Hite, that they sometimes experience a vaginal ache— the desire for vaginal penetration or to be filled up. Described as an intense pleasure/pain feeling, some find this quite nice, while others find it empty and unpleasant. The "hollow" feeling some describe is thought to come from the upper end of the vagina ballooning out. Many women feel that a penis "soothes" or diffuses the feeling.

In the Bedroom: A-Spot Potential

EXPLORE AN AREA of the woman's body called the "A-spot." Located midway between a woman's cervix and G spot, the A spot is the area on the anterior (front) wall of the vagina that is a patch of sensitive tissue at the inner end of the vaginal tube between the cervix and the bladder. Also known as the anterior fornix erogenous (AFE) zone, the A-spot has gained attention in recent years for its possible role in vaginal lubrication and erogenous qualities. The AFE Zone Stimulation Technique was originally introduced by A-spot researcher Dr. Chua Chee Ann to help women who complain of vaginal dryness. Yet such sex play is not reserved for those with such problems. By exploring the erogenous power of the A-spot during foreplay, her sexual response and vaginal lubrication may improve.

In finding the A-spot, make sure your lover's legs are bent and tucked toward her body. This is best achieved in a squatting position or by having her lean her back against a support. Then, do the following:

1. Insert your entire lube-covered index finger into her vagina, while she maintains this position, gently stroking the inner (upper) half of her anterior vaginal wall.

2. As she begins lubricating, bring your finger out to stroke both the spongy area that is at the outer (lower) half of her anterior vaginal wall, as well as the AFE zone (vaginal sponge area). Your strokes should be long, repetitive, in-and-out finger motions covering the entire length of the anterior vaginal wall.

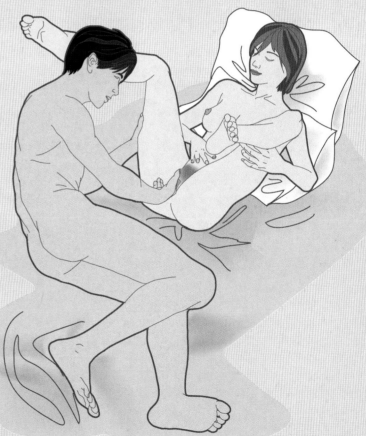

G spot Orgasm

G spot orgasms are the product of G spot stimulation. Activating this area triggers the pelvic nerve and hypogastric pathways, which stimulates areas deep inside the body. These climaxes involve contractions of your entire uterus, vagina, and pelvic region, with women describing a "pushing down" sensation from this type of vaginal orgasm. They produce a "fuller" feeling from the uterus, since it is pulled up when the G spot is played with. Explosive and pulsating, G spot orgasms often take longer to attain than clitoral orgasms, but the reverberations they send throughout the body may be well worth the effort.

THE SCIENCE OF Sex

The clitoris, pelvic floor muscles, urethral opening, and G spot are part of what's referred to as the "orgasmic crescent." This entire area swells up with stimulation, producing a sort of female erection.

In the Bedroom:
Stimulating the G Spot

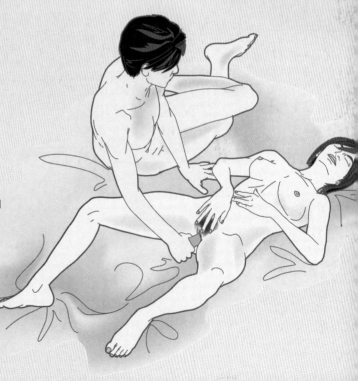

INSTEAD OF USING your fingers to find the G spot, try using a vibrator that is specifically made for such stimulation. Once your lover is lying on her back, use lube as you caress the genitals, building her arousal before performing the following:

1. Slowly insert the vibrator into the vagina.

2. Gently rub it against the G spot area on the front vaginal wall.

3. Check in with your lover to find out how the area feels (e.g., does it feel like it's swelling?). Ask her if she would like the vibrator to be turned on for more stimulation, starting with a low setting.

4. Like your finger, "hook" the dildo gently onto the G spot area, gently tugging it toward the vaginal opening.

5. Ask your lover if this feels good. Would she like more or less pressure? Would she like the vibe turned up?

6. Begin thrusting the vibrator as though you were having intercourse. Ask her to tighten her PC muscle, breathing deeply, as you increase the speed of the thrusting.

Cervical Orgasm

Another type of internal orgasm realized via vaginal penetration is the cervical orgasm. Despite containing relatively few nerve endings, the cervix is responsive to pressure, activating the pelvic, vagus, and hypogastric nerves. The orgasms that result from the tip of a penis, long fingers, or sex toy stimulating the cervix are described as deep, heavy, and involving the whole body. The vagina feels "fuller" during climax since the uterus pushes downward. While some women love having their cervix stimulated via pounding, tapping, or circling, others have no reaction or find it awfully painful, particularly during deep, hard thrusting.

Nipple Orgasm

While the occasional fellow may orgasm from nipple stimulation, some females can climax from nipple play alone. Some require such stimulation in order to reach orgasm in general. In exploring your nipple's potential, try arousing this erogenous zone in addition to other types of hot spot stimulation that normally works for you.

In the Bedroom:
Exploring the Cervix

SOME WOMEN MAY already know if they're keen on cervical stimulation, based on the sensations that the head of the penis can provide when hitting against it during intercourse. But if you and your lover would like to explore the pleasure potential of the cervix, take the time to do the following using a dildo:

1. With the woman lying on her back, caress the genitals for sexual excitement.

2. Once she is aroused, insert the dildo into the vagina, moving it to the deepest part of the front wall of the vagina. You will feel a knobby surface at the upper part of this wall. Pressure against the cervix may create a slight cramping sensation at first.

3. Move the dildo around the cervix using a circular motion, noting if one part of it feels better than the other areas.

4. For more stimulation, begin to stimulate the clitoris as you thrust the dildo against the cervix.

Penile-Triggered Orgasm

For men, orgasm from penile stimulation is by far the most common and frequent type of climax. This sensory activity actually originates from your prostate via the hypogastric nerve, eventually moving into the penis and testicles, for a possible total body experience. While almost always accompanied by ejaculation, the emission response of semen is a separate function from orgasm, which is the involuntary contraction of the pelvic muscles among other sensations. This reaction can happen sans emission for a dry orgasm (and vice versa).

Prostate-Triggered Orgasm

Stimulation of the prostate, most effectively accomplished via the rectum, can result in the prostate-triggered orgasm. Described as deeper, fuller, more implosive, and longer-lasting, this orgasm may be accompanied by ejaculation that is released in spurts versus a steady stream.

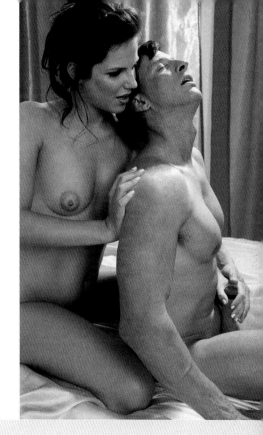

In the Bedroom:
Vibrating for His Pleasure

WHILE SOME MEN are curious about vibrators, they are often shy about such sex play given that these toys are typically regarded as female-only. Yet plenty of men love to use a vibrator on their scrotums, thighs, or the base of the penis to enhance their orgasm. So, using a hand vibrator, perform the following:

1. Once he is aroused, use the vibrator on the shaft of the penis at a low setting.

2. As you take your time stroking the penis, using slow, long strokes, be sure to breathe, tune into the sensations, and relax.

3. To tease him, occasionally run the vibe down his inner thigh, across his buttocks or scrotum, or press into his perineum.

Anal Orgasm

Stimulation of the anus can trigger nerve pathways for a deeper orgasm. This includes the direct stimulation of the prostate in the male and the indirect stimulation of the female's G spot during anal penetration.

Blended Orgasm

Blended orgasm is the result of you or your partner—or both of you at the same time— stimulating two (or more) of your hot spots simultaneously. In the female, for example, stimulating the G spot and clitoris at the same time triggers both the pudendal and pelvic nerves, resulting in an even stronger, more explosive, longer-lasting reaction. Such double stimulation allows you to mix unique sensations into one big peak for a possible longer, deeper orgasm. Women report feeling immobile, as if they were going to burst, consumed with intense electric jolts during this full-body spasm. Males may experience equally powerful reactions in having their prostate and penis stimulated at the same time. In both sexes, adding rectal stimulation in addition to other hot-spot play can increase the quality of an orgasm in its complexity, intensity, and pleasure.

In the Bedroom: Incorporating the Prostate

IN GETTING MORE out of his prostate, perform the following the next time you make love, in a position where his perineum is easily accessible (you can also use a dildo or vibrator for better reach).

1. Bring the thrusting to a slow and leisurely pace so that eventually your pelvises are grinding against each other as you remain merged.

2. She is to then use her lubricated finger or a sex toy to massage the perineum, checking in with him as to the rhythm and pressure he would like as she presses up against his prostate.

3. As he becomes more aroused, resume more of a thrusting motion. Allow the stimulation to mimic the pace and fervor of the thrusting.

Sexercise 13.1 Focus Your Attention on Erogenous Zones

Make a list of all of your favorite erogenous zones. Then together, strategize different ways that you and your lover can stimulate at least two of these areas during lovemaking. As you consider various combinations, keep in mind that the way to have a blended orgasm is to become partially aroused, as you would normally. Then switch to another method of stimulation before revisiting your original hot spot. You may need to alternate several times, firing up both erogenous zones to react at the same time.

Nocturnal Orgasms

Otherwise known as wet dreams, nocturnal orgasms are climaxes you may experience as you sleep. The brain is able to generate orgasm independent of the genitals, taking you through the entire sexual-response cycle. For men, this can result in ejaculation. While women don't have the same "evidence" men do, research published in the *Archives of Sexual Behavior* has found that during nocturnal orgasm, a woman's heart rate doubles, shooting up to one hundred beats per minute; her respiration goes from twelve to twenty-two breaths per minute; and she experiences increased blood flow. People who have nocturnal orgasms tend to have them several times per year.

Emotional Orgasm

Physical reactions aside, many lovers emphasize the emotional responses that come from being sexually intimate. With or without any of the other types of orgasm, they describe an "emotional orgasm" from the feelings of love, communion, and connection with another that reaches climax with intense feelings, such as the feeling of their lungs being in their throats, wanting deeper penetration or merging, and their chests swelling. An "orgasm of the heart," this type of climax, as described by Hite, involves the release of emotions.

Sexercise 13.2 Describe Your Orgasm Through Drawings

Using crayons and construction paper, draw your orgasm. If you feel that you are unable to do this or want to enhance your picture, write the words you would use to describe your emotional orgasm. Share your project with your lover, being sure to give detail as to what everything means.

THE SCIENCE OF *Sex*

In many ways the exception to the rule, spontaneous orgasms are orgasms that happen unexpectedly from genital or nongenital sensory stimulation. They can be due to any number of things, such as engaging in a charged debate, making an intellectual discovery, listening to jazz music, exercising in certain positions, smelling certain fragrances, using deep breathing techniques, or brushing your hair. For example, one 44-year-old woman is reported in *The Lancet* as having experienced spontaneous orgasm while driving.

Spontaneous orgasms have also been attributed to people "thinking off." While orgasms without mechanical stimulation are rare in males (Kinsey and his colleagues found, in 1948, that only three or four male study participants reported such), there are documented cases of women who can think their way to orgasm. Research in the *Archives of Sexual Behavior* has confirmed bodily reactions that are forms of sexual response—increases in heart rate, blood pressure, pupil diameter, and pain threshold. The body can respond to thoughts in the same way it does physical touch. Sexy thoughts trigger the brain's sexual center, including the hypothalamus, which increases sexual arousal.

THE "BIG O" FOR HER: CLIMACTIC TRICKS TO INTENSIFY HER ORGASMS

No matter what kind of orgasm you typically have, there are plenty of ways to intensify your climax for what's truly a "Big O." So whether alone or with a partner, whether it's your private parts or his, be sure to incorporate the following tips in magnifying your orgasmic sensations . . .

Fantasize about the Sexual Encounter

Like so many other women, you may find that daydreaming about your desires—and a planned sexual rendezvous—gets you physically aroused. So allow yourself to think about what's to come hours or days before it happens. This will have you ready for action the second you can make your "dirty" thoughts a reality.

Tune into Your Environment

Look for the sensual around you. Love songs, sexy videos, or hot, scandalous sex stories can all help build your sexual energy and anticipation. Let them penetrate you to the core, awakening your libido and feeding your desire.

Slip into an Erotic State of Mind

Clear your mind, pushing away any thoughts that can ruin your mood. Focus on the pleasurable feelings, giving yourself permission to be nothing but sexual.

Lose Yourself in Fantasy

Imagine an erotic or romantic scene that can stir your libido. Don't be afraid to be "bad." Try not to censor your thoughts, as you may just surprise yourself when it comes to what can be arousing.

Stay in the Moment

If you find yourself thinking about work or the dirty laundry, tune into your body. Boost your physical arousal by honing in on what your lover is doing to you, physically or mentally, to turn yourself on.

Close Your Eyes

While many lovers like to gaze lovingly at one another as they make love, this can be distracting for some women.

THE
SCIENCE OF *Sex*

Researchers have proposed that orgasm for both sexes helps to reinforce their desire to engage in sexual intercourse, which promotes procreation. It may also be a significant factor in mate selection for males or females. Behavioral excitement during orgasm, such as movement and vocalizations, could influence mate selection, as well.

Allow Yourself to Make Noise

Get those vocal chords in on the act! Hear your verbal responses. Invite a loud sexual release!

Pay Attention to the Clitoris

According to The Hite Reports, only one-third of women orgasm during coitus with "no hands." Most who do experience orgasm during partnered sex climax either before penetration or later, thanks to oral, manual, or toy stimulation of the clitoris. So if you've been ignoring the clitoris during intercourse, give it some proper attention. Don't be afraid to touch yourself during sex with your partner in the same way you would when you're alone. Be sure to teach your lover all about what works for you, aiming for sexual positions that allow for easy clitoral play.

Get Sexy with Your Sheets

During intercourse, some women can attain orgasm by lying on the stomach and rubbing against the bed sheet. Alternatively, you can lie on your stomach, clasp your hands, and wiggle, press, grind, and rub on them in a circular motion for intense clitoral stimulation.

Communicate

Nobody is a mind reader, so communicate clearly and effectively about what you want, need, desire, and feel.

Don't Rush

Would you rush while getting a facial, massage, or manicure? It's likely that you wouldn't. So give yourself the time for sex play. Being sexually intimate in a positive relationship is one of the most healthful things you can do for yourself. So be leisurely about luxuriating in it.

Learn to Let Go

Practice having an orgasm, even if you've never had one. Rehearsing your orgasm can help you to relinquish control. So mimic signs of an orgasm, making your sex face, shrieking with delight, exaggerating muscle tension, and letting your body feel as though it's rippling. Do anything that you think will help to reduce your anxiety while boosting your comfort. But don't ever "fake it" with your partner, as this cheats both of you of the opportunity to realize orgasm.

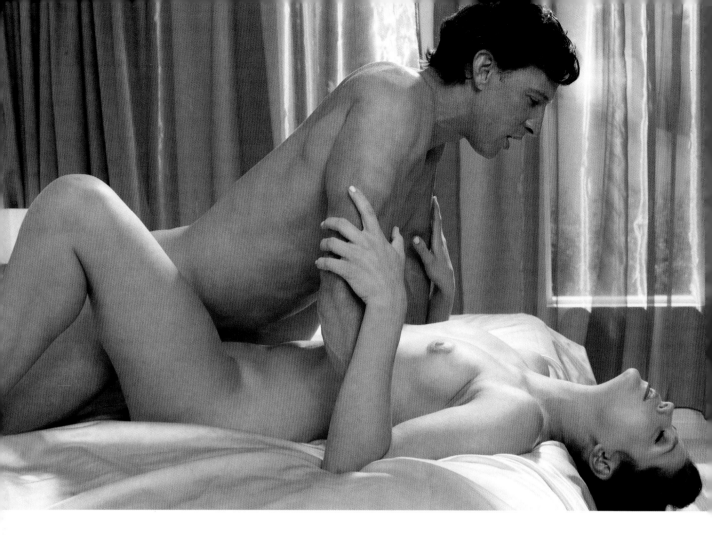

Try Hanging Your Head

Some women experience heightened arousal and sexual tension when they hang their head over the side of the bed.

Contract Your PC Muscle

Alternate tightening and relaxing your pelvic floor muscles, as instructed in Chapter 14, breathing into your sexual core as you do so. This alone can result in a climax!

Push Out

When a woman pushes out, her orgasm may become more intense. So push your pelvic floor muscles out, like there's something in your vagina you want out. This will lower your vaginal walls, making your G spot more accessible for an easier orgasm, if this is an erogenous zone for you.

Maintain Stimulation

It's tempting to go from one position to the next, hitting one erogenous zone after the next. But to better your chances of attaining orgasm, you want to stick with one position that's stimulating your biggest hot spots and stay there until you climax.

Use Toys

Sexual enhancement products can intensify stimulation and enhance sensation for a quicker climax. So use a small handheld vibrator during sex on your hot spots. You also have hands-free vibrator options. Remember, with vibrators, less is more at first. Don't put the vibe on the clitoris immediately, since this can numb it. You may also want to use a cloth between your vulva and the vibe if the sensations are too intense or if they're making you orgasm faster than you would like.

SEXUAL Q&A: DID SHE ORGASM?

How can I tell if my girlfriend has had an orgasm? I really want her to have one!

If you think there are certain signs that show that a person definitely experienced orgasm, like writhing or arching of the back, then you're out of luck. Most people don't show any obvious sign of having climaxed. Some people are quite active when they peak, while others don't move at all. While you could look for things such as a sex flush (blushing of the skin, especially of the chest), a sedated look, or muscle clenching, these are not guarantees that she has climaxed. So the best way to find out if your girlfriend is having an orgasm is by simply and nicely asking her. Explain to her that it's really important to you that she's sexually satisfied and that she should let you know how you can better help her attain orgasm. She'll be flattered that you're so concerned. However, be very sensitive about not putting pressure on her—something that almost guarantees she'll have trouble reaching orgasm.

THE "BIG O" FOR HIM: CLIMACTIC TRICKS TO INTENSIFY HIS ORGASMS

Whether you're taking matters into your own hands or are having sex with your partner, strive for the following pointers in intensifying climax:

Get Mentally Turned On

Some men tend to get so wrapped up in the physical part of sex that it's possible to disconnect from the mind, heart, and soul. If you want more of a body-gripping, all-consuming orgasm, allow yourself to tune into everything else you're feeling beyond physical pleasures.

Fantasize

Use mental imagery to intensify the experience, while still staying connected to your partner. For example, picture yourself having sex where you shouldn't be.

Stay Present

Take your time and don't rush to the "goal" of orgasm. Allow yourself to patiently enjoy the journey, focusing on every detail of what's taking place between you and your lover.

Get Noisy

Some men may be afraid to make noise during sex because they think it's a sign that they're losing control or not very manly. But typically people love to hear a lover's pleasure. So let your sexual response be known through your moans and groans!

Communicate

Let your partner know what you need, want, feel, and desire, and in explicit detail. Describe the kind of stimulation you need and where—the rhythm, pressure, and motion that will have you aroused like nothing else.

Squeeze Your Bum

Some men feel that the muscle tension derived from flexing their buttocks during climax heightens the experience.

THE
SCIENCE OF *Sex*

Men's orgasms are controlled by an "orgasmic center" near the brain stem. This area, the hypothalamus, is also the center for primal, uncontrolled reflexes and basic impulses, such as hunger and thirst. Women's orgasms, on the other hand, are the result of a much more complex sequence of events in the brain.

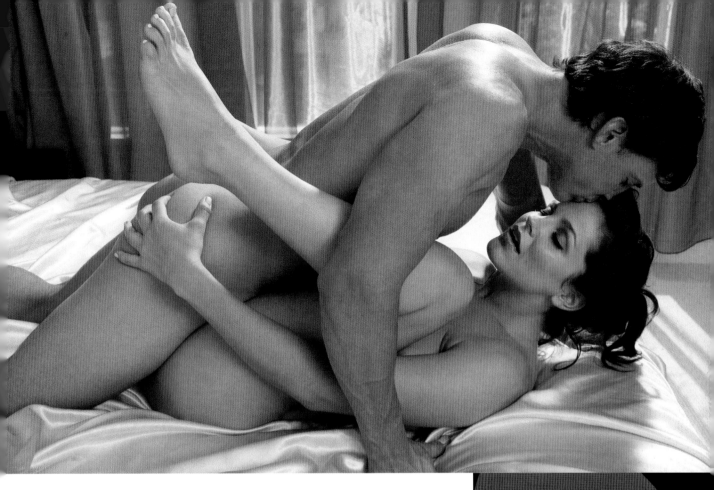

Contract Your PC Muscle

As we'll see in the next chapter, squeezing your pelvic floor muscles can not only help to make your orgasm better, but also may result in multiple orgasms!

Breathe Into Your Sexual Core

Channel your breath down into your perineum. This will help you to stay in control while enriching your pelvic muscles with fresh oxygen for a more mind-blowing experience.

Play with the Perineum

Press up on the prostate by massaging the perineum for more sensations.

*Sex*PERTISE

In adapting to their sexual response with age, men over forty still have the potential to experience better orgasms. This is accomplished when they learn to revel in the process of lovemaking, focusing on sensations, and not just the end point.

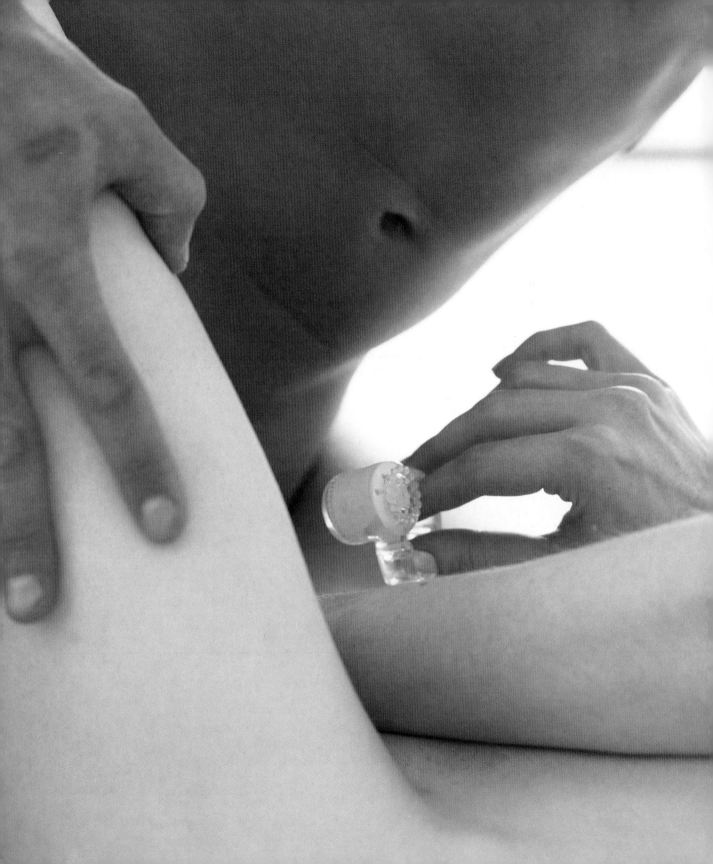

Tease Other Hot Spots

A male or his partner can play with his other erogenous zones as he reaches orgasm. His lover can, for example, bite or pinch his nipples.

Ask Her to Squeeze

To intensify his orgasm, a man's lover should grab his butt with dramatic pause, using her pelvic floor muscles to draw him deeper into her vaginal canal.

Consider Your Relationship

Males are likelier to have the type of orgasm they desire if they are in a committed, monogamous relationship with an interested lover. This is because of the level of comfort such a relationship provides, especially compared to that in other sexual encounters such as one-night stands. If this doesn't describe your sex life, you may want to consider how you can develop the comfortability within your relationship(s).

Use a Penis Ring

While there are plenty of sex toys to enjoy, the penis (or love) ring is in many ways the most effective one for him. Even if it's not more than a finger and thumb, squeezing the veins on the shaft prevents blood from leaving the penis. The tightness and pressure that results can boost the intensity of your orgasm. (A love ring that also goes around the scrotum can also help.)

Spend a Little Bit of Time Apart

Research out of Florida Atlantic University has found that men experience a 10 percent increase in sexual desire for their partner for every one hundred hours they spend apart. (Evolutionary theory would suggest that this is because a man becomes concerned that his partner is having sex with other men when he can't account for her whereabouts.) Spending some time apart before sex may increase your emotional reactions to coitus, possibly making for a more intense orgasm.

THE
SCIENCE OF *Sex*

Sex is good for male heart health. Results from the "Massachusetts Male Aging Study" showed a relationship between levels of DHEA (dehydroepiandrosterone), which is released in the bloodstream at orgasm, and a decreased risk of heart disease.

 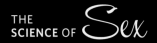

Don't Masturbate Beforehand

Not having sex on your own before lovemaking provides a physiological buildup that will intensify sexual sensations. What's more, psychologically, you'll feel more lust during sex.

Aim for Variety

Don't get locked into the same old routine with foreplay and sex. Encourage your lover to try new adventures. Your justification: Korean researchers found that the rigidity of erections decreased by almost 15 percent in forty-five men from the first time they watched an erotic video to the third time they watched the exact same flick. To stay excited and maintain the intensity, you may just need to change your stimuli!

EXPLORE YOUR ORGASMIC POSSIBILITIES TO SEAL YOUR SEXUAL BOND

The word "orgasm" comes from the Greek word orgasmos, which comes from "organ," meaning "to grow ripe, be lustful." Orgasms vary from lover to lover and from sexual experience to sexual experience. This is in large part because orgasm is a biopsychosocial experience, meaning your climax is dependent upon your physical and mental states. It's also affected by messages you've been fielding from your immediate environment and the world at large, about your sexuality and sexual activity. So there are many issues that can either shut down your climactic reactions or prevent you from realizing the best of orgasms.

In exploring your orgasmic possibilities, you and your lover need to make sure that you're in a healthy place, sexually speaking. This not only makes for better sex, but also helps to seal your bond. The following are among the most valuable strategies the two of you can employ for better, stronger, more explosive orgasms:

Avoid Being Goal-Oriented

Couples have the tendency to be very goal-oriented when it comes to sex. In wanting to feel like her sex "hero," many men will be more consumed with "giving" her an orgasm than enjoying the experience. Making things worse, many men expect their partner to climax every time they have sex, and, chances are, she won't. Don't work toward orgasm as a set goal. Just surrender to the sensations and be in the moment.

THE SCIENCE OF *Sex*

Pleasure comes in many forms. You don't have to climax from every sexual move to enjoy it. For example, according to *The Hite Report*, an overwhelming 87 percent of women like vaginal penetration even if they've never climaxed from penetration alone.

Take Responsibility for Your Own Pleasure

Nobody "gives" anybody an orgasm. You need to take responsibility for your own pleasure, overcoming any anxiety and tension. You need to put yourself in the driver's seat of your orgasm, exploring the realm of ideas we're covering in this book to realize better sex.

Be Open-Minded

As we have seen, orgasm comes in many forms. So don't get stuck on a fixed idea of what orgasm is or how it's supposed to be. Let your orgasms surprise you.

Stop Trying to Have an Orgasm

The anxiety and distraction this provokes can actually shut down your sexual response and the eroticism of the moment. Don't put pressure on yourself by focusing on the outcome. Focus on the pleasure, and it will "cum!"

Love What You're Doing

Orgasm is not the be-all and end-all of satisfying sex. You can have amazing sex because you're into the moment, you adore your partner, and you love the sharing—and not climax. Sex is a time to express affection and to feel close. Don't chalk it up as something purely physical, or else that's all it will ever be.

Don't Feel Like Damaged Goods

Just because you don't respond a certain way, sexually speaking, doesn't mean that there's something wrong with you. Never think that you're not man, a woman, or sexual enough. Women especially worry about if they're experiencing orgasm the "right" way or if their sexual response is good enough or too much. They often feel guilty in asking for the stimulation they need or are unable to give it to themselves. Know that there is no correct pattern of sexual response. Do whatever feels good for you.

THE SCIENCE OF *Sex*

Men Have Emotional Needs, Too.
"The Sex in America" study found that 75 percent of men and 29 percent of women always reach climax with their partner.

$\mathcal{S}$ex PERTISE

Surveys have found that some 30 percent of men and more than 70 percent of women fake orgasms. Most feel that they have plenty of good reasons to do so. Women and older men feel great pressure to perform and have an orgasm, so they just want to get it all over with. Lovers can also be tired, feel disconnected from their lover, are afraid to offend, or are on medications that inhibit their response.

While such sexual "white lies" may be a little less than angelic, they serve rather practical purposes in many respects. When faking becomes a pattern, however, you are ruining your best sex efforts. If you find yourself faking orgasm, be honest and direct about your needs with your lover. Otherwise you not only let the problem fester, you also deny both of you the opportunity for greater intimacy. Exploring better sex is a truly bonding experience, and figuring out ways to make yourself experience orgasm and/or sexually satisfied is something both you and your lover deserve.

Take On Your Issues with Sex

Many factors may foil our sex efforts. We get lots of mixed messages about our sexuality, with our response greatly influenced by cultural mores and norms, such as, "Don't feel desire or lose control," "Don't look silly," "Don't feel sexual . . . ." All of these can affect the quality of your sex life. Never let these factors get the best of you. Evaluate the way you've been conditioned to think about sex. Retrain yourself to become the sexual person you want to be. Allow yourself to be desirable and to desire.

Talk about It

If you expect to have super sex without addressing the vulnerability, anger, and trust issues that haunt your relationship, you may be just kidding yourself. Many of us need to have our emotional needs met in order to climax. And we're not just talking about women. Men don't necessarily orgasm every time they have sex, either. So think about what you need out of your relationship to feel secure when making love. Then set out to guarantee those needs—and attain orgasm.

Mind Your Health

You boost your chance of orgasm if you're exercising, eating properly, are drug-free, including nicotine-free, and well-rested.

WHEN SHE DOESN'T ORGASM

Despite the best of intentions in bed, many women do not experience orgasm during sexual intimacy. A couple of major surveys have found that that about one-third of American women do not orgasm at all. Formerly referred to as anorgasmia, preorgasmia is a lack of orgasm from certain types or all forms of sexual activity. This may be a preorgasmic primary condition, where they have never experienced climax, or it may be a preorgasmic secondary condition, meaning that they were able to reach orgasm until reaching menopause, for instance, or until being cheated on. Either condition may be due to the following factors, identified by studies reviewed by Elizabeth A. Lloyd in The Case of the Female Orgasm:

- Psychological issues, such as obsessive/compulsive personality
- Interpersonal factors in the relationship
- Various fears

- Performance anxiety
- Drug/alcohol abuse
- Nerve disorders
- A rigid, sexually repressive upbringing
- Childhood sexual abuse
- Shaming experiences related to one's sexuality
- Ignorance about the body and sex
- A lack of privacy during intimacy
- Genetics
- Lack of trust
- Fear of intimacy
- Inability to let go
- Unskilled lover
- Insufficient mental arousal
- Pattern of faking orgasm
- Lack of permission to be with partner
- Sexual ignorance
- Poor communication skills with partner

In dealing with this disorder, a woman should get a thorough physical exam and work with a sex therapist to carefully review her sexual and psychological history. In therapy, she will work to identify pleasure blocks; to reframe her right to experience eroticism; to face the truth about her current sexual relationship; and to map out strategies for improving her current relationship situation. With body coaching, she can also learn to masturbate, feel empowered, and become more educated about her sexuality and sexual response.

WHEN HE TAKES "TOO" LONG TO ORGASM

Just as men can climax too quickly, they can take "too" long to experience orgasm. Also known as inhibited ejaculation or ejaculatory incompetence, delayed ejaculation is a condition where a male experiences orgasm and/or ejaculation only after a great deal of time and effort. Some may never orgasm or ejaculate at all, a condition called anejaculation. For those who can, most say that it takes them a minimum of 30 minutes before they feel release. More common in men over 50 (about one out of every 8 men), there are a number of reasons why this sexual disorder occurs:

Organic: Physiological reasons for this lack of response include retrograde ejaculation (a condition where semen goes back into the bladder instead of out of the urethral opening), diabetes, nerve damage, vascular disease, medications (including antidepressants), fatigue, spinal cord injury, alcohol/drug addiction, excessive masturbation, and hormone factors.

Mental: Psychological reasons for delayed response include mood disorders, guilt, depression, stress, anxiety, performance pressures, strict religious upbringing with negative views about sex, sexually transmitted infection fears, past traumatic events, relationship or sexual orientation issues.

Relational: Problems in a couple's relationship can also impact his response, including anxiety over emotional intimacy, pressures to conceive, lack of attraction for his partner, infidelity, lack of stimulation for adequate arousal during sex, and not wanting to surrender to a woman.

In resolving this issue, a man should be thoroughly checked out by a healthcare provider in determining any organic causes, including prescriptions, and any medical interventions to treat such. You can also help him climax if you:

- Use more erotic fantasies, which will increase subjective arousal
- Help him to become more aware of orgasm triggers and to go with the flow
- Teach him to make requests for erotic stimulation
- Focus on stimulating his hot spots

In pursuing the orgasm of your dreams, it's important to remember that the connection sex invites is by and large much more important than the end result. For example, research published in the Journal of Counseling and Development found that the most satisfying sexual experience for many women involved being connected to someone and not just orgasmic satisfaction. So in your better sex quest, don't lose sight of what can truly make for amazing sex. Emotional satisfaction is what in many respects makes the moment, with or without an orgasm to complement it.

"*We are molded and remolded by those who have loved us.*"

—FRANCOIS MAURIAC

Sexual Homework

While we covered a plethora of ways to enhance any of the orgasms you may experience, there's always more fun to be had. In losing yourself in the following homework, you may end up losing yourself in orgasm.

Penetration Pleasures: While women are told that it can take them several minutes, if not a great deal longer, to have an orgasm during intercourse, some can experience climax upon penetration. In getting aroused, practice the following in exploring this type of climactic reaction.

1. Pleasure yourself with your partner's penis for up to twenty minutes, all the while staying in the moment and not worrying about where you're hoping things will go.

2. As you caress your lover's genitals, focus on your own sensations, staying relaxed and breathing deeply.

3. Rub your clitoris and labia against his penis, but do not insert it into the vagina.

4. Alternate this action with other forms of penile stimulation that turn you on, like oral sex. This helps to maintain his arousal while helping you to tease yourself as you build your arousal.

5. As you use his penis to stimulate your clitoris with rhythmic direct or indirect presses, allow your breath to get faster as you become more and more excited.

6. Just at the point you are about to orgasm, slide the penis into your vagina.

7. Begin thrusting, especially if you do not orgasm right away. Be sure to squeeze your PC muscle around the shaft as you do so.

Sexperimenting: Challenge the way you've come to know intercourse—namely, that it requires an erect penis—and explore the wonders of flaccid insertion, also known as "stuffing" or "quiet vagina." Take your time to enjoy the following . . .

1. In the side-by-side position, face one another. She should have one leg between his and the other leg on top
of his top leg.

2. Using lots of lube on the penis, gently part her vaginal lips, and apply even more lubrication.

3. She should then gently push the base of the penis into her vagina. (The penis head will naturally fold in as well.)

4. Once in, breathe and relax, noticing the wetness and warmth.

5. Tune into the erection. Has it changed?

6. Stay connected without moving, cuddling, talking, or kissing.

7. If desired, eventually begin to move so that you can have a stronger erection for intercourse.

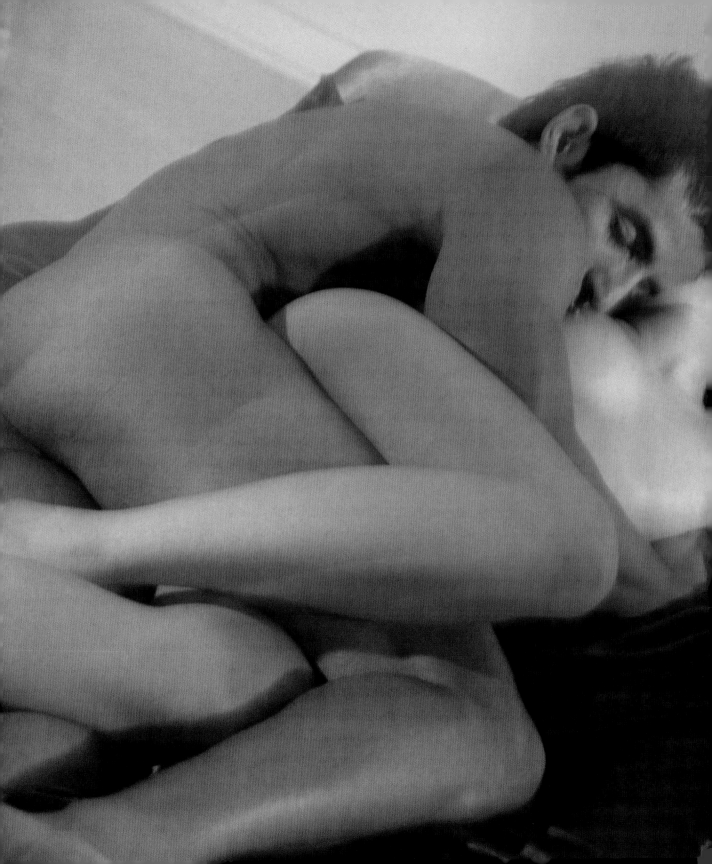

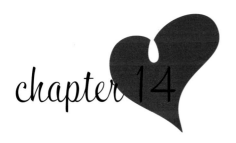

chapter 14

Reaching the "Big O" Again and Again: The Art of Multiple Orgasms and Lasting Longer

WHEN IT COMES to satisfying sex, you can never have too much of a good thing. And when it comes to good things, many might say you can never have too many orgasms. Yet while many people want to attain bliss again and again, many of us don't know how to extend our lovemaking to realize multiple orgasms. The good news is that every person—male and female—has the potential to experience multiple orgasms. Every person has the potential to experience different types of multiple orgasms, as well!

Some lovers are lucky enough to be multiorgasmic with relatively little effort, while others have to work at it. Thankfully, such work is play—and involves attending to your own natural sex toy, no less. You actually come pre-equipped with the most effective tool to better, more orgasmic sex. As mentioned earlier in this book, it's right between your legs and is known as your PC muscle. Our mission in this chapter is to strengthen it for the sex you desire!

"Two souls with but a single thought; two hearts that beat as one."

—FRIEDRICH HALM

MEET YOUR PC MUSCLE

The best way for both men and women to explore their multiorgasmic potential is to develop the strength of their pubococcygeus muscle (PC muscle). The PC muscle is actually a collective term for your pelvic floor muscles. This sex muscle runs from the front to the back of the pelvis in both sexes, holding your pelvic organs in place. You likely know it as the muscle group you contract when stopping the flow of urine. Many studies show a direct correlation between orgasmic sensation and a well-toned pubococcygeus muscle for both sexes. This is in part because your pudendal nerve, which runs through the PC muscle, triggers most of its reactions, detecting genital and anal stimulation. The pudendal nerve lets your brain know that you're experiencing arousal. Your brain, in turn, induces the rhythmic contractions that are associated with your most common types of orgasms.

REASONS YOU WANT A STRONG PC MUSCLE

Getting your PC muscle into shape holds enormous benefits, including the fact that:

- You'll get aroused more quickly and be more receptive to sensations, delighting in more and stronger contractions
- You'll experience increased stamina and have the energy to last longer. Men with a strong PC muscle have better erections and shorter refractory periods
- You'll experience increased pleasure and greater sexual sensations from arousal to orgasm
- Your orgasms will likely be much more satisfying and deeper, with a toned PC muscle contracting more forcefully with powerful spasms as you reach climax. Pulsations resonate throughout your entire body for much longer orgasm
- You'll be able to engage in more positions and be able to hold them for a longer period of time

For her: Having a strong PC muscle will enable a woman to experience a greater response to vaginal stimulation, allowing for the constant contact needed to stimulate her when certain sexual positions, such as missionary, or thrusting styles do not provide enough friction.

For him: The benefits realized by a man for having a strong PC is covered extensively in Chapter 14. But there are myriad benefits for him if she has a strong PC. For instance, her ability to squeeze with every thrust will deliver more pressure around his penis for greater intensity. This better grip allows her to control the depth and speed of his thrusts and the amount of friction lovers enjoy during sex. Furthermore, clamping down on the tip of his penis can stop his climax. When he ejaculates, it's much more intense.

Given all of the above, you'll both experience increased sexual desire, wanting more and more of each other.

PRACTICING YOUR KEGEL EXERCISES

When it comes to gratifying sex and better single and multiple orgasms, much of your physical experience comes down to PC muscle control. PC muscle exercises, also known as Kegel exercises, involve the rhythmic clenching and unclenching of your pelvic floor muscles. Last century, when Dr. Arnold Kegel developed Kegel (pronounced "KAY-gul") exercises as a way to help women

In the Bedroom: PC Exercises for Her

AS WITH ANY WORKOUT ROUTINE, you never want your interest to waiver. Fortunately, there are plenty of different PC exercises to keep you mindful of your practice. As your PC muscle becomes stronger, go ahead and show off your new talents. Ask your lover to stick a finger or two between your legs for a test run of what you can do during sex!

OPTION 1: Do intervals of 1 squeeze every 5 seconds, aiming for 10 squeezes at first, 2 times per day. Over time, work your way up to 25 squeezes, then up to 50 squeezes.

OPTION 2: Start with 10 squeezes, 3 times per day, holding each squeeze for 10 seconds. Over time, work your way up to 20 squeezes per session.

OPTION 3: Do 10 repetitions, holding each clench for 3 seconds and then relaxing for 3 seconds. Work your way up to a series of 50, 3 times daily.

You may also want to try the Pelvic Connecting Crunch, which uses your transverse abdominals and inner thighs to work the PC muscle even more. Lie on your back, knees bent, feet flat on the floor. Place a ball between your inner thighs, and squeeze your PC muscle as you lift your thighs up and back. Lift your head and shoulders off of the ground, holding this position for 10 seconds.

who suffer from urinary incontinence, he found that these pelvic floor muscle exercises were beneficial in other ways, too. Not only did they help women to push more efficiently during childbirth, but they also ultimately increased pleasure during intercourse, boosting sexual desire, intensifying orgasms, and helping women become multiorgasmic! Whether you're male or female, part of what makes Kegels so effective is that, any time you work out a muscle, you increase your overall blood flow to that part of the body. This heightens sensitivity in that area.

$\mathcal{Ex}$ercise 14.1 Methods for Strengthening Your PC Muscles

In beginning PC muscle exercises, you first need to identify the muscle group to be developed. The next time you need to urinate, try holding back the urine stream. For the full effect, don't contract your buttocks, thighs, or abdominals. You want to isolate your PC muscle, taking care not to contract other muscle groups. Squeeze your pelvic floor muscles to stop the flow of urine. (Note: Use this technique only to identify the PC muscle. Do not continue doing such in place of PC exercises since this can eventually affect the brain's normal control of the bladder sphincter.)

If you can do this, then you have found your PC muscle. Women can also identify the PC muscle by inserting a finger or two into the vagina and then clamping the vaginal walls around it. Once you've identified your PC muscle, you can do Kegel exercises presented in this chapter anytime, anywhere, including while you masturbate.

In practicing your pelvic floor routine, you may not only get turned on, but you may also feel the need to release the sexual tension you've created with some good old-fashioned masturbation. Many PC muscle enthusiasts have no qualms exploring their PC potential while self-pleasuring, saying it adds a whole new element to the exercise routine. Furthermore, playing with yourself while working the muscle can help you to develop the strength, endurance, and coordination needed to enhance your performance with your lover. Contracting your PC muscle while you masturbate in positions that replicate the rhythms of sex with your partner, for example, allows you to reap the benefits of your toning exercises while making them even stronger. You'll notice your pleasurable sensations growing stronger and deeper with each pelvic flex.

As you do the exercises in this chapter, be sure to inhale as you contract, and exhale as you release. After four to six weeks of spending up to five minutes per day on these exercises, you'll notice a change in your sensations and abilities in bed.

ENHANCEMENTS FOR A STRONGER PC MUSCLE

In further mastering PC muscle control, you may also want to use a sex toy specifically designed for strengthening your sex muscle. Research from the Karolinska Institute in Sweden found that training with cones greatly improves a woman's PC strength (versus exercising without cones). These weighted devices are inserted into the vagina; the PC muscle is then contracted around it for a short period of time. Other PC contraction devices include:

Vaginal Barbells: Often made of metal, these weight-resistance devices have balls on either end to easily grip (plus stimulate the G spot). Ideally, you want to strengthen your PC to the point that you can have the heavy end of the barbell inside of your body while standing, without it falling out.

Vaginal Beads: Modeled after traditional "geisha balls" or Ben Wa balls, pleasure/fitness systems such as vaginal beads seek to increase your muscle resistance over time. Using lots of lube, insert each bead, one at a time. Leave in place until your partner starts to orgasm, then pull them out slowly, one at a time, for more sensation.

GyneFlex: This tool has plastic tongs that provide resistance against the PC muscle when it's squeezed.

SEXUAL Q&A: PC MUSCLE EXERCISES

What are the health benefits, if any, from my husband and I doing PC muscle exercises?

PC muscle exercises have a number of health benefits for both sexes. For men, a strengthened PC muscle is beneficial in that it helps to keep his prostate healthy, possibly reducing the risk of prostate cancer. When it comes to women, strengthening your PC can boost your health by:

- Making you less prone to vaginal prolapse, which is when the vaginal wall gets pushed forward by one or more of the pelvic organs such as the uterus or bladder
- Supporting your bladder, helping to prevent any urine leakage when you cough or sneeze
- Aiding in proper placement of a diaphragm for birth control
- Reducing your chance of a vaginal infection, since more blood is sent to the vaginal lining

PC exercises also increase the flow of white blood cells to the pelvic area, helping to fight against illness-causing viruses and bacteria. Increasing the circulation of the pelvic area is also believed to get rid of toxins.

In testing your new strength, flex your PC as your partner thrusts during sex, squeezing down on the most sensitive part of his penis—the rim around the head. With time, you may notice that you're able to move your partner's penis deeper inside of you. While in woman-on-top position, do your Kegels in sync with your movements. As you rise, clench his penis for a second or two. As your partner ejaculates, literally "milk" his ejaculation out of him to boost his release. Or as you hit orgasm, rapidly flutter your PC, flexing it as fast and as shallow as you can, for a more intense orgasm.

In the Bedroom:
Tantric Stone Eggs

A SECRET OF ancient Chinese queens and concubines, this egg (not to be mistaken for real ones) has been used to keep women of all ages tight, resilient, and healthy. Using a clean, small (recommended for beginners) or large jade egg, stand with your feet slightly wider than hip distance apart, and insert the device into your vagina, large end first, bending your knees slightly. Feel free to use a water-based lubricant, water, or saliva if you don't feel lubricated.

In performing the egg exercise, follow these steps:

1. Once the egg is inserted, pull it up by contracting your PC muscle.

2. Squeeze the vaginal muscles at your vaginal opening around the egg so that it doesn't slip out.

3. As you inhale, contract the vaginal muscles closer to your cervix.

4. As you exhale, push the egg back down toward your vaginal opening.

5. Repeat this up-and-down movement for up to thirty-six repetitions or until you tire.

6. To finish, forcefully push down to expel the egg.

You may find it easier to have two eggs in your vaginal canal, with your squeezing effect pushing them toward one another. (Note: Be sure to wash your egg with warm water and soap after every use to avoid infection. Furthermore, be sure to dry it well and keep it in a dry place.)

Another type of egg that you can use is a stone egg with a small opening at each end for a string to slip through with a weight, such as a fishing weight (under 1 lb.). To insert this egg, make sure that you're kneeling, with the weight resting, as you insert the egg into your vagina, large end first. As you contract your muscles to hold the egg in place, slowly rise to a stance with legs slightly hip distance apart. Now swing the weight from front to back. As you contract your perineum, inhale as the weight swings backward between your legs. Exhale as it swings forward and pull it up into you. Repeat up to three times daily for one week, slowly increasing repetitions to 60 counts.

MAKING HIM ORGASM . . . AGAIN AND AGAIN

Male multiple orgasms have been written about since as early as 2,968 BC in China, in texts from Taoism, Tantra, Vishranti (ancient India), Imsak (Arab), Chira in the *Kama Sutra*, and more. Some men learn that they have this multiorgasmic ability by accident and are able to capitalize on it for the rest of their lives, while others must learn this later and often with guidance. Basically, male multiple orgasms involve remaining in a state of sexual excitement after the first feeling of orgasm. They are the phenomenon of experiencing more than one climax during the same erection. Instead of having one orgasm, often accompanied by ejaculation, followed by the loss of erection, a man can have one of several things happen:

- He has more than one orgasm before ejaculating.
- He has an orgasm and stays erect, going on to experience another orgasm or more a couple of minutes later.
- He has small ejaculations with each orgasm or one big ejaculation, after a series of climaxes, at the end.

In exploring his multiorgasmic potential, a man must have two skills: a well-toned PC muscle and an understanding of the two parts of ejaculation, namely, emission and expulsion. The emission (or contractile phase) is when the prostate contracts, emptying semen into the urethra. At this point, you reach the point of ejaculatory inevitability, where you must decide if you want to go

SEXUAL Q&A: TRAINING WITH STONE EGGS

I've gotten pretty serious with my PC muscle training, since the payoffs are huge; I'd like to use a stone egg—only I'm afraid that it will get stuck. What should I do if this happens?!

Stringless eggs may occasionally feel stuck. If this happens, stay calm, squat and try bearing down on the egg to push it out. If it doesn't come out, go do something else that will relax you, which will help the egg to move out on its own. If you're not keen on this option, ask your partner to insert a lubricated finger into your vagina to help the egg along. Avoid this situation entirely by using an egg with a string.

Se*X*PERTISE

Ensure that you're doing your PC exercises correctly, so you don't waste your efforts. To do so, insert a finger into the vagina, and squeeze. It should feel like an elevator, with your PC moving up with the squeeze, then going back down as you release. (To confirm that you're flexing as you should, consider visiting a continence specialist for personal training with the guidance of a biofeedback program that isolates the muscle.) Don't overdo your Kegel routine, since this can cause your PC to spasm to the point where you could have trouble urinating. An ideal number is 60 to 80 squeezes, performed in sets of 10 to 20, throughout the day. You want to hold each squeeze for 4 seconds, then relax for 4 seconds, while remembering to breathe.

for the immediate release and satisfaction that comes with ejaculating or if you should hold off. If you want to discover your multiorgasmic potential, slow your pace to avoid entering the expulsion phase, which is when semen shoots down your urethra and out of the penis. You can slow down your pace by:

- Squeezing your PC muscle around your prostate. Visualize the process—see yourself squeezing your prostate, in total control of what's often an involuntary process.
- Pushing on your perineum while contracting your PC to stop the ejaculatory reflex. (This will also cause a nicer throbbing sensation as more blood is forced into the penis.)
- Breathing energy from your groin and up your spine. (Visualizing the breath as you're doing this may make this more fluid—a skill made even easier with a dedicated meditation practice.)

In the Bedroom:
Exercises for Him

FLEXING THE PC MUSCLE isn't just for women. Men should also aim to develop their PC muscles for deeper orgasms and possibly multiple orgasms. Doing so can also help them to postpone ejaculation, which helps to prolong sex. This is because two to three inches of the penis are rooted in the PC muscle. In strengthening the PC, a man can learn to separate his orgasm from his ejaculation response, helping him to become multi-orgasmic. Let's first look at how you should strengthen your PC. We'll later get into how you can explore your multi-O potential!

As you do these exercises, breathe deeply with every squeeze. Visualize the semen contracting back into your body while squeezing tighter and tighter.

OPTION 1: At first, aim for 10 clenches, squeezing each repetition for 10 seconds before releasing. Slowly, work your way up to 30, and then to 100 repetitions.

OPTION 2: Aim for long, slow squeezes, holding each clench for 20 counts, and then resting for 30 seconds. Repeat 5 times.

OPTION 3: Squeeze your PC muscle 25 to 50 times for 1 count each. Do two sets per day, letting each clench get longer over time. Masters will eventually be able to do 300 repetitions per day for life. Such aspirations are well worth it. A Belgian study involving 178 men with minor erection problems found that, after a four-month program, 74 percent showed erection improvements with Kegels, and 43 percent were totally cured of their sexual disorder.

In doing any or a combination of these, you'll delay ejaculation. Thus, you'll stay in the emission phase, hovering on the brink of orgasm—relishing the mild or intense prostate contractions, known as "contractile-phase orgasms" or "pelvic orgasms." Just stay in control of your arousal here, welcoming all of the sensations you might experience, such as tingling, cooling, or warming. This will be challenging, but there are payoffs. This effort builds sexual tension as you pull back several times before orgasm, preparing your body for one orgasm after the next.

Know that all of this is much more easily said than done. These practices take a lot of time and patience and are best combined with the tips given later regarding how to last longer in bed. You may have to stop arousal altogether before reaching the emission phase if you tend to ejaculate easily. Also, if you do ejaculate, don't get frustrated or disappointed. Stick with your practice. Everything will get easier and better with time.

$\mathcal{S}ex$ercise 14.3 Techniques for Moving Your Sexual Energy

Get in touch with your sexual energy to learn how to draw it up the spine. Practicing the following by yourself can eventually help you during masturbatory practices, as well as during sex with your lover.

1. Cup your scrotum with a warm hand to bring them to life with a stirring or slight tingling.

2. As you inhale, squeeze your PC and anal muscles, drawing them up as you imagine that you are drawing this energy from your scrotum to your perineum. Envision this sexual energy moving onto your anus and tailbone.

3. As you exhale, relax your muscles, maintaining your attention on the rising sexual energy.

4. Continue inhaling and exhaling with the same pulling motion, until you can feel a warming or tingling of the perineum.

5. At this point, tuck your chin in and suck the sexual energy up your spine to the base of your skull.

6. Keep drawing the energy from your scrotum up through your spine until you feeling light or tingly in the head.

7. Touch the roof of your mouth with your tongue about a half inch behind your front teeth. This will help to channel the energy down the front of your body to your navel.

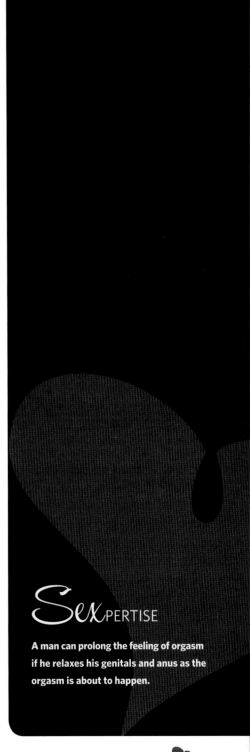

$\mathcal{S}ex$PERTISE

A man can prolong the feeling of orgasm if he relaxes his genitals and anus as the orgasm is about to happen.

I've been suffering from premature ejaculation, and I don't know what to do about it. Why do I have this problem, and how can I hold out longer? Help!

At different points in their lives, especially in their younger years, males may find themselves dealing with early ejaculation or feel that they're finishing too soon. Since every male's definition of "early" is different, it can be hard to determine who has an issue with premature ejaculation versus who is putting unrealistic pressure on himself when it comes to stamina. Early ejaculation is considered a problem when a male doesn't last for more than a couple of minutes when sexually intimate, and when this is recurrent and persistent before, upon, or shortly after penetration. This sexual disorder may be due to a several things, including a man's:

- Age
- Masturbation style (rushing to finish)
- Shyness or overexcitement in being with a partner
- Performance or general anxiety
- Health conditions
- Stress and fatigue levels
- Use of medications/drugs
- Excitement over sex play and overstimulation
- Personality type
- Interpersonal problems

Thankfully, there are ways to deal with this disorder. First, realize that the "average" sex session is anywhere from fifteen to forty-five minutes, with two to twelve minutes of that being actual intercourse. Second, retrain your ejaculatory response using pelvic floor muscle exercises using the Stop-Start Technique, explained later in this chapter, when masturbating or having intercourse with your partner. This involves becoming more aware of your sensations as you approach orgasm. Identify your level of excitement, and keep it at that level. Recognize when you're almost at the point where there's no turning back, and relax, taking a thirty- to sixty-second break. You'll do the same thing when you're with your lover, eventually working your way to slowing down or changing what you're doing instead of stopping.

As you work with your lover on this issue, start out with manual stimulation, gradually moving onto oral stimulation, and then to coitus, which may take weeks to do successfully. When you start having sex again, have her be on top so that you can relax while she does most of the thrusting. If you have trouble at any point, stop all movement and use the Squeeze Technique. Here, you or your lover squeeze your penis for three to four seconds, using the thumb and first two fingers as a penis ring at the base of your shaft or at the ridge on the head of the penis. No matter how you're enjoying yourselves, make sure that you're diffusing any sexual tension you feel before stimulation resumes.

MAKING HER ORGASM . . . AGAIN AND AGAIN

Most studies on multiple orgasms report that about 15 percent of women have experienced multiple orgasms, whether via self-stimulation or intercourse. So it's not too surprising that The Hite Report found that many women didn't know about multiple orgasms. For those who had experienced such, it was rarer for them to have orgasms with no break in between. Many women who experience multiple orgasms need to be re-stimulated for sequential orgasms, which often involves waiting for a few minutes for the next climax. Research has found, however, that some women are able to have orgasms in rapid succession, with some orgasms lasting anywhere from twenty to sixty seconds. In 1966, for example, Masters and Johnson documented an orgasm that lasted forty-three seconds. So, you see, you have the potential to experience a wide range of orgasmic responses, all of which could prove themselves to be absolutely fantastic! In making sure that you get your orgasmic fill, be sure to consider the following:

Don't Foil Your Game: If you think that you can have only one, that's likely all you'll have. So get in the right state of mind. Don't switch yourself "off" when you reach the first climax; rather, expect another orgasm and leave yourself open to more arousal. Your body will follow your mental lead.

Let Your Lover Know Your Hopes: While you certainly don't want to invite any performance pressure, let your lover know that you may experience multiple orgasms by extending sex. Ask him to draw things out for as long as he can. Work with him on his own multiorgasmic efforts, which involve delaying his gratification (which makes for your greater gratification). Remember, stay fun-focused, and go where your journey takes you instead of worrying about getting "there."

Start with Oral Sex: Any effort to get the body geared up for climax will help you to respond to vaginal stimulation during sex. Many women climax from cunnilingus—and more than once, at that. Many increase their chances of multiple orgasms when they've already had an orgasm. A lover's tongue can serve you well in mimicking a vibrator, giving intense repeated stimulation to your genital hot spots. Ask your lover to use the tip of his tongue to rapidly flick the clitoris, and ride the sensations as they envelope you.

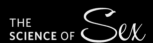

THE
SCIENCE OF *Sex*

At the point of orgasm, a woman's sense of touch may be enhanced.

Don't Stop After the First One: Don't think that sex is over after you've had an orgasm. You could be in for more. Continue stimulation as you're experiencing your first climax. If he can, ask that your partner keep thrusting, and give into the sensations that come for more explosive reactions. If you're feeling hyper-sensitive after the first orgasm, wait ten to fifteen seconds before resuming stimulation of the pelvic region. In the meantime, be sure to keep other parts of your body on high sexual alert.

Focus on the G spot: Get into positions that stimulate this erogenous zone, such as rear entry, to allow for deeper penetration, where the head of the penis can hit up against the G spot. Place a pillow under your lower back, or have your partner lift your pelvis for a more elevated vagina. Stimulating the G spot while playing with the clitoris can give you blended orgasms.

Squeeze Your PC: Contracting your pelvic floor muscles increases blood flow to your groin, which can result in a repeated series of pulses.

Stimulate More than One Spot: Research has found that women are likelier to have more than one orgasm if several body parts are being stimulated at the same time. So play with your nipples or neck as he toys with your nether region.

$\mathcal{S}$exercise 14.4 Breathing Your Way to Better Orgasms

In experiencing multiple orgasms, you may want to aim for deeper orgasms by practicing the following exercise.

1. Imagine what your uterus looks like, allowing yourself to feel connected to this part of the body.

2. Get in touch with your uterus by, while standing, placing your thumbs together at your navel and making a triangle with your index fingers (your index fingers will fall on the area that is approximately level with your uterus).

3. Take a deep breath and as you exhale, contract your mouth and eyes gently, feeling your cervix contract, as well. With practice, you may feel a slight orgasmic sensation in doing this.

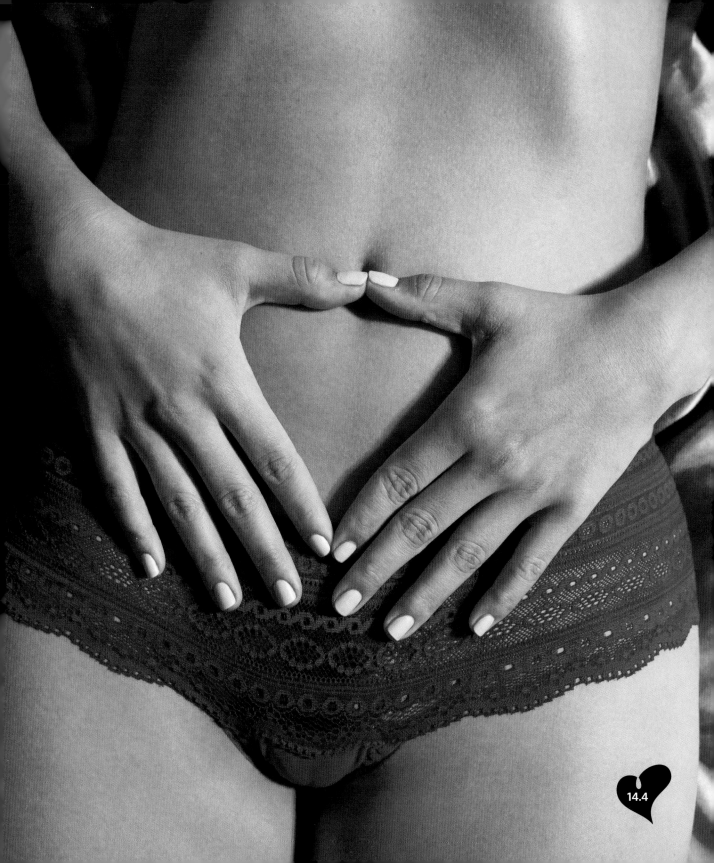

MAKING SEX LAST LONGER

Couples often daydream of having longer sex for bigger and better pleasures. Such longings should not go unanswered—because extended sex is what opens the door to more orgasms for both women and men. Being intimate longer can also help bring you together, as you enjoy the whole lovemaking process and your responses even more. Here are some tips to last longer:

- You can "break" in the middle of sex and just tease each other.
- You can change positions, which often slows down sexual response, since re-stimulation is often required.
- You can use a male or female condom, which can reduce the physical sensations that trigger orgasm.
- You can use a topical numbing cream to desensitize the penis head.

THINK ORGASMIC THOUGHTS

Envision yourselves having long-lasting sex, with you in total control. Imagine yourself gliding into your lover, feeling her moisture, her heat, her PC squeezing around your shaft . . . and that you've just been captured in time. Don't move, but just fantasize that you're inside of her for a few seconds before you slowly start to thrust. As you calmly increase your pace, on occasion, see yourself slowing down before you resume gradually increasing your pace again. As you build up to the point that you're about to climax, see yourself stopping all movement. Allow yourself to satiate the sensations before you slowly start to resume your movement, this time letting your body do what it's longing to do. Whenever you're ready, fantasize about your most amazing emission, feeling your body ricochet from the red-hot reactions. Rehearse these scenarios again and again to prepare yourself for actual sex.

MORE CONTROL TIPS AND TRICKS

Here are a few more recommendations designed for lasting longer when you're pleasuring yourself or when you're with your lover:

Breathe Properly: Being short on breath isn't going to work. You want to be cool, calm, and collected—think James Bond. You can do this by taking deep breaths that ease the tension that comes with sexual excitement. Breathe into the bottom of your lungs, and deeper, sending the breath down into your sexual core. Hold it there until your urge to ejaculate subsides. This type of breath control will also help you to experience more of a total body orgasm when you do decide to orgasm, enabling you to expand sensations throughout the body.

In the Bedroom:
Stroking to Last Longer

THE KEY TO longer-lasting sex is mostly in the man's court—in his ability to have control over his ejaculatory response. In developing ejaculatory control, a man should do the following Stop-Start Technique exercises a minimum of three times per week:

1. With a dry hand, masturbate, focusing on your groin or penis. Tune into your arousal and sexual tension, staying relaxed.

2. As you reach the point of ejaculatory inevitability, stop stimulating yourself, and breathe into the sensations racing through your body.

3. Resume stimulation when your sexual excitement and muscle tensions have dropped quite a bit (which can take anywhere from ten to sixty seconds).

4. Repeat the exercise at a later time, this time using a lubricant or massage oil.

When you've been able to do these exercises using lubricant a couple of times with only one or two stops, move on to change your stimulation technique. This may involve slowing your pace, focusing on a different part of the penis for maximum stimulation, or varying your stroke. Experiment with only one change at a time, seeing what works best for you. Repeat at a later time using lubricant. Make the dry and wet exercises even more challenging with some visualizing.

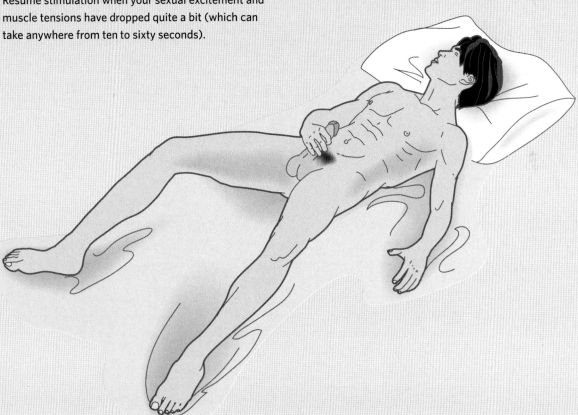

Concentrate: It's easy to get carried away with sexual fantasies, or with what you're seeing, or with what you want to do next, or with whatever is feeding your hunger for more and more, faster and faster . . . . Don't run away with yourself. Learn how to control a wandering mind. As you have sex, count to one hundred without getting caught up in other thoughts, giving each breath one count. Notice how this helps you to slow everything down.

Tune into Your Sensations: As you become aroused, pay attention to the stimulation and the rate of it. If you need to slow down, and even back off, do.

Plan Your "Stop" Activity: If you need to temporarily halt all activity because you're so aroused, stop, and sing the first verse of your favorite song. Or talk to your lover while you take several breaths. Think about how can you stay physically connected and not ruin the mood, even as you calm down.

Create Your Own Love Ring: Place your first two fingers and thumb at the base of the penis, and squeeze when you get too excited. For further assistance, pull down on your scrotal sac. Ask your lover to do these things as you're having sex.

In the Bedroom:
Partner Stroking for Longer Sex

BEFORE STARTING, come up with a word you will use to stop stimulation, and one you will use to start it. Staying relaxed and comfortable, ask your lover to manually stimulate your penis in ways that always feel good. Use your "stop" word to have her slow down when you get too aroused. When you feel in control of your sexual response again, use your "start" word to have her resume stimulation.

Eventually, do this exercise having her use lubricant or lotion. With time, you can graduate to having your lover slow the pace of her stimulation instead of stopping all action for ejaculatory control. Alternatively, she can change the stroking technique. Be sure to make this transition first with dry hands, then with lubricated ones.

In developing even more control, repeat these exercises with your lover orally pleasuring you. When you feel ready to practice ejaculatory control during intercourse, apply everything that you have been practicing on your own and with your lover. The first couple of times you want to climax, stop all action or slow down, then slowly resume. Over time, you'll be able to last longer between these couple of stops. Eventually, you won't need to stop at all.

Stay Positive: Don't trump your own game by putting yourself down or thinking that something isn't possible. You will last longer. It may just take time, dedication, and practice.

Strengthen Your PC Muscle: If you haven't already, start exercising your pelvic floor muscles as we discussed earlier in this chapter. Being able to squeeze your PC around the prostate voluntarily will help you to control your ejaculatory response.

In developing ejaculatory control for longer lovemaking with your partner, know that your sex sessions are going to feel a bit like doing homework. Only this homework is much more fun! Communicate with each other about the following exercises and your expectations. In the beginning, you will not be able to focus on your lover's arousal, since this may prove too much of a distraction for you. Stay focused on your own excitement and tension levels. No worries: Both of you will eventually be well-rewarded for your efforts.

CLIMAXING TOGETHER: ENJOY THE ULTIMATE BONDING EXPERIENCE FOR COUPLES

On many couples' wish list is the desire for mutual orgasm. For 25 percent of men and 14 percent of women, mutual orgasm is a must, according to *The Janus Report*. Yet it's important to realize that simultaneous orgasms are relatively rare, given men and women's different sexual-response rates. Moreover, while climaxing together can be perceived as "mind-blowing," it is equally wondrous to see your lover caught up in an orgasm right after or before you've had your own.

Still, for those on a simultaneous sex mission, there are ways to better your chances of realizing this goal:

Longer Foreplay: Since women often need more time to get warmed up, devoting more time to foreplay before sex will enable you better synchronize your sexual-response rates.

PC Your Way to O: A woman can use perineal squeezes to expedite her sexual response for simultaneous climax.

Vibrator: Using a vibrating sex toy can hasten a woman's sexual response, helping her to climax faster when she's intertwined with her lover.

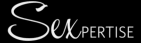

Much of Taoist sexuality focuses on the male essence, or jing. Taoists believe that men can live longer and increase their vitality by avoiding the exhaustion and loss of energy that follows ejaculation. Male and female satisfaction is equally emphasized, with the texts teaching men to fully satisfy their lovers without depleting their semen—their jing—through prolonged sex without the loss of semen.

Taoist sex also relies upon coitus reservatus, where a man attempts to stay in the Plateau phase of the sexual-response cycle. This is achieved through anal constriction combined with breathing and meditation. Taoists believe that such practices return jing up to the brain via the spine. This leads to spiritual illumination. Yet perhaps what makes the Taoist approach the most renowned worldwide is its encouragement of delaying ejaculation in hopes of experiencing multiple orgasms.

How do couples go about having sex in the CAT position?

The CAT (Coital Alignment Technique) position is designed to correct a potential flaw of the missionary position: that a man may end up thrusting about an inch below her clitoris, bypassing her hottest pleasure zone entirely. With CAT, he angles his pelvis so that it's slightly higher than his lover's. This happens when the man slides his body up higher than in regular missionary, so that the base of the shaft of his erection ends up rubbing over her clitoris. The woman then wraps her legs around his thighs, resting her ankles on his calves. She then leads on the upward stroke, which pushes his pelvis backward, while he, at same time, gives counter-pressure on her clitoris with the body of his penis. He then leads with downward stroke, pushing her pelvis downward, while she provides resistant counter-pressure in pushing the clitoris against the base of the penis. As both lovers keep their pubic bones connected, you want to maintain a rocking with the pelvic thrusts more so than a thrusting. This way, his penis will be able to stimulate her clitoris for maximum genital contact. (Note: His thrusts will be shorter, and since his stimulation is decreased, he should be able to last longer.)

Whether your hope is to last longer, have multiple orgasms, or experience simultaneous orgasms, your best starting point is taking the time to learn and observe how your body responds and how it feels at various stages of the sexual-response cycle. In all of these situations, you want to make sure that you are making love in a relaxed, positive atmosphere. Sex needs to be leisurely, not rushed or stressed, and involve the entire body. Building upon your natural foundation, you can stay in control of your pleasuring as you slow down, change the stimulation, or squeeze your PC muscle in addition to a whole host of other techniques we just covered. More than anything, enjoy the journey. Make the destination secondary. Staying in the present often lends itself to some of the sweetest of sexual surprises.

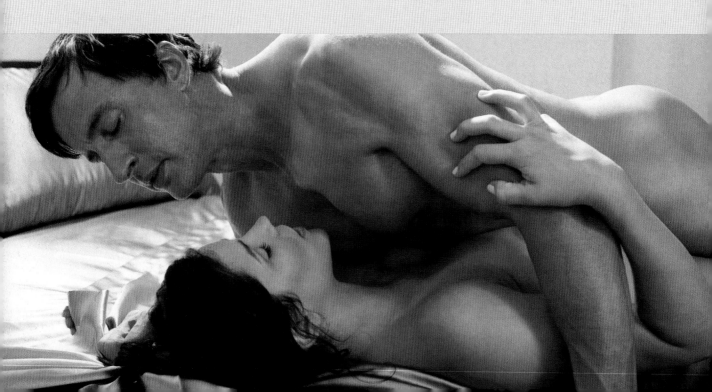

Deeper Thrusting: Couples should aim for positions that allow him to go deep, since a man's pubic bone can come in direct contact with more of her clitoral area. Rubbing against this area can also trigger orgasm when couples are ready to climax into the cosmos. (Note: Despite being known for this, the Coital Alignment Technique position, explained below, is somewhat controversial and is not widely accepted by all experts.)

"Sometimes the heart sees what is invisible to the eye."

—H. JACKSON BROWN, JR.

Sexual Homework

No matter what your orgasm is like, one curiosity many lovers have is how to expand their climax for a full-body sensation. So this sexual homework provides you with some key ingredients to doing just that.

Ecstatic Response: In capturing what you've learned throughout this book, seek to combine relaxation with high energy. This ecstatic response involves relaxing into the excitement so that your energy rises as it spreads throughout the body. To do this, you relax certain muscles and breathe slowly and deeply to impact your orgasmic release.

Instead of focusing on the sensations of the sex organs rubbing against one another, using the breath and movement to expand sexual energy can result in a full-body orgasm. In order to send vibrations through-out your body, pursue the following:

Releasing Tension: For twenty minutes, in a warm space and wearing little or no clothing, cleanse the body of tension by shaking each part gently, then more intensely. This brings energy and awareness to every part, sending tingly, warm sensations throughout the body. Take your time thinking about the body part, what you're doing, and how it responds. As you breathe in, imagine that you are sending the breath to this tense area, giving it new life. In finding a rhythm, you may want to add music.

Streaming Energy:

1. For fifteen minutes, close your eyes and stand in what's known as the Basic Stance (as though skiing, but with your arms hanging at your sides).

(continued on page 314)

2. Stay relaxed, allowing the energy to stream through your pelvis as you tune into the self, becoming aware of your inner sensations.

3. Rock back and forth on the balls of your feet, five times, holding yourself at the brink in either direction and breathing slowly.

4. Stop and "listen" for the tremors that may be felt around the knee and ankle joints.

5. Start rocking again, noting the trembling sensations (if you don't experience any, fake it until you do). Let the vibrations travel up your body, through your pelvis and abdomen, while breathing into these body parts.

6. Expand the sensations by focusing on all of these areas, envisioning them shaking.

7. Breathe deeper and make noise as you allow yourself to drown in the moment.

8. Sway your hips to intensify your reaction. Remember to stay relaxed at the same time.

9. Now visualize the vibrations moving from your groin and abdomen, all the way to the top of your head (which should not be tilted back).

10. Amplify the sensations as you relax into them, allowing yourself to be vibrated by your energy.

11. Finally, visualize the energy streaming back through your body to your feet.

12. After you've grounded your energy, take a few deep breaths and slow down till you're still. This is what you want to do during sex.

Instead of holding your breath, stopping all movement, or disrupting arousal with orgasmic response, you want to be able to surrender to the feelings. Allow yourself to be vulnerable and open with your lover. This is true intimacy. Thus, the next time you perform the aforementioned exercises, plan to have sex. Practice combining the sexual bonding you've learned, with PC muscle control, with channeling your streaming energy as you make love. Most importantly, do not put pressure on yourselves for instant results in your first few tries. All of this requires effort, time, and patience. So remember to enjoy the ride, relaxation, and union that comes with this kind of lovemaking.

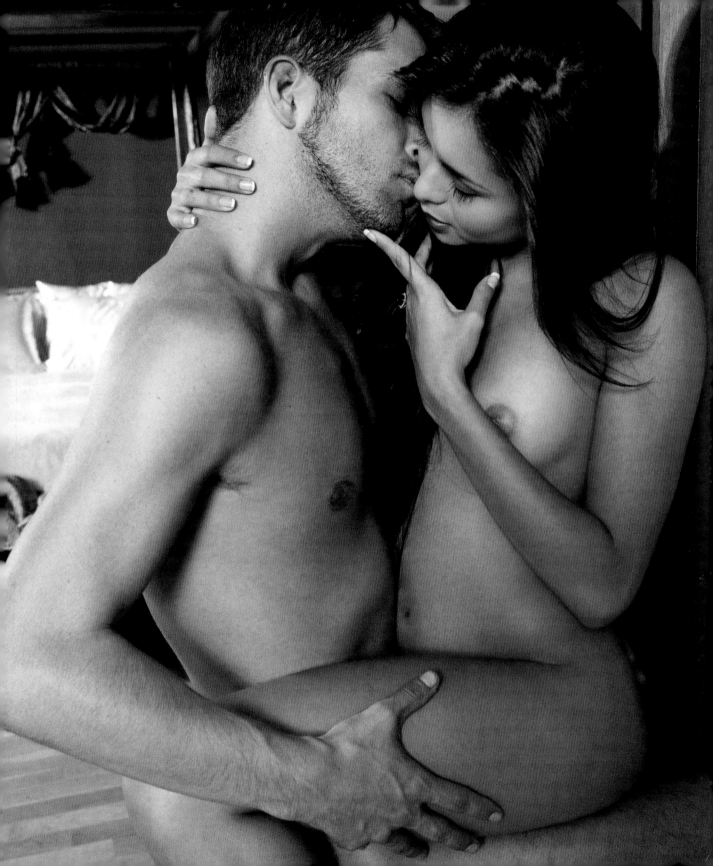

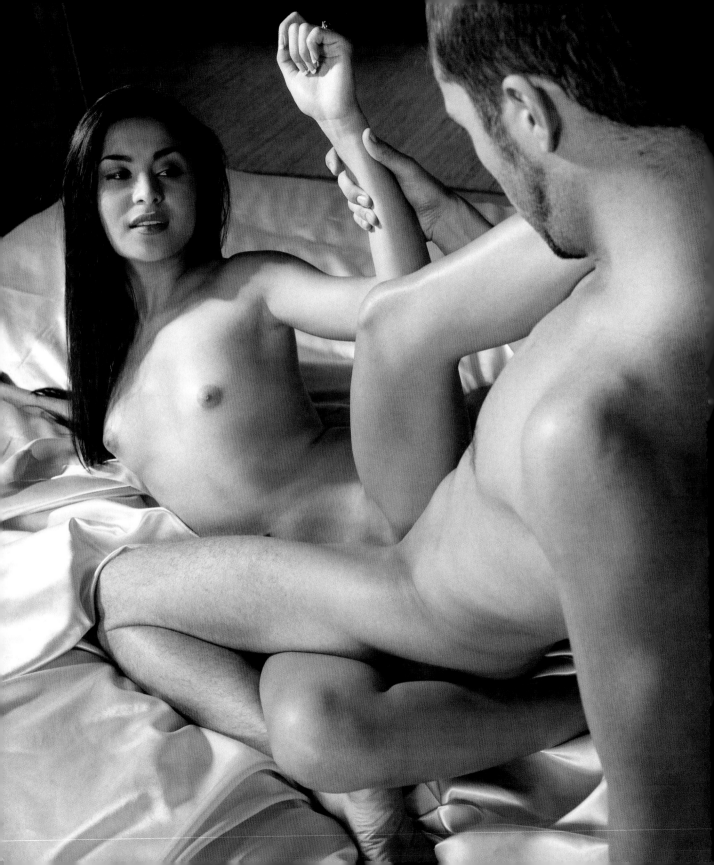

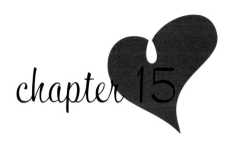

chapter 15

Ancient Wisdom for Modern Couples: Keep Your Sex New, Fresh, and Fun with These Sexual Classics

THE "SACRED SEX" teachings from the East, such as Tantric sex and the Kama Sutra, appeal to couples looking to connect with each other, the universe, and/or a higher power. With these approaches to better sex as your guide, you can supersede orgasm, possibly even realizing transcendent sex. In these ancient teachings, sex becomes a mystical, spiritual experience. Research on transcendent sex by Jenny Wade, Ph.D., has found that accidental and intentional realizations of such involve things such as:

- Paranormal powers
- Seeing visions, whiteness, or God's face
- Being visited by gods
- Time travel

"Now join your hands, and with your hands your heart."

—WILLIAM SHAKESPEARE

- Reliving past lives
- Feeling possessed by spirits
- Experiencing heat/light/energy waves throughout the body
- Suspension of time and being
- Lack of sensory channels as a sense of reality is lost
- Not recognizing the lover or feeling like the self
- Enlightenment

Whether you seek transcendent sex or simply sensational sex, the ancient approaches of Tantric sex and the Kama Sutra can help you have the most meaningful sex of your life. All involve applying special techniques to sensual acts, with an emphasis on:

- A "sex-is-good-and-important" attitude
- Sexual intelligence, which is learned over a lifetime
- Emotional intelligence, a critical component of which is effective communication
- Female sacred sexuality, with her satisfaction a must
- Making time for love
- Energy, especially effective breathing techniques
- Sensory development, increasing sensual play for increased arousal
- Going beyond orgasm to union and pleasure
- Expressing what you like
- Body freedom—letting go of negative messages to meet your biological, emotional, and spiritual needs
- A willingness to surrender
- Honoring the yoni (vagina) and lingam (penis)

Most importantly, sex is a gateway to sexual and spiritual enlightenment, where male and female energies are joined. Feminine energy is celebrated and honored. It is considered the catalyst for sexual and spiritual transformation. A male is to honor his lover's sexuality, surrendering himself to its limitless power. Neither partner, however, can be selfish. As we reviewed in Chapter 14, the male is encouraged to prolong lovemaking, making it sensitive and sensual so that a woman can reach the pinnacle of her pleasuring. The ultimate result: Your sexual experience is more energetic, spiritual, and emotional.

MARATHON SEX THAT BLOWS YOUR MIND, BODY, AND SOUL

In beginning our exploration of Eastern approaches to sex, let's take a closer look at the sensual traditions of Tantra and the *Kama Sutra*, both of which inform the other.

TANTRIC SEX

The sexual practices of Tantric sex are based on ancient teachings in sacred Hindu texts, dating as far back as 7,000 to 5,000 BCE. In these texts, the gods Shiva and Shakti joyfully couple, thereby creating and sustaining the universe. Like Shiva and Shakti, Tantric sex involves the connection between each lover's higher self, which combine for a divine union.

In Tantra, lovers seek to bridge the gap between the physical and spiritual worlds through their bodies and breaths. You unite Shakti and Shiva, and in doing so, experience bliss and happiness a millionfold times that of what you feel in regular physical intercourse. The ancient Hindus also believed that passionate loving in this life would lead to eternal bliss in the next. Tantra, Sanskrit for "woven together," is designed to help lovers achieve this eternal bliss through sexual intimacy.

KAMA SUTRA

The *Kama Sutra* is the original, classic guide, written around 350 AD, to having great sex. This Indian book was an effort to help prevent divorce. More than simply a manual of impressive sexual positions, special maneuvers, and sex tips, the *Kama Sutra* is also a prescription for living. Recognizing that good sex makes for happier couples, the *Kama Sutra* gives instruction on matters such as:

- Oral sex
- Creating a sensual environment
- Sacred sex
- Passionate loving
- Expressing emotions
- Attracting your lover with sex toys
- Magic spells
- Aphrodisiacs
- Courtesan behaviors

Both Tantric sex and the *Kama Sutra* encourage lovers to respect and appreciate one another while staying in the moment and freely expressing themselves. You learn to relax and to take time for lovemaking as you celebrate your sexual union, liberate your souls, and enjoy your own private sensual space together.

SEXUAL Q&A: CARNAL KNOWLEDGE OF THE TAO

My understanding of Taoist sex is that it involves meditation, breathing exercises, bathing rituals, and sexual gymnastics. So what makes Taoist sex practices different from Tantric sex practices?

Taoist sexuality began as a branch of Chinese medicine—but for the past five thousand years it has been regarded as an ecstatic sexuality. Sexual arts, in addition to meditation, breathing exercises, medicines, and a host of other practices, are regarded as means to immortality and longevity. In short, you harness your sexual energy to achieve enlightened bliss. This requires the harmonizing of our dual energies—think yin and yang, god and goddess, darkness and light. While much of this mirrors Tantric sex, there is a slight distinction. The Taoists use sex to boost longevity and health. Certain sexual positions will stimulate chi (energy) and harmoniously join male and female. The "healing love" of sex helps you become one with the universe.

Taoist sexual techniques stem from fang shu (a.k.a. fang zhong or fang zhong shu), meaning "inside the bedchamber" or "the art in bedroom." A number of experts developed intercourse techniques, with the key being to control ejaculate for both sexes. The practice finds it desirable for one's partner to climax without having orgasm yourself.

Sexual satisfaction without ejaculation is also emphasized in the Taoist belief system.

The Taoists believe that sex is something to be studied and understood. Sexual acts are considered vital and energizing and critical to balancing positive and negative energies. Taoism teaches us that we are to respect our masculine/feminine differences or else they'll be at odds with each other. Good sex is nourishment for the whole self.

Taoist sexual techniques give a great deal of attention to mastering sex differences in sexual arousal while harmonizing lovers' sexual wills and desires. Sex is to activate and liberate the female while relaxing the male. The man is to stay in control while getting her sexually excited. In keeping himself in control, the man remains detached, avoiding her caress, even when his lover performs sex acts. When she is ready for penetration, the male seeks to control his breath, control ejaculation, and achieve sexual satisfaction without emission.

PREPARING FOR SACRED SEX

Sex is sacred in relationships where lovers honor physical, emotional, and spiritual intimacy. The Eastern traditions set the stage for sacred sex by ritualizing it. Here are the elements that go into making a sacrament of sex:

Ambiance: Tantric lovers seek to create a sensual environment with pictures, plush oriental rugs, ornate pillows, tapestries, candles, bells, bowls, fruit, and shells. Attention is given to creating a harmonious, tranquil, warm, comfortable space using color, lighting, fabrics, and scents. Violet is seen as representing female sexual energy, while red is known to stimulate male and female vitality and life force. Both can enhance a space with silk, chiffon, or muslin fabrics that can be hung. You may also want to have music, such as New Age or Tantric titles (which have special rhythms to facilitate your practice, create harmony, work with breathing, and activate the body). You can also use chants or chimes to charge your connection.

Altar Offering: Set up an altar in your bedroom or a special part of your home that only you and your lover can touch. Decorate it with special objects, such as a poem, incense, candles, or fresh flowers. Place objects that represent the lingam, including crystals, wands, or bananas, and the yoni, such as triangles, almonds, horseshoes, or fresh apricots. Place a stone on a velvet cushion. A dark cushion should have a light stone on it, while a light one should have a dark stone. Stones to consider are ruby for a very deep, passionate love affair; diamond for everlasting love; garnet for sexual pleasure; red jasper for warm, sensuous love; and pearls for long-lasting love.

Anointing the Other: You want to honor the body as a temple of your spirit. Your aim is to offer the body as a gift to each other and the universe. This is often done using essential oils mixed with an oil base, such as pure vegetable oil. You can, for example, anoint each other's hearts with a rose or geranium essential oil, or your third eye, the area between your eyebrows, with a sandalwood essential oil.

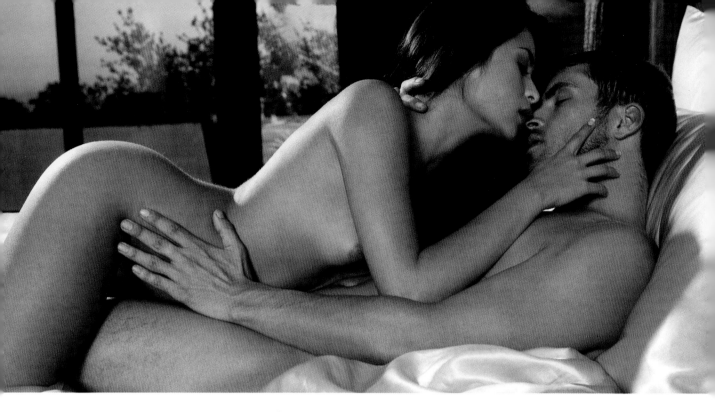

$\mathcal{S}$*exercise* 15.1 Seduce Each Other with Talk

Have verbal intercourse, seducing each other with love talk as you share your innermost feelings about love and sex. Allow yourselves to be flirtatious and playful as you hold hands, gaze lovingly into each other's eyes, and express yourself from the heart in asking to make love.

Energy Meld: Unite your energies by lying down on top of each other, using pillows for support. Relax and let your weights sink. Feel your energies flowing as one field combined with your joint aura. Breathe in rhythm, breathing in the aromas you've just anointed, and breathing out any negative energy. Do this for fifteen minutes or until you feel light.

Ritual Bath: Care of the body is important, so take a sensuous bath together, scattering the water with rose petals. Once clean, you may want to dress up in robes if that feels even better to you.

Food Ritual: In clearing any blockages in the body, becoming more aware of your energy, and in bonding, feed each other as a part of foreplay. You're not only making offerings to one another but also sharing an offering for the gods. Fruits are especially popular, chased with a small amount of wine.

$\mathcal{S}\ell\mathcal{X}$ercise 15.2 Consider Your Food Choices

Brainstorm foods for pleasing your palates, keeping in mind that your offerings need to be:

A. Light—heavy food will make you sleepy, and alcohol can suppress your libido.

B. Enticing—The foods should appeal to all of your senses, in their texture, smell, taste, and presentation.

C. Easy to prepare—You don't want to waste your energy in the kitchen when you can be in the bedroom!

D. Seductive—Think of foods that can be devilishly delicious in how they can be sucked, slurped, licked, and, especially, fed to your lover.

Caressing Meditation: Also referred to as the "Tantric Touch," connect with your own inner heart-center. Then caress your partner with delicate touch using a feather, then fingertips, honoring every part of the body equally as you show your love and deep appreciation. Your whole skin will feel alive and tingly as your sense of touch expands and your other senses become heightened.

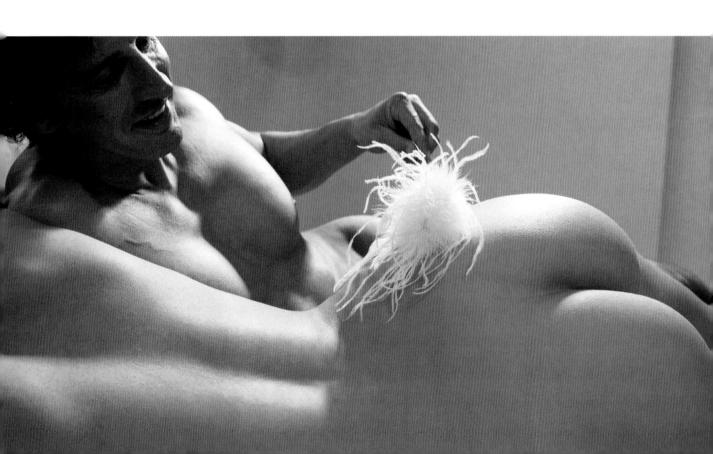

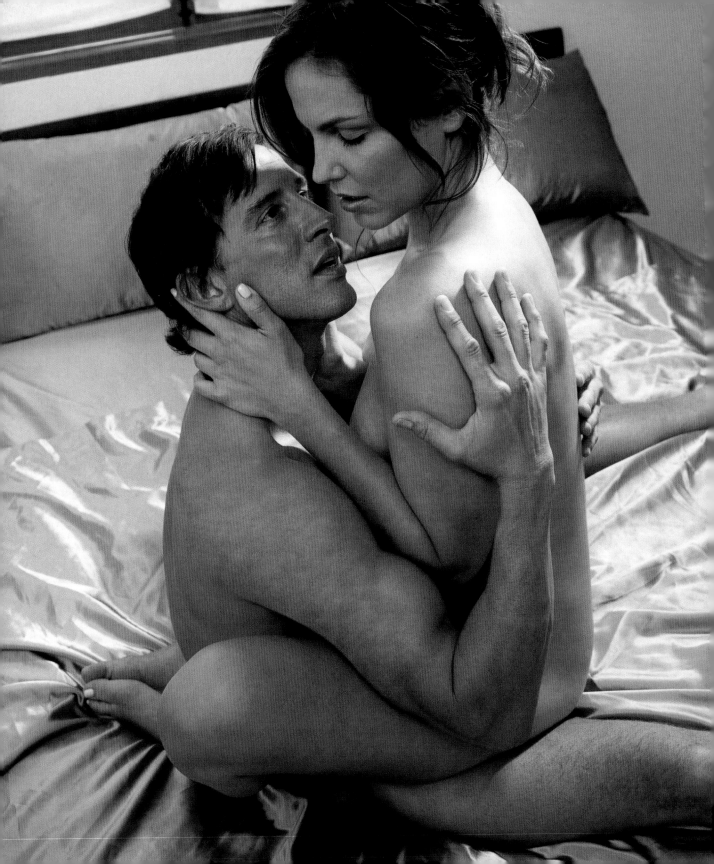

Balancing Male/Female Energy: The act of intercourse is regarded as a harmonious union of the male and female principles in us all. One of the ways to approach the union of opposites is through the Yab-Yum position. Here, the man sits cross-legged, with the woman straddling his lap, legs wrapped around him; this allows the two of you to look into each other's eyes as you align your hearts, giving easy access to your bodies.

Attend to Your Breathing: Prana, the breath, is your life force—a vital conduit between flesh and spirit. Learning to channel the breath through the body using breathing and visualization practices is considered important in harmonizing your spirit and flesh, especially as you balance your masculine and feminine energies. The breath gives your body life and the spirit energy for lovemaking. Thus, there are many breathing exercises for lovers that, as stress-busters, energy-boosters, and mood enhancers, make for enlivening sex.

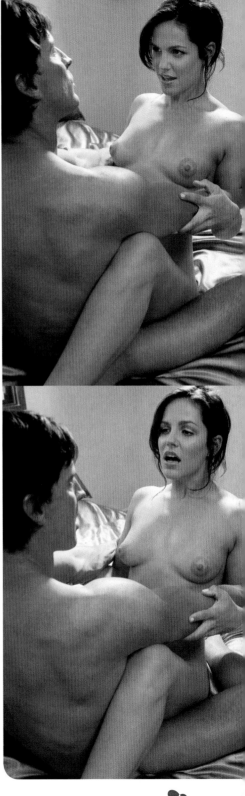

Exercise 15.3 Practice Rhythmic Breathing

Ujjayi, Sanskrit for "victorious uprising," is one way to prepare your breath for lovemaking:

1. Close your mouth, and inhale through your nose, allowing your rib cage to expand sideways, shooting for a count of 4.

2. Fill the lungs from the bottom up, keeping your shoulders motionless.

3. Pause at the top of your inhale for at least 2 seconds.

4. Exhale through your mouth or nose for a count of 4.

   Do this rhythmic breathing slowly and deliberately. Should you need help concentrating, imagine a balloon filling with air as your inhale. Feel the calmness spreading throughout your body and being.

Synchronize Your Breaths: This form of foreplay sets a rhythm, one you'll want to maintain during sex. Synchronizing the breath also lowers the risk of injury during advanced sexual positions.

$\mathcal{S}ex$ercise 15.4: How to Synch Your Breathing with Your Partners'

To harmonize your breaths:

1. Sit back-to-back, cross your legs, and lean against each other.

2. Unless it causes strain, hold each other's hands.

3. Repeat the ujjayi instructions, inhaling and exhaling together, communicating only through the breath.

4. Strive for elongating each breath, matching the duration of your inhale and exhale.

$\mathcal{I}n$ the Bedroom:
Honoring Her Yoni

WITH FEMALE PLEASURING front and center in Tantric and *Kama Sutra* sex practices, lovers are highly encouraged to honor her yoni with the following climax-inducing maneuvers:

Pressing Yoni Kiss: As your hands explore her body, kiss her vaginal lips like you would a plump set of lips.

Outer Yoni Tongue Strokes: Explore her inner lotus flower (vulva) with your lips, using slips of your tongue on occasion.

Inner Yoni Tongue Strokes: As she stands, kneel before her and open her outer labia to kiss and lick her inner labia.

Kissing Yoni Blossom: As she sits or stands, give the labia long licks up to the clitoris. If she can handle it, you can add a bit of sucking.

Flutter of Butterfly: With a stiffened tongue, flick the clitoral shaft as though you were fluttering butterfly wings.

Sucking Yoni Blossom: With your mouth over her clitoris, suck, gently pulling with your mouth. Intermittently use a few tongue strokes.

Kiss of the Penetrating Tongue: Part her yoni, and push your tongue into her vaginal opening, pushing farther and farther.

During sex, I sometimes wet the bed—at least I think I do. Only, the fluid doesn't smell like urine, which baffles my husband and me. Any thoughts on what's going on?

You're likely not wetting the bed but rather experiencing female ejaculation, a.k.a. "ambrosia." Described as "drinking from the fountain of life" by Eastern sex practitioners, who encourage her lover to drink her juices, this phenomenon is the reaction of a woman being highly aroused. Most often due to G spot, or "Sacred Gate," stimulation, female ejaculation involves the emission of a prostatic-like fluid during orgasm, mostly via the urethra. This perfectly normal sexual response can happen every time a woman experiences great sexual arousal, sometimes, or never. Yet, in not knowing that a woman is capable of ejaculating, some lovers mistake female ejaculate for urine.

Sometimes salty, sweet, or earthy in smell and taste, female ejaculate varies according to a woman's menstrual cycle, the type and amount of stimulation she's getting, the strength of her PC muscle, and her comfort with this bodily reaction. The volume of ejaculate released can range from 3 to 16 ccs, which is about a teaspoon. Anything more than that, as seen in erotic adult films that show up to one liter of fluid, is regarded by the scientific community as urine in addition to the ejaculate. The fluid, which may be clear or more like the color of skim milk, may have traces of urine, even slightly smelling or tasting like such at times, but it is not urine. In fact, its levels of urea and creatinine, the two main ingredients of urine, are very low.

Perhaps the biggest controversy when it comes to female ejaculation is around the existence of a "female" prostate and if such a gland is the source for female ejaculation. Most recently, ultrasound imaging, biochemical studies of the ejaculated fluid, and an endoscopy of the urethra have been used to identify the female prostate. High-definition perineal ultrasound images show a structure consistent with gland tissue surrounding the entire length of the female urethra. Fluid emitted during orgasm, biochemically, had all of the parameters found in male prostate plasma. Chemical analysis further shows that the fluid contains high levels of prostatic acid phosphatase (a chemical the prostate gland secretes that is found in semen), plus prostatic specific antigen (PSA). It is also composed partially of glucose and fructose, both of which are forms of sugar.

MASTER EXOTIC POSITIONS TO KEEP YOUR SEX EROTIC

The best known part of the Kama Sutra is "The Rules of Love." It emphasizes a relationship in its wholeness, appealing to our desire for connection, sexual satisfaction, and intimacy, as well as our spiritual hunger. What follows is some of its most celebrated advanced lovemaking techniques.

Natural/Upasripta

With this churning technique considered our most instinctive sexual maneuver, upasripta involves stroking the yoni with the lingam while using gentle forward motions. You want to press your pelvic bone against her clitoris to stimulate her, varying the depth, rhythm, and speed according to her liking.

In the Bedroom:
Honoring His Lingam

JUST AS WE HONOR THE YONI, we honor the lingam for his pleasuring. The following are regarded as some of the most effective ways to bring him bliss:

Nominal Congress: For a warm-up, hold his lingam with one hand, and place it between your lips, letting your mouth move about it.

Biting the Sides: Cover the end of his lingam with your fingers. Then press the sides of it with your lips, actually using your teeth, as well.

Outside Pressing: Press the end of his lingam with your lips, which are pressed together, and kiss his penis as though you're drawing something out.

Inside Pressing: Put his lingam farther into your mouth, and press it with your lips before taking it out.

Rubbing: Touch his lingam everywhere with your tongue, then pass the tongue over the head.

Sucking a Mango Fruit: Put half of his lingam into your mouth, and then forcibly kiss and suck it.

Swallowing Up: Put the whole lingam into your mouth, and press it to the end.

Churning/Manthana

The lingam is held with a hand and is moved so that its head makes circles in her yoni.

Double-Blade Knife/Hula

With the man's body slightly higher than hers, the shaft is released so that the upper part of the yoni is struck with the lingam in sharp downward motions. This provides more stimulation for the clitoris.

Rubbing/Avamardana

Her hips are slightly lifted with a pillow. His hips are then thrust in upward motions to firmly rub against her clitoris. Every few seconds, keep the lingam inside of her in the Piditaka position (below).

Pressing/Piditaka

The yoni is pressed by the lingam (the lingam is kept deep inside the yoni without movement) over an extended period of time, with pressure applied to the clitoris.

Giving a Blow/the Buffet/Nirghata

The lingam is removed from the yoni at some distance to tease her with desire before forcibly striking it with a deep dive.

Blow of a Boar/Varahaghata

The lingam continuously rubs only one side of the wall of her yoni, switching sides after some time.

Blow of a Bull/Vrishaghata

Both sides of the yoni are rubbed with the lingam. The lingam is thrust wildly in all directions while her lover maintains steady pressure on her clitoris with his pelvis.

Sporting of a Sparrow/Chatakavilasa

The lingam moves up and down in the yoni frequently and without being taken out, bringing her to climax.

In the Bedroom:
Kama Sutra Sexual Positions

THE KAMA SUTRA is also known for its many sexual positions. While it would take an entire book (and there are many) or DVD, such as Sinclair's *The Tantric Guide to Better Sex* video, just to explore all of the positions that this sex bible has to offer, the following are among its most impressive recommended positions:

Turning Position

From missionary position, the man turns around, still enjoying his lover without leaving her. Not easily accomplished, the Turning Position—along with many Kama Sutra positions—may be best practiced in water, since it may be easier.

Suspended Congress

The man can support himself against a wall while holding his lover, who throws her arms around his neck and hugs his hips with her thighs. She can then move herself using her feet, which touch the wall.

Congress of Cow

A woman is on all fours, with her lover mounting her like a bull. The Kama Sutra encourages lovers to demonstrate the characteristics of different animals that also couple like this, such as the tiger, dog, and cat.

In performing any sexual position, don't lose yourselves in your genital reactions. Be sure to stay connected by:

- Kissing and caressing each other
- Gazing into each other's eyes
- Breathing in sync
- Exchanging words of love, adoration, and appreciation
- Taking things slow

Sacred sexual union is about celebrating your union using the joys of sensuality. Deemed the true state of enlightenment, sexual bonding joins sexuality with spirituality, allowing your energies to connect. Feeling merged on every level, couples can experience more passionate sex, losing themselves in the moment in a whole other world. In loving, appreciating, and showing respect for one another, lovers feel free to express themselves and more.

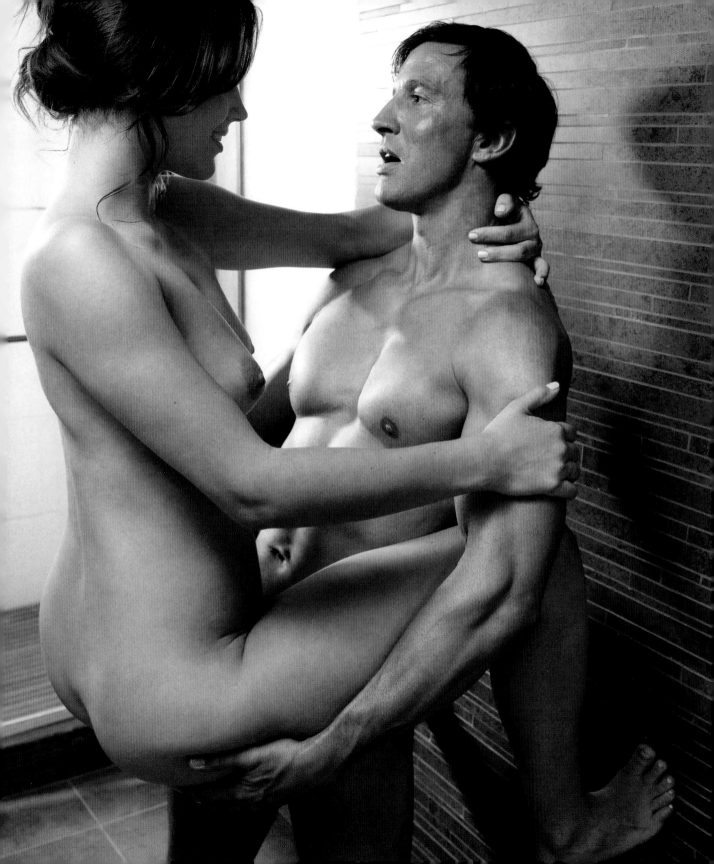

> *"Love is friendship set to music."*
>
> —E. JOSEPH COSSMAN

Sexual Homework

Khajuraho Meditation: Rooted in ancient Tantra, this essential Tantric method lasts one hour. The first stage is to be repeated four times and the second stage is to be repeated three times, over the course of seven days (or twice per week for three-and-a-half weeks). For the first stage, take twenty minutes to lie naked on your bed with your partner. The man is to close his eyes and visualize the position in which he would like to see his lover. Look at this vision, taking note of your thoughts and emotions. The woman should close her eyes, too, as she rests on the bed. She is to take note of her own thoughts and emotions as she becomes not herself, but the universal woman. After twenty minutes, the man is to call her "back."

For stage two, which lasts forty minutes, partners should make love, tuning into their thoughts and emotions. After sex, bow down to each other, touching your lover's feet with respect and thanks. In either step, do not discuss your meditative experience, as this is to remain private.

Relating Yin and Yang: Sit, facing your partner, and take each other's hands. For five minutes, do no more than gaze into each other's eyes, trying not to blink. Really examine your lover's face. After five minutes, close your eyes, but do not say anything. After a moment or two, look into your partner's face again for five minutes, only this time receiving the gaze. Allow yourselves to be vulnerable and exposed. Note your thoughts, and share your experience.

332   THE BETTER SEX GUIDE TO EXTRAORDINARY LOVEMAKING

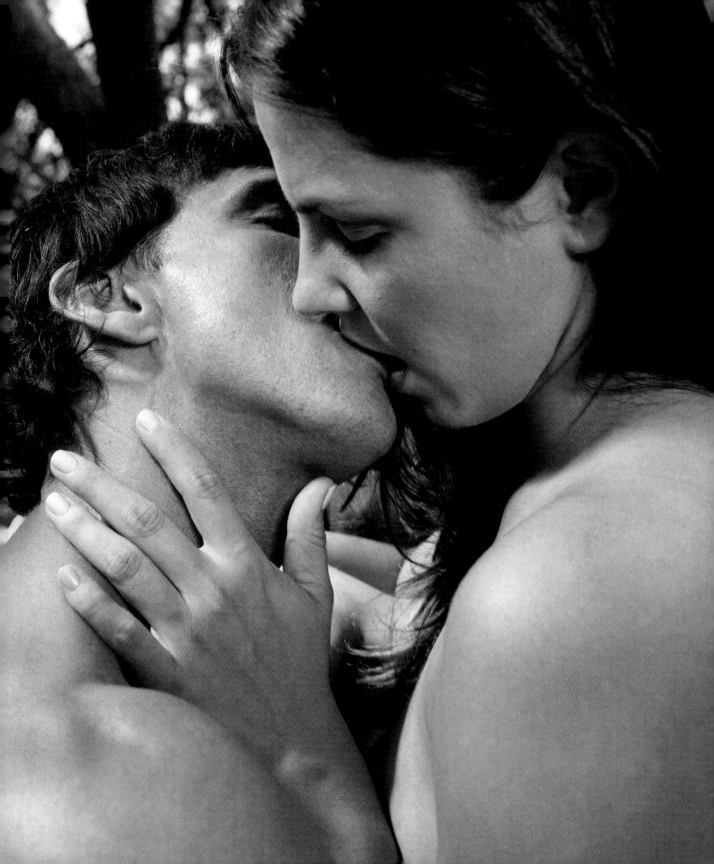

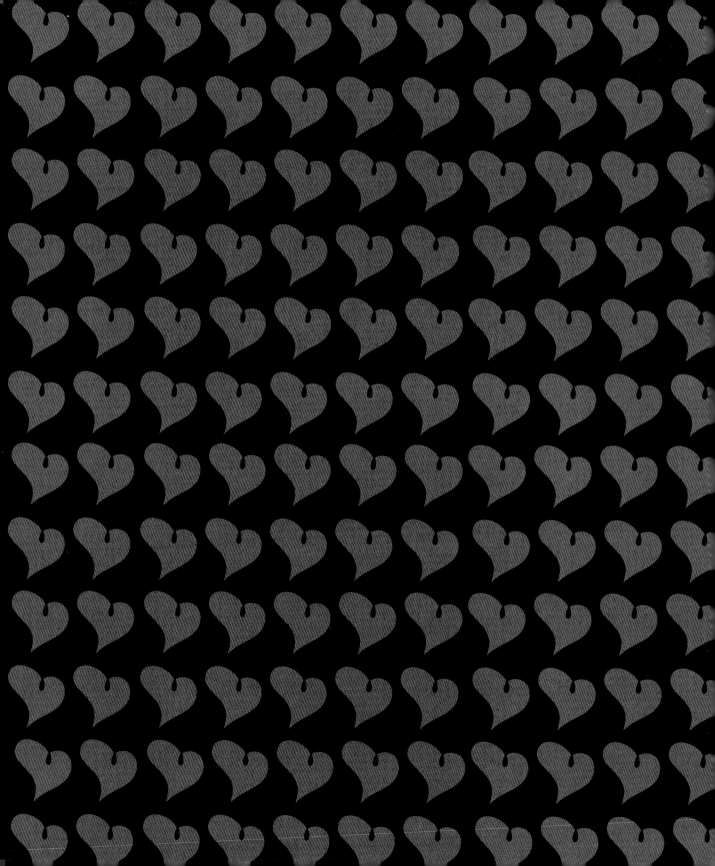

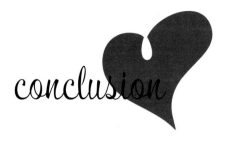

conclusion

A Better Sex Life Forever!

WHILE YOU MAY HAVE REACHED the end of this book, you have not reached the end of your sexual journey. In many ways, it is just the beginning. *The Better Sex Guide to Extraordinary Lovemaking* seeks to equip you with all of the information and skills you need for better lovemaking, and more. Realizing your full pleasure potential involves exploring the wide spectrum of ways to physically, emotionally, and spiritually connect with your partner.

Cultivating sexual intelligence is a lifelong journey. As all of us grow and evolve, both physically and emotionally, we need to, as lovers, continually revisit our means of realizing sexual fulfillment. We need to, on occasion, look at our sex lives in a whole new light—keeping it rich, erotic, and renewed. Emotional intelligence is a major component of the sexual satisfaction so many seek. Lovers who are open, honest, and present with each other are able to revel in even greater pleasures as they share their feelings, honor one another, and are simply there for each other in embracing sensual joys. With emotional smarts fueling sexual desire, couples are sure to set themselves up for a future of nothing more than a better sex life forever.

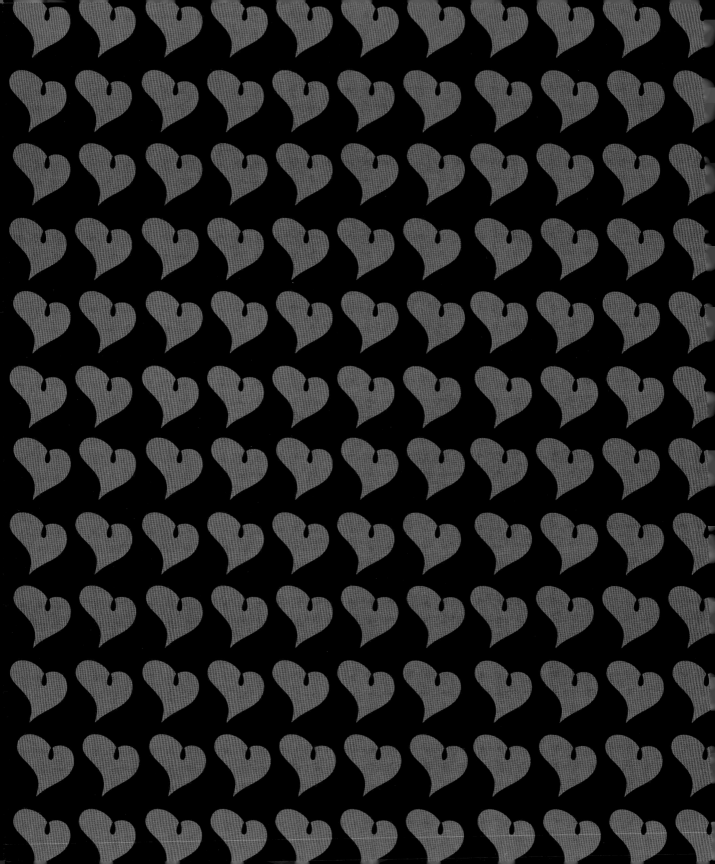

about the Sinclair Institute

SINCLAIR INSTITUTE is recognized as the leading source of sex education for adults who want to improve the quality of intimacy and sex in their relationships. Since 1991, the Institute has developed an extensive award-winning video library of over sixty programs with topics ranging from erectile dysfunction solutions to advanced sexual positions, as well as published numerous books on sexual health and wellbeing topics. The Institute's vast educational film library is sold in over twenty-four countries and includes the acclaimed Better Sex Video Series.

In 1993, The Sinclair Institute developed the Sinclair Advisory Council, which is composed of well-known sex educators, therapists, doctors, and researchers from across the country to help guide policies and program development, as well as to stay abreast of scientific and therapeutic trends in sexual health. The Advisory Council helps guide the development of Sinclair Institute products. The Sinclair Institute understands the need for quality sexual health education and is committed to helping couples overcome the wide range of barriers that affect the quality of sexual relationships.

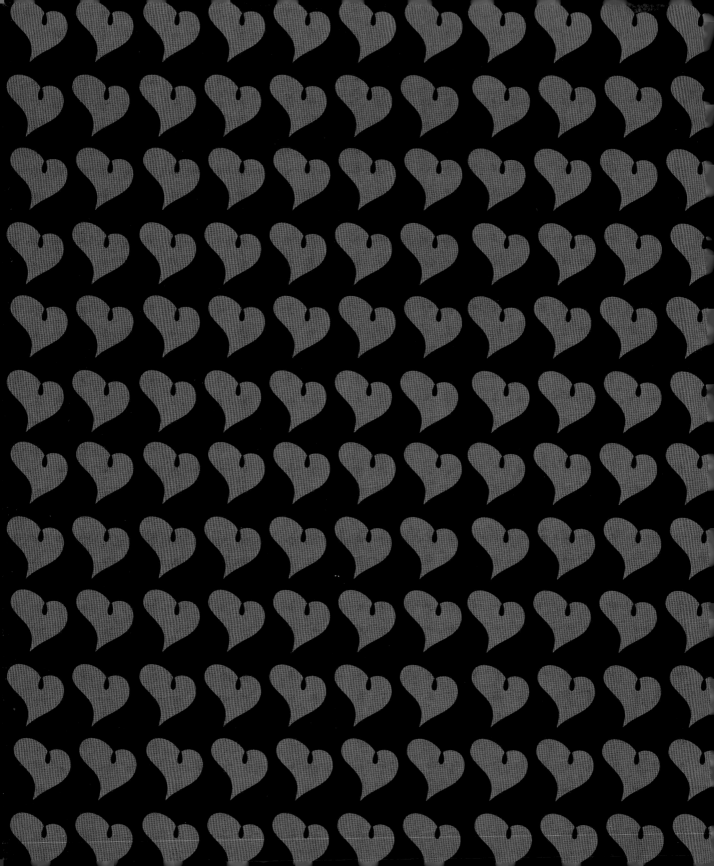

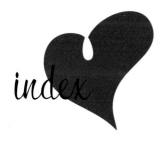

index

emotional arousal, 50

emotional intimacy, 73

emotional orgasm, 279

emotional security, 31

endorphins, 99

energy meld, 322

environment, 57

equality, 32

erectile dysfunction (ED), 99–101

erections, 99

erogenous zones, 152–155, 279

erotic dreams, 64–65

erotic imagination, 200–202

erotic power-play, 223–237

erotic visuals, 69

erotophilic, 43

erotophobic, 43, 44

ex, dreams about sex with, 65

excitement, 81–82, 130

exercise, 52, 72, 84, 104, 105

exhibitionism, 69, 237–238

exotic positions, 249, 328–331

face caress, 118

faceless lover dream, 64

facial cues, 68

famous people, dreams about sex with, 64

fantasies, 59–63, 129

fatigue, 35, 103

feet, 155

fellatio, 171, 173–175

female arousal, 82, 152

female body parts, 78–79

female ejaculation, 327

female genitals, 78–79, 133

female masturbation, 132–137

female orgasm, 271–276, 280–283, 290–291, 305–307

female sexual arousal disorder (FSAD), 101–102

female sexual desire, 69, 71, 72

female sexual psychology, 70–73

fertility cycle, 24–25

fetishes, 218–223

fitness, 104

flavored lubricants, 126

flirting, 67

food, 222, 323

food ritual, 322

foreplay, 107, 147–165, 152

  for anal sex, 261

  erogenous zones for, 152–155

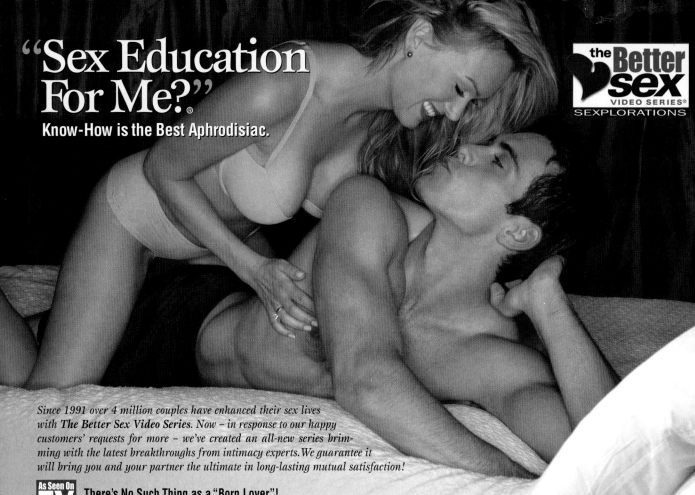